Essential Neurosurgery

Essential Neurosurgery

Andrew H. Kaye MBBS, MD, FRACS
Department of Neurosurgery, Royal Melbourne Hospital, Melbourne,
Australia

CHURCHILL LIVINGSTONE
EDINBURGH LONDON MELBOURNE AND NEW YORK 1991

CHURCHILL LIVINGSTONE
Medical Division of Longman Group UK Limited

Distributed in the United States of America by Churchill
Livingstone Inc., 1560 Broadway, New York, N.Y. 10036, and
by associated companies, branches and representatives
throughout the world.

First edition 1991

ISBN 0-443-04350-7

British Library Cataloguing in Publication Data
Kaye, Andrew
    Essential neurosurgery.
    1. Man. Nervous system. Surgery
    I. Title
    617.48

Library of Congress Cataloging in Publication Data
Kaye, Andrew, 1950–
    Essential neurosurgery/Andrew H. Kaye. — 1st ed.
        p.   cm.
    Includes bibliographical references.
    Includes index.
    ISBN 0-443-04350-7
    1. Nervous system — Surgery. I. Title.
    [DNLM: 1. Central Nervous System — surgery. 2. Neurosurgery. WL
368 K23e]
    RD593.K28   1991
    617.4'8 — dc20
    DNLM/DLC
    for Library of Congress

90–1982
CIP

Produced by Longman Singapore Publishers (Pte) Ltd.
Printed in Singapore

Preface

Clinical neurosurgery requires an understanding of the art of neurology and of the principles of the neurosciences, particularly neuropathology and neurophysiology. In the past the mystique of neurosurgery has inadvertently prevented both medical trainees and physicians from a proper appreciation of even basic neurosurgery and consequently has created a rather nihilistic view of neurosurgical illnesses. The improvements in medical technology have markedly improved the accuracy of the diagnosis, the efficacy of neurosurgical treatment and the range of diseases that can be diagnosed and treated. In particular, the exciting advances in neuroradiology have simplified the diagnostic process and made neurosurgery more accessible.

This book is intended as an introduction to neurosurgery. It is hoped that it will be useful for physicians in training, neurosurgical trainees and medical students. The book is not intended to be an exhaustive coverage of neurosurgery but rather concentrates on the more common neurosurgical problems and only briefly mentions rare entities.

The neurological principles, pathological basis and relevant investigations that form the basis of the diagnosis are emphasised. The neurosurgical management is outlined but the surgical techniques are only briefly mentioned, so that the reader will understand the postoperative problems likely to be encountered in the management of the patient. Modern neurosurgery has evolved principally from North American and European practises and there are often significant differences in the philosophical approach in the management of clinical problems. The author has in general described his own practice, which hopefully utilises the best of both systems.

The references have been chosen for their general coverage of the topics, ease of access, historical interest and, in some cases, because they will provide thought provoking alternatives that give a different perspective to the subject.

It is not possible to list and acknowledge all the many people who have helped in the preparation of this book, both knowingly and as a result of their influence on my own neurosurgical practices. However, the late John Bryant Curtis was the major initial influence not only on my own neurosurgical education but on that of many other Australian neurosurgeons. I particularly acknowledge the help of my neurological and neurosurgical colleagues at the Royal Melbourne Hospital in the preparation of this book. Stephen Davis and Christine Kilpatrick have provided chapters on their own areas of expertise. Professor Brian Tress, Director of Radiology at the Royal Melbourne Hospital, has always been accessible and helpful and I am indebted to him for his expert teaching over many years and for assistance with the details on magnetic resonance imaging. His department supplied most of the X-rays. Dr Meredith Weinstein, neuroradiologist at the Cleveland Clinic, kindly provided magnetic resonance scans (Figs 7.9, 12.7, 13.5). Professor Colin Masters, Department of Pathology, University of Melbourne and Dr Michael Gonzales, neuropathologist at the Royal Melbourne Hospital, gave assistance with the pathology details and illustrations. My residents and registrars at the Royal Melbourne Hospital have always provided stimulating advice and criticisms. I particularly acknowledge the assistance of Drs John Laidlaw and Michael Murphy, registrars in neurosurgery, who proofread the manuscript and offered constructive criticism. I thank Sue Dammery for the many hours spent preparing the manuscript and Richard Mahoney for the illustrations.

The book would not have been possible without the guidance and stimulus from Peter Richardson at Churchill Livingstone.

I am especially grateful to the encouragement and patience of my wife Judy and son Ben.

Melbourne, 1990   A. K.

Contents

1. Neurological assessment and examination

An accurate neurological assessment is fundamental for the correct management of the patient. The basic aim of the neurological examination is to solve the following four questions:

1. Is there a neurological problem?
2. What is the site of the lesion (or lesions) in the nervous system?
3. What are the pathological conditions that can cause the lesions?
4. Having ascertained the neuro-anatomical site and the pathological cause from the history, what is the most likely diagnosis?

Answering these four questions in turn will indicate the type of investigation necessary to confirm the diagnosis.

The neurological assessment involves:

- The history of the illness
- Clinical examination
  a. of the nervous system
  b. general examination.

THE NEUROLOGICAL HISTORY

As in general medicine and surgery the neurological history is the key to the diagnosis. The history involves not only questioning the patient but also careful observation. Many neurological illnesses can be diagnosed just by observing the patient. The patient's general manner, mood, posture, gait, facial expression and speech are all vital clues to the final diagnosis. In addition, patients who do not have an organic disease may present in a characteristic manner, particularly with an exaggeration of the complaint.

The history and examination commences with observation, and this should begin when first meeting the patient and while taking the history. The way in which the patient walks into the examination room, sits on the chair, answers questions and climbs on to the examination couch will provide vital clues in the search for the diagnosis. Initially it is important to allow the patient adequate opportunity to explain their symptoms in an unstructured and unprompted manner. Direct questioning should then follow.

The questions concerning neurological symptoms are in essence a verbal examination of the neurological system. It is not just the content of the answer that is important but the way in which the patient responds to the questions. The following is a general classification of neurological symptoms.

1. General neurological symptoms
   a. headache
   b. drowsiness (decreased conscious state)
   c. vertigo
   d. seizures, blackouts
2. Symptoms of meningismus
   a. headache
   b. photophobia
   c. neck stiffness
   d. vomiting
3. Symptoms related to the special senses
   a. vision
   b. hearing
   c. taste
   d. smell
4. Symptoms related to speech and comprehension
5. Motor symptoms
   a. power
   b. coordination
6. Sensory symptoms
7. Symptoms of other systems which may relate to diseases of the nervous system.

Careful questioning will ascertain the important details concerning each symptom. These include:

— The **time, mode of onset, progression and duration** of the symptom. The mode of onset is a valuable clue in discerning the pathological process. Sudden onset of a neurological disturbance is usually due to a vascular or epileptiform cause; a sudden severe headache is characteristic of subarachnoid haemorrhage whereas a slowly progressive headache is more in keeping with a cerebral tumour. Similarly, the abrupt onset of a hemiplegia may result from a vascular catastrophe and the slowly progressive weakness may be due to a compressive or infiltrative cause.
— What factors result in **alleviation** or **exacerbation** of the symptom? Headache from raised intracranial pressure is characteristically worse in the morning and on coughing and straining. The hand pain associated with carpal tunnel syndrome is often worse at night and alleviated when the patient shakes their hand over the side of the bed.
— Is there a **past history** of any similar event?

It is often helpful to obtain details of the history from the patient's relatives or a witness; it is vital to do this if the patient is a child or if there is impairment of conscious state or memory disturbance. Details of the nature of epileptic seizures should always be obtained from a relative or friend who has witnessed an event.

A thorough understanding of the nature of the illness and symptomatology should have been obtained before the examination is commenced.

NEUROLOGICAL EXAMINATION

The formal neurological examination should be undertaken in a systemic fashion in the following order:

1. a. Mental state
   b. Speech
2. Cranial nerves
3. Examination of limbs and trunk
   a. posture
   b. wasting
   c. tone
   d. power
   e. reflexes
   f. sensation
   g. coordination and gait.

Mental state

Examination of the mental state involves an assessment of:

- Conscious state
- Orientation in time, place and person
- Memory
- Emotional state
- Presence of delusions or hallucinations.

A correct assessment of the mental state is essential prior to the evaluation of the other neurological signs. The remainder of the neurological examination will be undertaken within the context of the patient's mental state. The assessment of conscious state is particularly important in neurosurgical problems and the evaluation of the level of consciousness using the Glasgow Coma Scale is described in the chapter on head injuries (Ch. 4). Imprecise terms such as 'stuporose' should be avoided and the examiner should objectively assess and describe the patient's response to specific stimuli. **'Drowsiness'** — a depressed conscious state — is the most important neurological sign and indicates major intracranial pathology. As with all neurological symptoms and signs it is essential to obtain an assessment of the progression of the drowsiness by questioning the patient's friends or relatives. **A deteriorating conscious state is a neurosurgical emergency.**

Memory disturbances should be tested formally for both short-term and long-term preservation. Short-term memory should be tested by listing a name, address and type of flower and asking the patient to recall it after five minutes. Loss of short-term memory with relative preservation of memory for long-past events is typical of dementia, e.g. Alzheimer's disease. In Korsakoff's psychosis the disturbance of recent memory and disorientation may be so severe that the patient will make up stories to provide a convincing answer to the questions. This is **confabulation** and is classically associated with alcoholism, although it may rarely be seen as a result of anterior hypothalamic lesions due to trauma or following subarachnoid haemorrhage and vasospasm.

Speech disorders

There are four main speech disorders:

1. Mutism
2. Dysphonia
3. Dysarthria
4. Dysphasia.

Mutism

Mutism is characterised by the patient being alert but making no attempt to speak. It may result from lesions affecting the medial aspect of both frontal lobes, classically occurring as a result of vasospasm following subarachnoid haemorrhage from a ruptured anterior communicating artery aneurysm.

Aphonia

Aphonia is said to occur when the patient is able to speak but is unable to produce any volume of sound. It is due to a disturbance of the vocal cords or larynx. If the patient is able to cough normally then it is usually hysterical.

Dysarthria

Dysarthria is due to impaired coordination of the lips, palate, tongue and larynx and may result from extrapyramidal, brain stem or cerebellar lesions. The volume and content of the speech will be normal but the enunciation will be distorted.

Spastic dysarthria. This is due to bilateral upper motor neuron disease due to pseudobulbar palsy, motor neuron disease or brain stem tumours.

Ataxic dysarthria. This is due to incoordination of the muscles of speech, the words are often staccato or scanning and the rhythm is jerky. This type of dysarthria is seen in cerebellopontine angle tumours, cerebellar lesions, multiple sclerosis and phenytoin toxicity.

Dysarthria may result from lesions of the lower motor neurons and the muscles, such as occur in palatal palsies or paralysis of the tongue.

'Rigid dysarthria'. This is characteristic of Parkinson's disease. In severe cases the phenomenon of palilalia is seen, in which there is a constant repetition of a particular syllable.

Dysphasia

Dysphasia may be either expressive or receptive. Patients with expressive dysphasia can understand speech but cannot formulate their own speech. Patients with receptive dysphasia cannot understand the spoken or written speech. Although one type of dysphasia may predominate there is frequently a mixture of the two patterns of disability. Dysphasia results from lesions of the dominant hemisphere which is the left hemisphere in right handed people as well as in a high proportion of left-handed people.

Expressive dysphasia. This is due to a lesion affecting either Broca's area in the lower part of the precentral gyrus (Fig 1.1) or the left posterior temporoparietal region. If the latter region is affected the patient may have a **nominal dysphasia,** in which the ability to name objects is lost but the ability to speak is retained.

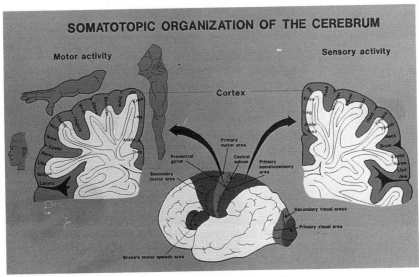

Fig. 1.1 Major areas of somatotopic organisation of the cerebrum.

Receptive dysphasia. This results from lesions in Wernicke's area, which is the posterior part of the superior temporal gyrus and the adjacent parietal lobe.

Alexia

Alexia is the inability to understand written speech. Alexia with agraphia (inability to write) is due to a lesion in the left angular gyrus. The patient is unable to read or write spontaneously and the condition is often accompanied by nominal dysphasia, acalculia, hemianopia and visual agnosia. **Gerstmann's syndrome** consists of finger agnosia for both the patient's own finger and the examiner's finger, acalculia, right/left disorientation and agraphia without alexia. It is found in lesions of the dominant hemisphere in the region of the angular gyrus.

Examination of the cranial nerves

Olfactory nerve

The sense of smell should be tested by the patient sniffing through each nostril as the other is compressed. The common causes of anosmia are olfactory nerve lesions resulting from head injury, and tumours involving the anterior cranial fossa, especially olfactory groove meningiomas. It is important to use non-irritant substances when testing olfaction, as irritating compounds (e.g. ammonia) will cause stimulation of the nasal mucosa.

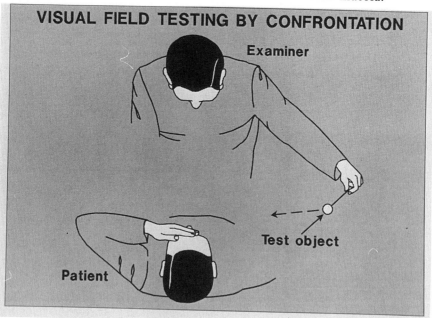

Fig. 1.2 Visual field testing by confrontation.

Optic nerve

The optic nerve should be tested by:

- Measuring the visual acuity and colour vision
- Charting the visual fields
- Fundal examination with an ophthalmoscope
- The pupillary light reflex.

Visual acuity. The visual acuity should be tested using the standard Snellen type charts placed at 6 metres. The acuity is recorded as a fraction, e.g. 6/6 or 6/12, in which the numerator indicates the distance in metres from the chart and the denominator the line on the chart that can be read. 6/6 is normal vision. Refractive errors should be corrected for by testing with the patient's glasses or by asking the patient to view the chart through a pinhole.

Visual fields. The visual fields can be charted by confrontation, with the patient facing the examiner and objects of varying size being moved slowly into the visual field (Fig. 1.2). Formal testing using perimetry should be undertaken in all cases of visual failure, pituitary tumour, parasellar tumour, other tumours possibly involving the visual pathways, demyelinating disease or if there are any doubts after confrontation that the fields may be restricted.

Perimetry can be performed using either a tangent screen, such as a Bjerrum screen (Fig. 1.3), or a Goldmann perimeter. The Bjerrum screen

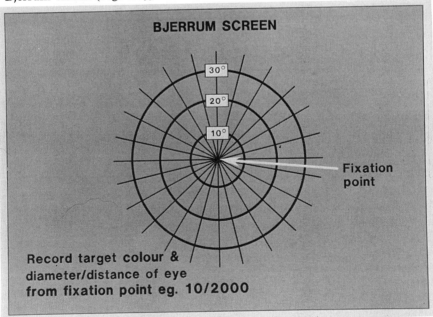

Fig. 1.3 The Bjerrum screen.

records the central field of vision. By enlarging the central area out to 30° it is easier to detect scotoma and to measure the blind spot and, provided a small enough target is used, the tangent screen provides an accurate representation of the peripheral fields.

The pattern of visual field loss will depend on the anatomical site of the lesion in the visual pathways (Fig. 1.4):

- Total visual loss — optic nerve lesion
- Altitudinous hemianopia — partial lesion of the optic nerve due to trauma or vascular accident
- Homonymous hemianopia — lesions of the optic tract, radiation or calcarine cortex
- Bitemporal hemianopia — optic chiasm lesions such as pituitary tumour, craniopharyngioma or suprasellar meningioma.

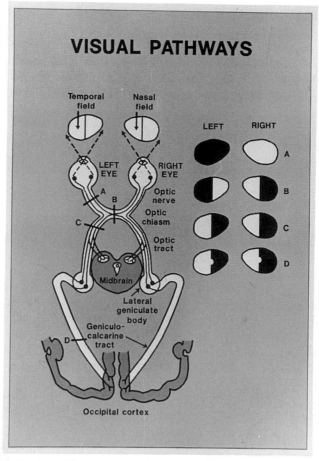

Fig. 1.4 Diagrammatic representation of visual pathways, the common sites of lesions and the resulting field defects.

Fundal examination. The fundus should be examined using the ophthalmoscope with particular attention to the:

- Optic disc
- Vessels
- Retina.

A pale optic disc is due to optic atrophy which may be either primary, as a result of an optic nerve lesion caused by compression or demyelination, or consecutive, which follows severe swelling of the disc. Papilloedema is due to raised intracranial pressure and is evident by:

- Blurring of the disc margins
- Filling in of the optic cup
- Swelling and engorgement of retinal veins, with loss of normal pulsation of the veins
- Haemorrhages around the disc margin (if severe).

Third, fourth and sixth cranial nerves

As these cranial nerves are all involved in innervation of the extraocular muscles they are usually examined together. This examination involves assessment of:

- The position of the eyelids
- The pupils
- Extra-ocular movements.

Position of the eyelids. **Ptosis** is due to paralysis of the levator palpebrae superioris as a result of a 3rd cranial nerve lesion or due to weakness of the tarsal muscle due to a sympathetic lesion (Horner's syndrome).

The pupils. An assessment should be made of the **pupil size, shape** and **equality.** The pupils' reaction to light should be tested by shining a beam into the eye and noting the reaction in that eye, as well as the consensual response in the opposite eye. The reaction to convergence and accommodation for near vision should be tested by asking the patient to fix on a distant object and then placing a pen approximately 12 cm in front of the bridge of the nose.

A unilateral **constricted pupil (myosis)** often indicates a lesion in the sympathetic supply to the pupillary dilator muscle.

Horner's syndrome, in its complete state, consists of myosis, ptosis, enophthalmos and dryness and warmth of half of the face. It is due to a lesion of the sympathetic supply such as results from an intracavernous carotid artery aneurysm, or a Pancoast's tumour of the apex of the lung.

A **dilated pupil (mydriasis)** results from paralysis of the parasympathetic fibres originating from the nucleus of Edinger–Westphal in the mid-brain, and is therefore seen in a 3rd nerve palsy. The possible causes are an enlarging posterior communicating artery aneurysm causing pressure on these fibres in the 3rd cranial nerve (Ch. 9) and tentorial herniation resulting from intracranial pressure with the herniated uncus of the temporal lobe compressing the 3rd nerve (Ch. 5).

The **Argyll-Robertson pupil** is a small, irregular pupil not reacting to light, reacting to accommodation but responding poorly to midriatics; it is usually caused by syphilis.

The **myotonic pupil (Holmes–Adie)** usually occurs in young women and presents as a unilateral dilatation of one pupil with failure to react to light. The pupil shows a slow constriction occurring on maintaining convergence for a prolonged period. In the complete syndrome the knee and ankle jerks are absent.

Ocular movement. The following are the general actions of the extra-ocular muscles:

- Lateral rectus (6th nerve) moves the eye horizontally outwards
- Medial rectus (3rd nerve) moves the eye horizontally inwards
- Superior rectus (3rd nerve) elevates the eye when it is turned outwards
- Inferior oblique (3rd nerve) elevates the eye when it is turned inwards
- Inferior rectus (3rd nerve) depresses the eye when it is turned outwards
- Superior oblique (4th nerve) depresses the eye when it is turned inwards.

The patient should be tested for diplopia, which will indicate ocular muscle weakness before it is evident on examination. The following rules help determine which muscle and cranial nerve are involved.

- The displacement of the false image may be horizontal, vertical or both
- The separation of images is greatest in the direction in which the weak muscle has its purest action
- The false image is displaced furthest in the direction in which the weak muscle should move the eye.

Disorders of eye movement may be due to **impaired conjugate ocular movement.** The centre for the control of conjugate lateral gaze is situated in the posterior part of the frontal lobe, with input from the occipital region. The final common pathway for controlling conjugate movement is in the brain stem, particularly the median longitudinal bundle. A lesion of the frontal lobe causes contralateral paralysis of conjugate gaze (i.e. eyes deviated towards the side of the lesion) and a lesion of the brain stem causes ipsilateral paralysis of conjugate gaze (i.e. eyes deviated to side opposite to the lesion).

Nystagmus should be tested by asking the patient to watch the tip of a pointer. This should be held first in the midline and then moved slowly to the right, to the left and then vertically upwards and downwards.

Jerk nystagmus is the common type consisting of slow drift in one direction and fast correcting movement in the other.

Horizontal jerk nystagmus is produced by lesions in the vestibular system which may occur peripherally in the labyrinth, centrally at the nuclei, in the brain stem or in the cerebellum. In peripheral lesions the quick phase is away from the lesion and the amplitude is greater in the direction of the quick phase. In cerebellar lesions the quick phase is in the direction of gaze at that moment but the amplitude is greater to the side of the lesion. By convention the quick phase is taken to indicate the direction of the nystagmus, so that if the slow phase is to the right and the quick phase to the left the patient is described as having nystagmus to the left.

Vertical nystagmus is due to intrinsic brain stem lesions such as multiple sclerosis or brain stem tumours. The so-called 'downbeat' nystagmus, which is characterised by a vertical nystagmus exaggerated by down gaze, is particularly evident in low brain stem lesions as caused by Chiari syndrome, where the lower brain stem has been compressed by the descending tonsils (Ch. 11).

Trigeminal nerve

The 5th cranial nerve (trigeminal nerve) is tested by assessing facial sensation over the three divisions of the cranial nerve; corneal sensation should be tested using a fine piece of cotton wool. The motor function of the 5th nerve can be tested by palpating the muscles while the patient clenches their jaw, testing the power of jaw opening and lateral deviation of the jaw (Fig. 1.5).

Facial nerve

The facial nerve is tested by assessing facial movement. In an **upper motor neuron** facial weakness the weakness of the lower part of the face is very much greater than the upper, with the strength of the orbicularis oculis being relatively preserved. This is due to a lesion between the cortex and the facial nucleus in the pons. **Lower motor neuron** weakness is evident by equal involvement of the upper and lower parts of the face and is due to a lesion in, or distal to, the facial nerve nucleus in the pons.

The chorda tympani carries taste sensation from the anterior two-thirds of the tongue and this should be examined using test flavours placed carefully on the anterior tongue.

Vestibulocochlear nerve

The 8th cranial nerve consists of:

• the cochlear nerve — hearing
• the vestibular nerve.

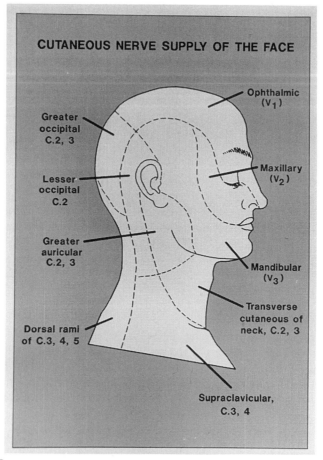

CUTANEOUS NERVE SUPPLY OF THE FACE

Ophthalmic (V$_1$)

Greater occipital C.2, 3

Maxillary (V$_2$)

Lesser occipital C.2

Greater auricular C.2, 3

Mandibular (V$_3$)

Transverse cutaneous of neck, C.2, 3

Dorsal rami of C.3, 4, 5

Supraclavicular, C.3, 4

Fig. 1.5 Cutaneous nerve supply of the face, scalp and neck.

The cochlear nerve. Hearing can be examined at the bedside by moving a finger in the meatus on one side, to produce a masking noise, and repeating words at a standard volume and from a set distance in the other ear. Differentiation between conduction and sensory neural deafness can be aided using tests with a tuning fork.

The **Rinne's test** involves placing a vibrating tuning fork in front of the external meatus and then on the mastoid process. In nerve deafness both air and bone conduction are reduced, but air conduction remains the better. In conductive deafness the bone conduction will be better than the air conduction.

In **Weber's test** the vibrating tuning fork is placed on the centre of the forehead. In nerve deafness the sound appears to be heard better in the normal ear but in conductive deafness the sound is conducted to the abnormal ear.

Formal audiometry should be performed if there are symptoms of impaired hearing.

The vestibular nerve. The simplest test of vestibular function is the caloric test, which is usually performed in patients suspected of having a cerebellopontine angle tumour or as a test of brain stem function in patients with severe brain injury. The test is described in Chapter 4, page 66.

Glossopharyngeal and vagus nerves

The glossopharyngeal and vagus nerves can be most easily assessed by testing palatal movement and sensation from the pharynx and soft palate. If necessary the vocal cords (vagus nerve) can be examined and taste from the posterior one-third of the tongue (glossopharyngeal nerve) can be tested.

Accessory nerve

The accessory nerve supplies the motor power to the upper part of the trapezius and sternocleidomastoid. The latter muscle can be tested by turning the patient's head against resistance and watching and palpating the opposite sternomastoid muscle. The trapezius muscle is best tested by asking the patient to shrug the shoulders and attempting to depress the shoulders forcibly.

Hypoglossal nerve

The hypoglossal nerve is responsible for movements of the tongue. The tongue should be inspected to detect wasting and movements from side to side should be observed to detect weakness. The tip of the protruded tongue will deviate toward the side of weakness.

Examination of the periphery

Posture and general inspection

The patient's posture may indicate an underlying neurological disability, or an abnormal posture may result from pain. A patient with sciatica will often lie on the opposite side with the affected leg flexed at the hip and knee. The decerebrate posture is discussed in the Chapter 4.

The limbs should be inspected to compare size and shape and to detect deformity; long-standing neurological lesions may result in impaired growth or wasting. Lesions of lower motor neuron in infancy, such as a brachial plexus palsy or poliomyelitis, will cause marked retardation in limb growth. Upper motor neuron lesions of long standing, such as acute infantile hemiplegia and cerebral birth trauma, will also cause retardation in growth, but of a lesser degree, with a hemiplegic posture and exaggerated reflexes.

Wasting

The limbs and shoulder girdles should be inspected to detect wasting and fasciculation. As well as palpating for specific muscle wasting in each limb the circumference of the limbs should be measured at clearly identifiable positions, such as 8 cm above or below the olecranon, 10 cm above the patella and 8 cm below the tibial tuberosity.

The pattern of wasting will be an important clue as to the underlying neurological disease.

Wasting of the forearm and small muscles of the hand. This results from lower motor neuron lesions affecting particularly the C7, C8 and T1 levels and may be due to lesions of the:

- Spinal cord — motor neuron disease, syringomyelia, cervical cord tumours
- Cervical nerve root — cervical disc prolapse
- Brachial plexus — trauma, cervical rib, axillary tumour
- Peripheral nerve — ulnar nerve compression at the elbow, carpal tunnel syndrome (median nerve).

Wasting of the muscles of the lower leg. This will result from compression of the cauda equina or lumbosacral nerve roots caused by a lumbar disc prolapse or tumour.

Muscular dystrophies. These are genetically determined degenerative myopathies and cause particular patterns of muscle wasting:

- Facioscapulohumeral dystrophy involves the face and shoulder girdle
- Proximal limb girdle dystrophy involves both shoulder and hip girdles
- Dystrophia myotonica involves the face, sternomastoids and quadriceps femoris. Myotonia (the failure of muscle to relax after contraction) is present, particularly in the peripheral muscles and tongue
- Peroneal muscular atrophy, with predominant involvement of the lower limbs, causes the 'inverted bottle appearance' with similar but less striking changes in the upper limbs
- Pseudohypertrophic muscular dystrophy occurs mainly in young boys and affects the arms and legs; the muscles have a pseudohypertrophic appearance.

Tone

The tone in the upper limbs should be tested using a flexion–extension movement of the wrist, by holding the patient's terminal phalanges and by pronation–supination of the forearm. The tone in the lower limbs should be tested by flexion of the hip, knee and ankle.

Decreased tone. This is due to:

- A lower motor neuron lesion involving the spinal roots or anterior horn cell of the spinal cord
- Lesions of the sensory roots of the reflex arc, e.g. tabes dorsalis
- Cerebellar lesions cause ipsilateral hypotonia
- Myopathies
- Spinal shock (the acute phase of a severe spinal lesion usually due to trauma).

Increased tone. This will be produced by any upper motor neuron lesion involving the corticospinal tracts above the level of the anterior horn cell in the spinal cord.

There are three major types of hypertonicity:

1. 'Clasp knife' spasticity, in which the resistance is most pronounced when the movement is first made. It is usually more marked in the flexor muscles of the upper limbs and extensor muscles of the lower limbs and is a sign of an upper motor neuron lesion
2. 'Lead pipe' rigidity, in which there is equal resistance to all movements. This is a characteristic feature of a lesion of the extrapyramidal system but is also seen in severe spasticity from an upper motor neuron lesion
3. 'Cog wheel' rigidity, in which there is an alternating jerky resistance to movement and which occurs in degenerative lesions of the extrapyramidal system, particularly Parkinson's disease.

'Clonus' is best demonstrated by firm rapid dorsiflexion of the foot and is indicative of marked increased tone.

Power

The power should be tested in all limbs, comparing each side. A systematic evaluation will enable the recognition of a particular pattern of weakness that will be in keeping with either a cerebral, spinal cord, plexus or peripheral nerve weakness. The major nerve and main root supply of the muscles are shown in Table 1.1.

The Medical Research Council classifies the degree of weakness by recording power, ranging from 0 to 5 (Table 1.2). It is apparent that there is a considerable range of power between the grades 4 and 5 and some clinicians make their own further subclassification in this region.

Weakness due to a **corticospinal tract lesion** is most marked in the abductors and extensors of the upper limbs and the flexors of the lower limbs. It is normally associated with increased tone and exaggerated reflexes.

Table 1.1   Nerve and major root supply of muscles

Upper limb	Spinal roots
Spinal accessory nerve	
Trapezius	C3, C4
Brachial plexus	
Rhomboids	C4, C5
Serratus anterior	C5, C6, C7
Pectoralis major	
clavicular	**C5**, C6
sternal	C6, **C7**, C8
Supraspinatus	**C5**, C6
Infraspinus	**C5**, C6
Latissimus dorsi	C6, **C7**, C8
Teres major	C5, C6, C7
Axillary nerve	
Deltoid	**C5**, C6
Musculocutaneous nerve	
Biceps	C5, C6
Brachialis	C5, C6
Radial nerve	
Triceps Long head / Lateral head / Medial head	C6, **C7**, C8
Brachioradialis	C5, **C6**
Extensor carpi radialis longus	C5, **C6**
Posterior interosseous nerve	
Supinator	C6, C7
Extensor carpi ulnaris	**C7**, C8
Extensor digitorum	**C7**, C8
Abductor pollicis longus	**C7**, C8
Extensor pollicis longus	**C7**, C8
Extensor pollicis brevis	**C7**, C8
Extensor indicis	**C7**, C8
Median nerve	
Pronator teres	C6, C7
Flexor carpi radialis	C6, C7
Flexor digitorum superficialis	C7, **C8**, T1
Abductor pollicis brevis	C8, **T1**
Flexor pollicis brevis★	C8, **T1**
Opponens pollicis	C8, **T1**
Lumbricals I and II	C8, **T1**
Anterior interosseous nerve	
Flexor digitorum profundus I and II	C7, **C8**
Flexor pollicis longus	C7, **C8**
Ulnar nerve	
Flexor carpi ulnaris	C7, **C8**, T1
Flexor digitorum profundus III and IV	C7, **C8**
Hypothenar muscles	C8, **T1**
Adductor pollicis	C8, **T1**
Flexis pollicis brevis	C8, **T1**
Palmar interossei	C8, **T1**
Dorsal interossei	C8, **T1**
Lumbricals III and IV	C8, **T1**

Table 1.1   Contd

Lower limb	
Femoral nerve	
Iliopsoas	**L1, L2**, L3
Rectus femoris	
Vastus lateralis	
Vastus intermedius ⎱ Quadriceps femoris	**L2, L3, L4**
Vastus medialis	
Obturator nerve	
Adductor longus	
Adductor magnus	**L2, L3**, L4
Superior gluteal nerve	
Gluteus medium and minimus	
Tensor fasciae latae	**L4, L5**, S1
Inferior gluteal nerve	
Gluteus maximus	**L5, S1**, S2
Sciatic and tibial nerves	
Semitendinosus	L5, **S1**, S2
Biceps	L5, **S1**, S2
Semimembranosus	L5, **S1**, S2
Gastrocnemius and soleus	S1, S2
Tibialis posterior	L4, L5
Flexor digitorum longus	L5, **S1, S2**
Flexor hallucis longus	L5, **S1, S2**
Small muscles of foot	S1, S2
Sciatic and common peroneal nerves	
Tibialis anterior	**L4**, L5
Extensor digitorum longus	**L5**, S1
Extensor hallucis longus	**L5**, S1
Extensor digitorum brevis	L5, S1
Peroneus longus	L5, S1
Peroneus brevis	L5, S1

⋆ Flexor pollicis brevis is often supplied wholly or partially by the ulnar nerve

Weakness due to **lower motor neuron lesions** is usually more severe than when the upper motor neuron is involved and is seen in the distribution of the nerve affected. It is associated with wasting, hypotonia and diminished reflexes.

Fasciculation is an irregular, non-rhythmical contraction of muscle fascicles which is most easily seen in the deltoid or calf muscles. It occurs classically in motor neuron disease but may also occur in lower motor neuron lesions, e.g in the lower limbs following long-standing lumbar root compression.

Reflexes

The deep tendon reflex requires the stimulus, sensory pathway, motor neuron, contracting muscle and the synapses between the neurons in order to elicit a response.

Reduced or absent tendon reflex. This may occur due to any breach in the reflex arc:

- Sensory nerve — polyneuritis
- Sensory root — tabes dorsalis
- Anterior horn cell — poliomyelitis
- Anterior root — compression
- Peripheral motor nerve — trauma
- Muscle — myopathy.

Increased deep tendon reflexes. Due to lesions of the pyramidal system, increased deep tendon reflexes may be excessively prolonged, with a larger amplitude in a cerebellar lesion. In myxoedema the relaxation phase of the reflex is retarded.

Each deep tendon reflex is associated with a particular segmental innervation and peripheral nerve as listed in Table 1.3.

The superficial abdominal reflex has a segmental innervation extending from T9 in the upper abdominal region to T12 in the lower area. The reflex may be absent in pyramidal lesions above the level of segmental innervation, particularly in spinal lesions. However, the reflex may also be difficult to elicit when the abdominal muscles have been stretched or damaged by surgical operations, or in a large, pendulous, obese abdomen.

Table 1.2 Medical Research Council Classification of power

0	Total paralysis
1	Flicker of contraction but no movement of limb
2	Muscle only able to make normal movement when limb is positioned so that gravity is eliminated
3	Normal movement against gravity but not against additional resistance
4	Full movement but overcome by resistance
5	Normal power

Table 1.3 Deep tendon reflexes, peripheral nerve and segmental innervation

Tendon reflex	Major segmental innervation	Peripheral nerve
Biceps jerk	C5(6)	Musculocutaneous
Supinator jerk	C5/C6	Radial
Triceps jerk	C7(8)	Radial
Flexor finger jerk	C6–T1	Median and ulnar
Knee jerk	L3/L4	Femoral
Ankle jerk	S1(2)	Medial popliteal and sciatic

Plantar reflex. This should result in the great toe flexing the metatarso-phalangeal joint. The Babinski response consists of extension of the great toe at the metatarsophalangeal joint, and usually at the interphalangeal joint, and indicates disturbance of the pyramidal tract.

Sensation

The modalities of sensation which should be tested are:

- Light touch
- Pinprick (pain)
- Temperature
- Position (proprioception)
- Vibration.

Sensory testing involves an accurate understanding of the anatomical pathways of sensation. All modalities of sensation travel by the peripheral nerve and sensory root to the spinal cord, or via the cranial nerves to the brain stem. The fibres for pain and temperature sensation enter the posterolateral aspect of the spinal cord, travel cranially for a few segments and then cross to the opposite anterolateral spinothalamic tract. This tract ascends to the brain stem and is joined by the quintothalamic (trigeminothalamic) tract in the pons. The fibres end mostly in the ventro-lateral nucleus of the thalamus and from here the sensory impulses pass through the posterior limb of the internal capsule to the postcentral sensory cortex (see Ch. 19, Fig. 19.1). Fibres carrying light touch, proprioception and vibration sensation ascend mainly in the ipsilateral posterior columns of the spinal cord on the same side to the nuclei gracilis and cuneatus. The fibres cross the midline to ascend through the brain stem in the medial lemniscus, to the thalamus and on to the sensory cortex.

The sensory loss involving nocioceptive stimuli (pain and temperature) should conform to a particular pattern:

- Peripheral nerve
- Dermatome (nerve root)
- Spinal cord — resulting in a sensory level
- 'Glove and stocking' due to peripheral neuropathy
- Hemi-analgesia — thalamic or upper brain stem
- Loss of pain and temperature on one side of the face and the opposite side of the body — lesion of the medulla affecting the descending root of the 5th nerve and the ascending spinothalamic tract from the remainder of the body.

Coordination

Coordination should be tested in the upper and lower limbs. In the upper limb it is best assessed using the 'finger nose' test and in the lower limb using the 'heel knee' test. It is important to determine whether abnormalities of coordination are due to defects in:

- Cerebellar function
- Proprioception
- Muscular weakness.

Gait

An essential part of the examination is to observe the patient's gait. This is best done not only as a formal part of the examination but also when the patient is not aware of observation. The type of gait is characteristic of the underlying neurological disturbance.

A hemiparesis will cause the patient to drag the leg and, if severe, the leg will be thrown out from the hip, producing the movement called **circumduction.**

A **high stepping gait.** This occurs with a foot drop (e.g. L5 root lesion due to disc prolapse, lateral popliteal nerve palsy, peroneal muscular atrophy). The patient raises the foot too high to overcome the foot drop and the toe hits the ground first. In tabes dorsalis the high stepping gait is due to a profound loss of position sense but a similar gait, of lesser severity, will result from involvement of the posterior column of the spinal cord or severe sensory neuropathy which interferes with position sense. The gait is worse in the dark and the heel usually strikes the ground first.

In **Parkinson's disease** or other extrapyramidal diseases the patient walks with a stooped, shuffling gait. The patient may have difficulty in starting walking and stopping. A slight push forward will cause rapid forward movement (protopulsion).

In the **ataxic gait,** the patient is unstable due to cerebellar disturbance. A midline vermis tumour will result in the patient reeling in any direction. If the cerebellar hemisphere is involved then the patient will tend to fall to a particular side.·

A **waddling gait** is associated with congenital dislocation of the hips and muscular dystrophy.

The hysterical gait is often bizarre and is diminished when the patient is unaware of any observation.

Following the clinical assessment, a presumptive diagnosis is made and further investigations can be performed to confirm the diagnosis. These laboratory investigations and radiological procedures are described in the following chapter.

BRAIN DEATH

The use of donor organs for transplantation and the advent of improved intensive care facilities have resulted in the necessity of medically and legally accepted criteria of brain death.

If there is irrecoverable brain stem damage and the tests described below show no evidence of brain stem function, then the patient is medically and legally dead. If artificial ventilation is continued the other organs may continue to function for some time. However, continued prolonged ventilation of the patient after the diagnosis of brain death is not only undignified for the dead patient and distressing to the relatives, but is also wasteful of expensive medical resources that are often in short supply.

The diagnosis of brain death relies on:

- Preconditions before testing can be performed
- Brain death tests.

The preconditions are that reversible causes of brain stem depression have been excluded, these include:

- Depressant drugs
- Hypothermia (temperature must be greater than 35 °C)
- Neuromuscular blocking drugs
- Metabolic or endocrine disturbance as a cause of the patient's condition.

If there is any doubt, brain death testing must be delayed until these preconditions are absolutely satisfied.

The tests for brain stem function are:

- Lack of pupil response to light
- Lack of corneal reflex to stimulation
- Lack of oculocephalic reflex
- Failure of vestibulo-ocular reflex (caloric testing)
- Failure of a gag or cough reflex on bronchial stimulation
- No motor response in the face or muscles supplied by the cranial nerves in response to painful stimulus
- Failure of respiratory movements when the patient is disconnected from a ventilator and the $PaCO_2$ is allowed to rise to 50 mmHg.

The tests should be repeated after an interval of 30 minutes and it is essential that they should be carried out by two doctors of adequate seniority and with expertise in the field.

FURTHER READING

Medical Research Council 1976 Aids to the examination of the peripheral nervous system. Her Majesty's Stationery Office, London

Walton J (ed) 1977 Brain. In: Diseases of the Nervous System, Oxford University Press, Oxford

Conference of Medical Royal Colleges and Their Faculties in the UK 1979 Diagnosis of death. British Journal of Medicine 1: 322

Harrington D 1974 The visual fields, 4th ed. C V Mosby, St Louis

Jennett B 1981 Brain death. British Journal of Anaesthesia 53: 1111–1119

Plum F, Posner J B 1980 Diagnosis of stupor and coma, 3rd ed. F A Davis, Philadelphia

Plum F 1980 Brain death. Lancet ii: 379

2. Neurosurgical investigations

Investigations to determine the exact diagnosis are nearly always necessary following the clinical examination. The following is a list of the more common investigations that may need to be undertaken:

- Cerebrospinal fluid (CSF) studies
- Radiological investigations
- Electroencephalography
- Nerve conduction studies
- Evoked potential studies
- Nuclear medicine investigations.

Some of these investigations will be described in this chapter. The others will be dealt with in the chapters dealing with the relevant neurosurgical problems.

CEREBROSPINAL FLUID INVESTIGATION

The CSF is produced by the choroid plexus at a rate of approximately 0.4 ml per minute. The fluid circulates from the lateral ventricles through the interventricular foramen (of Munro) into the 3rd ventricle, through the cerebral aqueduct of Sylvius into the 4th ventricle and into the subarachnoid space via the two laterally placed foramen of Luschka and a medial aperture in the roof of the 4th ventricle — the foramen of Magendie. The fluid circulates caudally into the spinal subarachnoid space, throughout the basal cisterns, up through the tentorial hiatus and then over the cerebral hemispheres. It is absorbed by the arachnoid villi of the dural sinuses, and especially by the superior sagittal sinus. Approximately 500 ml of CSF is produced each day. The total CSF volume is 140 ml; the lateral ventricles contain approximately 25 ml, the spinal cord subarachnoid space 30 ml and the remainder of the fluid is found in the basal cisterns. Table 2.1 shows the normal constituents of CSF.

The CSF glucose content is approximately 65% of the blood plasma level in the fasting state. There is a gradient for many of the constituents of CSF along the cerebrospinal axis (Table 2.2).

Table 2.1 CSF statistics (lumbar)

Volume	500 ml
Rate of production	0.4 ml/min
Pressure (recumbent)	10–15 cm of CSF
Cells	Less than 3–4 white cells/mm^3
Protein	0.15–0.45 g/l (15–45 mg/100 ml)
Glucose	2.8–4.2 mmol/l (50–75 mg/100 ml)
IgG	10–12% of total protein
Chloride	120–130 mmol/l

The values are expressed in SI (Système Internationale) units and the corresponding traditional units are in parentheses.

Table 2.2 CSF gradients along the cerebrospinal axis

	Ventricle	Cisternal	Lumbar
Protein (g/l)	0.1	0.2	0.4
Glucose (mmol/l)	4.5	4.0	3.4

The fluid is normally clear and colourless; it will appear turbid if it contains more than 400 white blood cells or 200 red blood cells per mm^3. Yellow discolouration, xanthochromia, is due to the breakdown products of red blood cells, these follow haemorrhage into the CSF.

CSF can be obtained by:

- Lumbar puncture
- Cisternal puncture
- Cannulation of the lateral ventricle.

The fluid is usually obtained by lumbar puncture. Cisternal puncture is performed if the lumbar puncture has failed due to technical difficulties, if there is local skin sepsis or, in some radiology investigations, where it is the preferred route of contrast administration for myelography. Ventricular puncture is usually only performed as an intra-operative procedure or for temporary reduction of intracranial pressure in an emergency.

Lumbar puncture

The most common indications for CSF examination by lumbar puncture are:

- Meningitis
- Subarachnoid haemorrhage
- Neurological diseases such as multiple sclerosis
- Cytological examination for neoplastic disease
- Radiological imaging (e.g. myelography) or radio-isotope investigations
- Measurement of intracranial pressure.

The most important **contraindication** to lumbar puncture is clinical evidence of **raised intracranial pressure**. Papilloedema is an absolute contraindication and a lumbar puncture should never be performed in a patient in whom an intracranial space-occupying lesion is suspected. If there is any doubt a CT scan must be performed prior to lumbar puncture. A lumbar puncture should not be performed if there is local infection.

Technique of lumbar puncture

The patient should be positioned on the side, the back vertical on the edge of the bed and with the knees flexed up to the chest. The iliac crest is palpated; this lies at the L3/4 level. The lumbar puncture can be carried out at this space or at the spaces immediately above or below. The area is prepared with antiseptic solution and draped. The procedure must be performed under completely sterile conditions. The interspinous area is palpated and the skin injected with 1–2 ml of 1% xylocaine local anaesthetic. The lumbar puncture needle is inserted between the two spinous processes, pointing in a slightly cranial direction. If performed carefully it is usually possible to feel the needle pass through the interspinous ligament and then through the dura. The stilette of the lumbar puncture needle is withdrawn and a manometer attached to measure the pressure. The fluid is drained into sterile containers and sent for examination.

Complications of lumbar puncture

If performed properly, with the appropriate indications, lumbar puncture is well tolerated and complications should be minimal. However, there are several potential hazards and complications, these include:

- Progression of brain herniation
- Progression of spinal cord compression
- Injury to the neural structures
- Headache
- Backache
- Infection — local and meningitis
- Implantation of epidermoid tumour (rare).

The potential risk of lumbar puncture worsening brain herniation can be avoided if the procedure is not undertaken in patients with raised intracranial pressure. Neurological deterioration may follow lumbar puncture and myelography in patients with spinal tumours where there is severe cord compression, but the procedure is usually necessary to make the diagnosis, although in some cases may be avoided by the use of MRI and CT scanning. Neurological deterioration requires prompt surgery, this is discussed in Chapter 15. Infection should be avoided by the use of scrupulous sterile techniques. If the procedure is performed at a level that is too high there is a risk of neural damage, particularly to the conus medullaris. Rarely, a nerve root may be injured by the improper placement of the needle. Injury to a spinal radicular artery may occasionally give rise to a spinal subdural or epidural haematoma; this risk is increased if the patient is taking anticoagulation therapy.

The traumatic effects of the lumbar puncture are responsible for minor, transient low back discomfort. Very rarely, frank disc herniation has been reported due to damage of the annulus fibrosus of the disc.

Headache. The most common complication of lumbar puncture is headache. In most cases this is due to low CSF pressure that results from persistent leakage of the fluid through a hole in the arachnoid and dura. It is generally recommended that patients should remain flat for 12 hours following a lumbar puncture to minimise the risk of this complication. The use of a narrow gauge needle (20 gauge or less) and avoiding multiple puncture holes in the meninges also decreases the chance of troublesome postlumbar puncture headache.

If the headache develops following mobilisation the patient should be instructed to lie flat for a further 24 hours and encouraged to drink large volumes of non-alcoholic fluids. Some clinicians advocate the use of 'blood patch' for the treatment of persistent postspinal headache. This technique uses the epidural injection of autologous blood at the site of dural puncture to form a thrombotic tamponade which seals the dural opening, but this is very rarely necessary.

CSF examination

The CSF should be examined immediately. If the fluid is blood-stained it should be spun down in a centrifuge and examined for evidence of xanthochromia, this being indicative of haemorrhage into the CSF.

Three major pigments derived from red cells may be detected in CSF; oxyhaemoglobin, bilirubin and methaemoglobin.

Oxyhaemoglobin is red, but after dilution it appears pink or orange. It is released by lysis of red cells and may be detected in the CSF within two hours of the release of blood into the subarachnoid space. It reaches a maximum in the first 36 hours and gradually disappears over the next 7–10 days.

Bilirubin is yellow and is the iron-free derivative of haemoglobin produced in vivo following the haemolysis of red cells. Bilirubin formation in the CSF probably depends on the ability of macrophages and other cells in the leptomeninges to degrade haemoglobin. It is first detected about 10 hours after the onset of subarachnoid bleeding and reaches a maximum at 48 hours. It may persist for 2–4 weeks after extensive haemorrhage.

Methaemoglobin is a reduction product of haemoglobin. It is a brown pigment that is dark yellow in dilution and it is characteristically found in encapsulated subdural haematomas.

Although it may be detected by spectrophotometry of the spinal fluid in patients with large encapsulations of this sort, the pigment is not usually observed in other xanthochromic spinal fluids.

Xanthochromic spinal fluid may also occur in jaundice, such as jaundice secondary to liver disease or in haemolytic disease of the newborn.

The fluid should be sent for microbiological and biochemical examination and, if clinically indicated, cytological examination for malignant cells.

The common abnormalities are shown in Table 2.3. Normal CSF contains no more than four lymphocytes or mononuclear cells per mm^3. Polymorphonuclear cells are never found in normal CSF but an isolated granulocyte, presumably derived from blood at the time of lumbar puncture, may be seen if the CSF has been cytocentrifuged. A granulocyte pleocytosis is the hallmark of bacterial infection; a granulocytic phase also occurs at the onset of a viral meningitis, prior to the development of a purely mononuclear reaction.

Eosinophils are not seen in normal CSF. The most common causes of prominent eosinophilic reaction are parasitic diseases, but eosinophilia may also occur in inflammatory diseases and in a range of other diseases, as shown in Table 2.3.

Table 2.3 CSF abnormalities

CSF abnormality	Disease suspected
Polymorphonuclear pleocytosis	Bacterial meningitis
Mononuclear pleocytosis	Viral meningitis Tuberculous meningitis Acute demyelination

Eosinophils	Parasitic infections
	    Trichinella and ascaris
	    Toxoplasma
	    Cysticercosis
	Inflammatory diseases
	    Tuberculosis
	    Syphilis
	    Subacute sclerosing panencephalitis
	    Fungal infections
	Other diseases
	    Lymphoma
	    Hodgkin's disease
	    Multiple sclerosis

Raised protein	CNS infection Spinal block (very high levels — Froins syndrome) Carcinomatosis of the meninges Spinal neurofibromas Acoustic neuromas Guillain–Barré syndrome
Low sugar	Bacterial meningitis
Low chloride (<110 mmol/l)	Tuberculous meningitis

CSF electrophoresis

Electrophoresis of the spinal fluid is useful in the diagnosis of patients suspected of having demyelination. An IgG of over 15% of the total protein
is suggestive of disseminated sclerosis but it may also be raised in auto-
immune states, such as Guillain–Barré syndrome and carcinomatosis. Electrophoresis of the cerebrospinal fluid may also demonstrate myeloma
protein.

In addition to the absolute increase noted in gamma globulins in inflammatory diseases of the system, qualitative changes in CSF gamma globulins
have been demonstrated in concentrated CSF with agarose gel electrophoresis and other gels. This technique demonstrates discreet bands in the
gamma globulin pattern which have been called **oligoclonal bands**. The
term describes a population of proteins, having identical electrophoretic
characteristics derived from the same population of immunocompetent cells.
A single antigen is presumed to give rise to a single band. Oligoclonal bands
are reported in about 90% of patients with multiple sclerosis and are frequently observed whenever CSF gamma globulin is increased due to a
variety of inflammatory disorders of the nervous system. In patients with
multiple sclerosis the band pattern seems to be unique for each patient, and
it remains stable over time.

Serological investigations for neurosyphilis should be performed on the
CSF if suspected.

RADIOLOGICAL INVESTIGATIONS

The major radiological investigations are:

- Plain X-rays
- Computerised tomography (CT) scan
- Cerebral angiography
- Myelography
- Magnetic resonance imaging.

Skull X-ray

The usefulness of the plain skull X-ray has been largely superseded by CT
scanning. However, it is still a helpful preliminary investigation in patients
with head injuries. The details of the use of this investigation in trauma are
discussed in Chapter 4.

The major abnormalities to look for on a skull X-ray are:

- Fractures
- Hyperostosis, e.g. meningioma
- Bone erosion due to skull vault tumours
- Midline shift of the pineal gland — from space occupying lesion

- Abnormal calcification, e.g. tumours such as meningioma, oligodendroglioma, craniopharyngioma or calcified wall of an aneurysm
- Signs of long-standing raised intracranial pressure — erosion of posterior clinoid processes
- 'Copper beating' of the skull vault. Enhanced digital markings are not uncommon under the age of 30 but may indicate long-standing raised intracranial pressure if present over the whole vault.

Plain X-rays of the spine

These are useful preliminary investigations for patients presenting with spinal pain. Particular note should be taken of:

- Vertebral alignment
- Presence of degenerative disease with narrowing of the neural foramen and spinal canal
- Evidence of metastatic tumour with erosion or sclerosis of the vertebral body, pedicles or lamina
- Enlargement of a neural foramen indicating a spinal schwannoma
- Congenital abnormalities such as spina bifida.

Computerised tomography scanning

Computerised tomography (CT) scanning was introduced in the 1970s and has revolutionised the radiological investigation of neurological disease. Over the past decade considerable technical advances have greatly improved the quality of scanning which can now be performed in both the axial (horizontal) and coronal planes. Sagittal reconstruction pictures can be obtained by computer manipulation of the data.

The CT scan is the initial investigation of choice in the investigation of nearly all intracranial diseases. Figure 2.1 shows the normal structures seen in axial CT scans at various positions through the cranium.

Intracranial calcification may be seen on the plain CT scan. Intracranial lesions that show calcification on the plain CT scan include:

- Meningioma — will also show hyperostosis of cranial vault
- Most oligodendrogliomas
- Astrocytoma — 30% of low grade tumours but infrequently in high grade tumours
- Ependymoma and subependymoma
- Craniopharyngioma
- Wall of giant aneurysm, arteriovenous malformations.

The pineal gland is usually calcified and calcification of the choroid plexus, basal ganglia and falx may occur in normal scans.

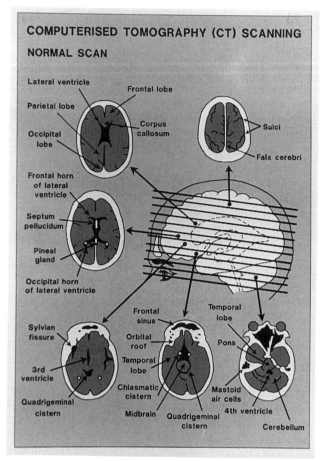

Fig. 2.1 Normal intracerebral and cranial structures on CT scan at various levels through the cranium.

Following a plain CT scan **iodine-based contrast medium** is administered intravenously; this will enhance areas with increased vascularity or with impairment of the blood–brain barrier. The non-ionic iodine agents have reduced the very small risk following intravenous administration of contrast, the most serious side-effect being an anaphylactic reaction. Intracranial lesions that enhance following contrast administration include:

- High grade cerebral gliomas
- Meningiomas
- Acoustic neuromas
- Large pituitary tumours
- Metastatic tumours
- Arteriovenous malformations.

Cerebral abscesses usually enhance with a peripheral ring. Low grade gliomas often have scanty, if any enhancement.

An intracranial mass will cause distortion of the lateral ventricles either as a result of the lesion itself or because of the associated **cerebral oedema**, which appears as an area of decreased density around the lesion.

CT scanning of the spine is valuable in the management of:

- Lumbar disc prolapse
- Degenerative disease of the lumbar spine
- Lumbar canal stenosis
- Cervical canal stenosis
- Spinal trauma
- Spinal dysraphism.

CT scanning, when combined with intrathecal iodine contrast, is the preferred imaging technique for cervical disc prolapse. This is discussed in Chapter 14.

Cerebral angiography

Angiography of the intra- and extracranial vessels is now usually performed using computerised digital subtraction angiographic techniques. The procedure is usually done under local anaesthesia in the adult patient. The catheter is inserted into the femoral artery and threaded up into the carotid or vertebral origin with the aid of an image intensifier.

Digital subtraction angiography has considerably reduced the complications of standard angiography, although there is still a very small risk of cerebral embolus from a clot or an atherosclerotic plaque broken off by the catheter tip.

The major indications for angiography are:

- Investigation of cerebral ischaemia due to carotid artery disease and intracranial atheroma
- Investigation of subarachnoid haemorrhage, e.g. cerebral aneurysm, arteriovenous malformation
- Investigation of venous sinus thrombosis
- Preoperative embolisation of meningioma.

Cerebral angiography is now only infrequently used in the investigation of intracranial tumours. The major intracranial vessels are shown in Figure 2.2.

Myelography

Myelography is used in the investigation of spinal disease which has resulted in compression of the adjacent neural structures. The technique, using

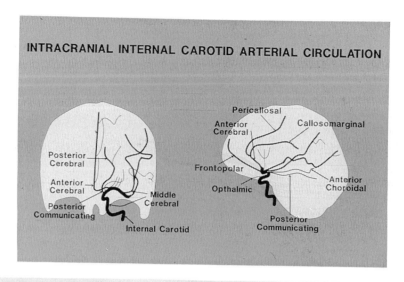

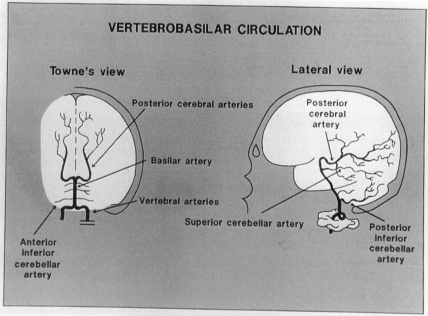

Fig. 2.2   The major intracranial vessels seen on cerebral angiography.

water-soluble contrast agents, is safer and produces higher quality imaging than was achieved with the previously used oil-based materials. In particular, the dreaded complication of postmyelography arachnoiditis does not occur with the water based material. Complications, which are now very uncommon, include epileptic seizures, systemic reactions to the contrast material and the risks of the lumbar puncture itself. The major indications for myelography are:

- Cervical disc prolapse
- Lumbar disc prolapse
- Spinal tumour
- Cervical canal stenosis causing cervical myelopathy
- Lumbar canal stenosis.

High quality CT scanning and the introduction of magnetic resonance imaging has considerably diminished the indications for myelography. Most lumbar disc prolapses and lumbar canal stenosis can be adequately assessed with the CT scan. Spinal tumours and most cervical spinal pathology are shown well with the higher quality magnetic resonance imaging, although at present posterolateral cervical disc prolapse is not adequately imaged. However, as magnetic resonance imaging is not yet readily available in most countries, myelography is still frequently indicated.

Magnetic resonance imaging

Magnetic resonance imaging (MRI) is a diagnostic radiological technique which utilises the magnetic properties of the body's hydrogen nuclei to produce cross-sectional images in any plane. A moving charged particle creates a small magnetic field. At equilibrium the multiple tiny magnetic fields created by the randomly spinning hydrogen nuclei (protons) within the body cancel each other out. If the body is placed within a strong external magnetic field, the protons tend to align themselves within that field. If energy, in the form of pulses of electromagnetic waves of precisely the right frequency and band width (usually in the FM radio range), is introduced into the body, the protons can be induced to spin in unison, or resonantly (Fig. 2.3). When the external energy source is removed, the energy from the excited protons is emitted in the form of a radio signal, which progressively dies away. Although faint, the decaying signal can be detected by sensitive antennae (receiver coils) placed strategically in relation to the part of the body being scanned. Initially, the strength of the signal is proportional to the distribution of the protons within the tissue. The rate of decay, or 'relaxation', is dependent upon two factors. First, the efficiency with which energy is transferred from the protons to their immediately adjacent molecular lattice, or framework, which is described by an exponential curve with time constant, T1. Although commonly named 'T1 relaxation time', other eponyms used include 'longitudinal relaxation time', 'spin lattice relaxation time' and 'thermal relaxation time'. The second factor contributing to signal decay is the destructive interference of the protons' spins with each other. Because the protons are exposed to minute differences in local magnetic field, their spins become out of phase, resulting in loss of

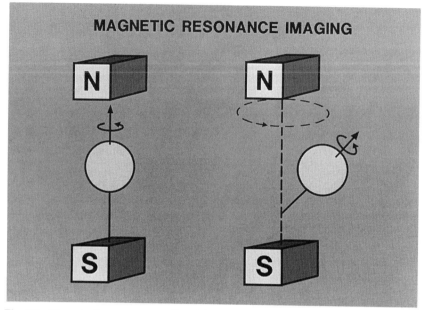

Fig. 2.3 The spinning protons are aligned in a magnetic field (left). An electromagnetic pulse displaces the protons (right).

synchronisation, or resonance. The rate of signal decay due to this factor is described by another exponential curve with time constant T2, which is commonly called 'T2 relaxation time'. It is also known as 'horizontal relaxation time' and 'spin-spin relaxation time'.

Contrast between different tissues in MRI images is due to differences in proton concentration, T1 and T2. These differences can be maximised by varying the rate of the pulses of electromagnetic energy (T_R or pulse repetition time) and the time interval following the pulses at which the signal is recorded (T_E, or echo time).

In MRI studies of the central nervous system the T1 scans show the anatomical structures in detail; the CSF is black. The T2 scans show intracranial pathological processes, all of which are associated with abnormal accumulations of water; the CSF is white.

Magnetic resonance imaging, or nuclear magnetic resonance, has considerable potential advantages over CT scanning including:

- No ionising radiation
- No bone artefact so that lesions around the skull base are clearly identified
- High resolution.

Intravenous contrast material using gadolinium compounds considerably enhances the value of MRI. These materials are water-soluble and cross the abnormal blood–brain barrier in a manner similar to the iodine-based, water soluble contrast material used in CT scanning. The paramagnetic compounds function by changing the local magnetic environment. The signal intensity of those hydrogen nuclei that are in direct contact with the paramagnetic compounds is altered. The consequent shortening of the T1 relaxation time results in an enhancement or brightening of the area.

The major disadvantage of MRI at present is its relative unavailability due to cost. It is a valuable investigation in the following neurosurgical conditions:

- Intracranial tumours — especially meningioma, acoustic neuroma, pituitary tumours, skull base tumours (with gadolinium contrast)
- CNS infection — cerebral abscess, herpes simplex encephalitis
- Arteriovenous malformations
- Venous sinus thrombosis
- Craniospinal abnormalities such as Arnold–Chiari malformation
- Syringomyelia
- Spinal tumours
- Lumbar disc prolapse
- Cervical cord compression — cervical myelopathy, cervical central disc prolapse.

RADIO-ISOTOPE STUDIES

Isotope brain scanning for the detection of tumours is now largely obsolete. However, radio-isotope cisternography is sometimes useful in the detection of the site of CSF leakage following a fracture of the skull base. The technique is also sometimes used to assess cerebrospinal fluid flow in patients with communicating hydrocephalus; reflux into the ventricular system, followed by slow clearance suggests communicating or normal pressure hydrocephalus. However, the technique has been largely superseded by intracranial pressure monitoring.

Other highly sophisticated techniques using radioisotopes, such as **single photon emission computerised tomography** (SPECT) or **positron emission tomography**, are used to measure cerebral blood flow or cerebral metabolism. At present they are useful experimental study techniques but are not in general use as investigations. Single photon emission computerised tomography utilises single photon-emitting radiopharmaceuticals which distribute in the brain according to regional blood flow. Imaging is performed using a gamma camera and computer analysis. Positron emission tomography utilises positron emitting isotopes which depend on a cyclotron for their production and, in general, their short half-life dictates that a cyclotron should be readily available. The scanning is of particular use in studying the relationship between cerebral blood flow, oxygen utilisation and extraction in focal ischaemia or infarction. It has also been used to study epilepsy and metabolic activity in brain tumours.

ELECTROENCEPHALOGRAPHY

Electroencephalography (EEG) records the spontaneous electrical activity of the brain. The details are described in the chapter on epilepsy (Ch. 21). The major indication for EEG recordings in neurological practice are:

- Suspicion of epilepsy in a new patient
- Assessment of epilepsy in a patient with recurrent seizures
- Assessment of the risk of epilepsy in a patient having undergone intracranial surgery or following a severe head injury
- Aid in the diagnosis of herpes simplex encephalitis and Creutzfeldt–Jakob disease.

NERVE CONDUCTION STUDIES/ELECTROMYOGRAPHY

The electrical activity within a particular muscle is recorded by needle electromyography. Nerve conduction studies measure the electrical activity occurring within a particular nerve.

In electromyography a needle is inserted into muscle and the electrical activity assessed; normal muscle is electrically 'silent' at rest. As the muscle contracts motor unit potentials appear. This activity, which is seen on voluntary contraction of the muscle, is known as the interference voluntary contraction of the muscle, is known as the **interference pattern**. Neuropathy or myopathy will produce characteristic abnormalities.

Spontaneous activity at rest

- Fibrillation potentials are due to single muscle fibre contraction and indicate active denervation, e.g. neuropathy, motor neuron diseases, some myopathies
- Fasciculation — spontaneous contraction of a bundle of muscle fibres
- Slow negative waves preceded by sharp positive spikes — known as 'positive sharp waves' — in chronically denervated muscle.

Motor unit potentials

- In neuropathy. Where there is significant denervation the surviving motor unit potentials are polyphasic with large amplitude and long duration
- In myopathy the potentials are polyphasic with small amplitude and short duration.

Interference pattern

- Neuropathy — reduced interference due to diminished motor units
- Myopathy — interference pattern normal.

Nerve conduction studies measure the latency from the stimulus to the recording electrodes (distal latency), amplitude of the evoked response and conduction velocity. The studies are useful in assessing:

- Peripheral nerve injuries (Ch. 17)

- Peripheral nerve entrapment (Ch. 17)
- Brachial plexus injury (Ch. 17)
- Neuropathy
- Myopathy (studies are normal)
- Muscular dystrophy (studies are normal).

EVOKED POTENTIALS

Visual, auditory and somatosensory evoked potential monitoring may be of value in the detection of neurological and neurosurgical diseases as well as providing a useful intra-operative recording. Stimulation of the sensory receptor will evoke a signal in the appropriate region of the cerebral cortex.

Visual evoked potential. This involves retinal stimulation using either a stroboscopic flash or an alternating checkerboard pattern. The evoked visual signal is recorded over the occipital cortex. It is particularly useful in the diagnosis of multiple sclerosis. Intra-operative visual evoked potential monitoring has been used by some neurosurgeons during pituitary surgery to detect subtle interference with the optic nerves and chiasm but the technique is not sufficiently developed for general use at this time.

Brain stem auditory evoked potential. This stimulates the auditory pathways in the vestibulocochlear cranial nerve and records the electrical activity in the auditory cortex. The technique has been used in the detection of small acoustic neuromas but has been largely superseded by high quality MRI. Intra-operative recording has been performed during acoustic tumour surgery and microvascular decompression operations but its use is limited.

Somatosensory evoked potential. This involves sensory evoked potential recording over the cortex in response to stimulation of a peripheral nerve and has been used in the detection of lesions within the sensory pathways, particularly the brachial plexus, spinal cord or brain stem. The technique is used in some neurosurgical units during complicated spinal surgery as an additional intra-operative monitoring technique.

FURTHER READING

DuBoulay G H 1965 Principles of X-ray diagnosis of the skull. Butterworth, London
Fishman R A 1980 Cerebrospinal fluid in diseases of the nervous system. W B Saunders, Philadelphia
McComb J G 1983 Recent research into the nature of cerebrospinal fluid formation and absorption. Journal of Neurosurgery 59: 369–383
Stevens J M, Valentine A R 1987 Magnetic resonance imaging in neurosurgery. British Journal of Neurosurgery 1: 405–426.
Taveras J M, Wood E H 1986 Diagnostic neuroradiology, 2nd edn. Williams & Wilkins, Baltimore

3. Raised intracranial pressure and hydrocephalus

INTRACRANIAL PRESSURE

Raised intracranial pressure is a major clinical feature of many neurological illnesses. It is the most important neurological symptom, requiring prompt diagnosis and often needing urgent treatment.

Pathophysiology

The mechanisms of raised intracranial pressure are best understood by considering the normal physiology of pressure within the intracranial cavity. The normal supine intracranial pressure is 10–15 mmHg, measured at a position equal to the level of the foramen of Munro. The intracranial pressure is directly related to the volume of the intracranial contents within the skull. The basis of the **Munro–Kellie doctrine** is that the cranial cavity is a rigid sphere filled to capacity with non-compressible contents. In 1783, Alexander Munro the younger (the son of the man who described the connection between the lateral and 3rd ventricles) published his observations on the intracranial contents. Forty years later, Kellie made observations that appeared to support Munro's hypothesis, although at that time neither was aware of CSF. Subsequently, the Munro–Kellie doctrine has been generally accepted but with the qualification that the craniospinal intradural space is *nearly* constant in volume and its contents are *nearly* incompressible.

The intracranial contents are:

- Brain
- CSF
- Blood.

The relative volumes of the contents are shown in Figure 3.1. Raised intracranial pressure may be due to:

- Increased volume of normal intracranial constituents
- A space-occupying lesion.

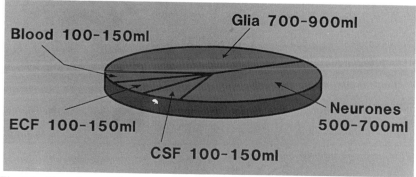

Fig. 3.1 The volume of the intracranial contents.

The increase in volume of normal intracranial contents may be due to:

- Brain
  a. cerebral oedema
  b. benign intracranial hypertension
- CSF — hydrocephalus
- Blood volume — vasodilatation due to hypercapnia.

The increase in volume of intracranial contents will determine the rise of intracranial pressure. Figure 3.2 shows the intracranial pressure–volume

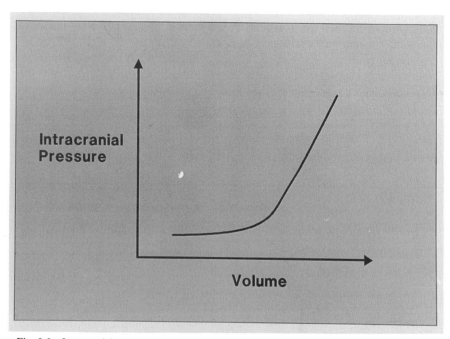

Fig. 3.2 Intracranial pressure changes related to the volume of the intracranial contents.

relationship. Initially, a small increase in the volume of the intracranial contents causes no rise in pressure; a small amount of CSF can move into the spinal subarachnoid space, which is very slightly distensible. However, the skull being a relatively closed container, a critical volume is soon reached when a small rise in intracranial volume will result in an exponential rise in pressure. The relationship of the **volume to pressure** is described in terms of **compliance** or **elastance** of the intracranial space. Compliance is expressed as **dV/dP** and is the amount of 'give' available within the intracranial space. Elastance is the inverse of compliance and is the resistance offered to expansion of a mass or of the brain itself. A brain that has a small degree of compliance, i.e. very little 'give' within the intracranial space, would be reflected by a small change in volume producing a large change in intracranial pressure. This is the situation on the vertical portion of the volume/pressure curve, where the compliance is said to be low and the elastance is high.

Experiments using Rhesus monkeys and involving the gradual expansion of an extradural balloon, showed that the vertical section of the curve could be shifted to the left with either more rapid inflation of the balloon or pathological changes, such as experimentally produced brain swelling, that reduced the amount of displaceable CSF before the balloon was expanded.

Depending on the cause of the raised intracranial pressure or the position of the intracranial mass, brain herniae may occur as shown in Figure 3.3. The three major herniations of the brain are described as:

1. Transtentorial
2. Foramen magnum
3. Subfalcine.

The transtentorial herniation involves displacement of the brain and herniation of the uncus of the temporal lobe through the tentorial hiatus, causing compression of the 3rd cranial nerve and mid-brain. The 3rd cranial nerve is affected, initially on the ipsilateral side, and in most cases compression of the pyramidal tracts in the crus cerebri causes contralateral hemiparesis. However, lateral displacement of the brain stem may result in the opposite crus cerebri being compressed on the tentorial edge (Kernohan's notch), causing an ipsilateral hemiparesis. Similarly, the posterior cerebral artery may be kinked, causing cerebral ischaemia resulting in a hemianopia. Brain stem compression will result in a deterioration of conscious state leading to coma, hypertension and bradycardia (the Cushing response) and respiratory failure, often being initially manifest by Cheyne–Stokes periodic breathing. (See Table 3.1).

Increased pressure within the posterior fossa will result in herniation of the cerebellar tonsils into the foramen magnum and compression of the medulla. If this is slowly progressive the patient may develop an abnormal neck posture and a child with a posterior fossa tumour may have a head tilt. Neck stiffness results from irritation of the dura around the foramen

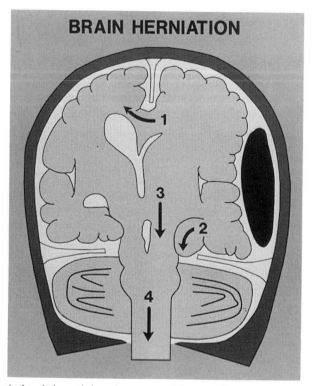

Fig. 3.3 Brain herniations. A lateral supratentorial mass will cause displacement of the lateral ventricles with (1) subfalcine herniation of the cingulate gyrus below the falx cerebri; (2) herniation of the uncus into tentorial hiatus; (3) caudal displacement of the brain stem. Raised pressure within the posterior fossa may cause herniation of the cerebellar tonsils into the foramen magnum (4). (Adapted from Jennett and Teasdale 1981. Reproduced with permission).

Table 3.1   Transtentorial herniation

Compression of 3rd cranial nerve — causing initial dilatation of the ipsilateral pupil

Compression of the mid-brain:
  Hemiparesis, usually contralateral
  Occasional compression of opposite crus cerebri causes ipsilateral hemiparesis
  Hypertension, bradycardia — Cushing response
  Respiratory failure

Compression of posterior cerebral artery

magnum. Compression of the medulla may cause rapid respiratory failure, which is manifest as apnoea or abnormalities of respiratory rate and rhythm, such as Cheyne–Stokes breathing. These may occur without significant impairment of conscious state. The pressure from the herniated tonsils may cause abrupt limb paresis and sensory disturbance.

Clinical symptoms and signs of raised intracranial pressure

The common causes of raised intracranial pressure are:

- Space occupying lesion — cerebral tumour (and oedema), abscess, intracranial haematoma
- Hydrocephalus
- Benign intracranial hypertension.

The clinical features will be determined in large part by the underlying cause of the raised pressure. However, some of the clinical symptoms and signs will be the same, no matter what the cause of the raised pressure. The major features are:

- Headache
- Nausea and vomiting
- Drowsiness
- Papilloedema.

Headache. The headache associated with increased intracranial pressure is usually worse on waking in the morning and is relieved by vomiting. Intracranial pressure increases during sleep, probably from vascular dilatation due to carbon dioxide retention. The cause of the headache in raised intracranial pressure is probably traction on the pain-sensitive blood vessels and compression of the pain-sensitive dura at the base of the cranium.

Nausea and vomiting. The nausea and vomiting is usually worse in the morning.

Drowsiness. As is often repeated in this book, drowsiness is the most important clinical feature of raised intracranial pressure. It is the portent of rapid neurological deterioration and must never be brushed aside as simply 'sleepiness', or disaster will almost certainly occur.

Papilloedema. The definitive sign of raised intracranial pressure, papilloedema is due to transmission of the raised pressure along the subarachnoid sheath of the optic nerve. The oedema of the nerve head, which may also be due to obstruction of axoplasmic flow, results initially in 'filling-in' of the optic cup and dilatation of the retinal veins. The experienced observer will be able to note that there is failure of the normal pulsations of the retinal veins. As the pressure rises the nerve head becomes more swollen and the disc margins will become blurred on fundoscopic examination. Flame-shaped haemorrhages develop, particularly around the disc margins and alongside the vessels. In severe papilloedema 'blob' haemorrhages and exudates appear. Long-standing papilloedema from prolonged raised intracranial pressure will subsequently develop into secondary optic atrophy.

Sixth nerve palsy, causing diplopia, may occur in raised intracranial pressure due to stretching of the 6th nerve by caudal displacement of the brain stem. This is a so-called 'false localising' sign.

In an infant, raised intracranial pressure will cause a tense, bulging fontanelle.

Other clinical manifestations of raised intracranial pressure may result from the brain herniation, as described above, and from the mass lesion that has caused the rise in pressure.

Measurement of intracranial pressure

Monitoring and recording the intracranial pressure was first described in the early 1960s by Lundberg and Langfitt and within a decade was being extensively used in clinical practice. The indications for monitoring the intracranial pressure vary considerably in neurosurgical practice. The most common indications are:

- Head injury (Ch. 4)
- Following major intracranial surgery, measurement of the intracranial pressure may help in the management of patients. In particular, after posterior fossa surgery early detection of a prolonged rise in intracranial pressure will indicate the need for a CSF shunt
- In the assessment of dementia and benign intracranial hypertension, described later in the chapter.

The major abnormalities in the pressure are:

- Elevation of the baseline intracranial pressure
- The development of pressure waves.

Normal intracranial pressure has a baseline between 10 and 15 mmHg, with small pulsations due to respiration and cardiac pulse. The normal amplitude of the combined cardiac and respiratory variation is approximately 3–5 mmHg. As the intracranial pressure increases the pulse pressure will increase. When the pressure is raised abnormal pressure waves may occur. 'Plateau' waves, described by Lundberg as 'A' waves, arise in pressures above 50 mmHg and last at least 5 minutes, but often up to 20 minutes. They are always pathological and are probably due to increased cerebral blood flow and blood volume. 'B' waves are smaller in height and have a short duration (1–2 minutes) (Fig. 3.4). If they are infrequent and of low amplitude they may be a normal finding.

The intracranial pressure may be recorded from the ventricle, brain substance, subdural or extradural space. The intracranial catheters are attached by a transducer to a continuous recorder. There are now numerous monitoring devices with various degrees of technical sophistication. Every method has its own particular advantages and complications and the type of monitoring performed will depend on the clinical situation (e.g. size of the ventricles) and the neurosurgeon's preference. The major complication from intracranial pressure monitoring is infection and the risk is directly proportional to the length of time of the monitoring.

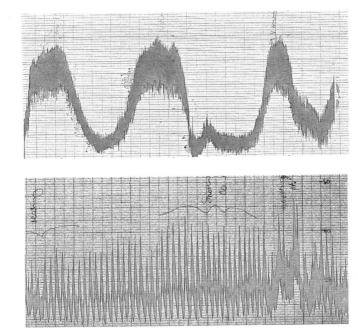

Fig. 3.4 Intracranial pressure waves. (A) 'A' waves, or plateau waves, are elevations of intracranial pressure above 50 mmHg lasting 5–20 minutes. (B) 'B' waves have a smaller amplitude and short duration.

Management of raised intracranial pressure

The treatment of raised intracranial pressure will depend on the underlying cause. The definitive treatment may involve removal of the space-occupying lesion, or in the case of hydrocephalus, a CSF shunt.

In an emergency situation, when the patient has become comatose and has failing respiration, it is essential that the patient's ventilatory state is urgently maintained and this will necessitate the passage of an endotracheal tube and ventilatory support. While the patient is being transferred for definitive treatment of the raised pressure it may be possible to temporarily lower the intracranial pressure by hyperventilation which will reduce arterial CO_2 and diminish vasodilatation, and by the administration of a diuretic such as mannitol or frusemide (Ch. 4).

HYDROCEPHALUS

Hydrocephalus is an abnormal enlargement of the ventricles due to an excessive accumulation of cerebrospinal fluid resulting from a disturbance of its flow, absorption or secretion. CSF is produced by the choroid plexus in the ventricles at a rate of 0.4 ml per minute. The CSF flows from the lateral ventricles through the foramen of Munro into the 3rd ventricle, via the aqueduct of Sylvius into the 4th ventricle and then into the subarachnoid space and basal cisterns. The CSF circulates throughout the spinal subarachnoid space and the basal cisterns up through the tentorial hiatus. It flows over the cerebral hemispheres and is largely absorbed by the arachnoid villi of the dural sinuses. There are a number of ways of classifying hydrocephalus but the most useful classification system is:

— Obstructive hydrocephalus — when there is an obstruction to the flow of CSF through the ventricular system
— Communicating hydrocephalus — when there is no obstruction to the flow of CSF within the ventricular system but the hydrocephalus is due to either obstruction to CSF flow outside the ventricular system or there is a failure of absorption of CSF by the arachnoid granulations.

The most common causes of hydrocephalus are:

1. Obstructive hydrocephalus
   a. Lateral ventricle obstruction by tumours, e.g. basal ganglia glioma, thalamic glioma
   b. 3rd ventricular obstruction, due to colloid cyst of the 3rd ventricle, glioma of the 3rd ventricle
   c. Occlusion of the aqueduct of Sylvius (either primary stenosis or secondary to a tumour)
   d. 4th ventricular obstruction due to posterior fossa tumour, e. g. medulloblastoma, ependymoma, acoustic neuroma
2. Communicating hydrocephalus
   a. Obstruction to flow of CSF through the basal cisterns
   b. Failure of absorption of CSF through the arachnoid granulations over the cerebral hemispheres.

The most common causes of communicating hydrocephalus are infection (especially bacterial and tuberculous) and subarachnoid haemorrhage (either spontaneous, traumatic or postoperative). Other uncommon causes are carcinomatous meningitis, increased CSF viscosity from a high protein content and excessive secretion of CSF due to a choroid plexus papilloma.

Presenting features

Hydrocephalus in infants

The incidence of infantile hydrocephalus is approximately 3–4 per 1000 births and most cases are due to congenital abnormalities. The incidence of hydrocephalus occurring as a single congenital disorder is 1–1.5 per 1000 births and hydrocephalus occurring with spina bifida and myelomeningocele varies from 1.5–2.9 per 1000 births.

The most common congenital cause is stenosis of the aqueduct of Sylvius. This is a major cause of hydrocephalus in children with spina bifida and myelomeningocele who also have a Chiari type II malformation (Ch. 11). Congenital atresia of the foramen of Luschka and Majendie (Dandy–Walker cyst) is a rare cause. The acquired forms of hydrocephalus result most frequently after intracranial bleeding, particularly in premature infants, meningitis and because of tumours. The marked improvements in the survival of very low birthweight premature infants has resulted in an increase in infants with hydrocephalus resulting from perinatal intracranial haemorrhage.

The major clinical features in infants are:

- Failure to thrive
- Failure to achieve milestones
- Increased skull circumference (compared with normal growth curves)
- Tense anterior fontanelle
- 'Cracked pot' sound on skull percussion
- Transillumination of cranial cavity with strong light
- When severe there is impaired conscious level and vomiting
- 'Setting sun' appearance due to lid retraction and impaired upward gaze from 3rd ventricular pressure on the mid-brain tectum
- Thin scalp with dilated veins.

Adult hydrocephalus

Adult patients with hydrocephalus may present with either:

- Acute onset and deterioration
- Gradual onset and slowly progressive deterioration.

Acute onset adult hydrocephalus. This type of presentation occurs particularly in patients with tumours causing obstructive hydrocephalus, although it may occur with any of the causes of hydrocephalus and an acute rapid neurological deterioration may occur in patients who have had long-standing chronic hydrocephalus.

The major presenting features are due to the signs and symptoms of raised intracranial pressure as described earlier:

- Headache
- Vomiting
- Papilloedema
- Deterioration of conscious state.

Upgaze will often be impaired due to compression of the 3rd ventricle on the superior colliculus of the tectum.

Gradual onset adult hydrocephalus. This type of onset occurs less frequently than the previous type in patients with obstructive hydrocephalus

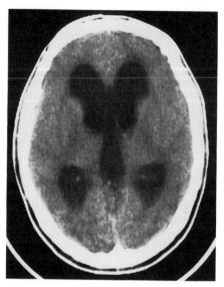

Fig. 3.5 Hydrocephalus of the lateral and 3rd ventricles due to aqueduct stenosis.

due to a tumour. The symptoms of raised intracranial pressure are only very gradually progressive and late diagnosis is common. Early features in the adolescent involve deteriorating school performance as a result of headaches, failing mental function, memory loss and behavioural disturbances. Endocrine abnormalities such as infantilism and precocious puberty can occur in association with chronic hydrocephalus in older children and adolescents due to disturbance of the hypothalamus and possible compression of the pituitary gland. If the condition is unrecognised progressive visual failure will occur, secondary to papilloedema and optic atrophy. As mentioned earlier, acute decompensation may occur and the patient may suddenly develop a rapid deterioration of conscious state.

In elderly patients a chronic form of hydrocephalus is called 'normal pressure hydrocephalus'; this is described later in the chapter.

Radiological investigation

The most important investigation is a CT scan of the brain (Fig. 3.5) which will show which ventricles are dilated. If the lateral ventricles and 3rd ventricle are all very dilated, and the 4th ventricle is small, it is likely that the obstruction is at the level of the aqueduct of Sylvius. An enhanced CT scan will help determine the cause, as it will better define the presence of an obstructing tumour. In a communicating hydrocephalus all the ventricles are dilated.

Magnetic resonance imaging. In the sagittal plane MRI is particularly helpful in showing aqueduct stenosis and lesions around the 3rd ventricle causing obstructive hydrocephalus.

Ultrasonography. Ultrasonography through the open anterior fontanelle is useful in assessing ventricular size in infants and may obviate the need for repeated CT scans.

Treatment

In general, the treatment of hydrocephalus is a CSF shunt. If there has been rapid neurological deterioration this will need to be performed as an emergency.

If the hydrocephalus is due to an obstructing tumour that is surgically accessible, resection of the mass may lead to resolution of the hydrocephalus and a shunt might not be necessary.

Arrested hydrocephalus. This is a state of chronic hydrocephalus in which the CSF pressure has returned to normal and there is no pressure gradient between the cerebral ventricles and brain parenchyma. It is uncommon and is most likely to occur in communicating hydrocephalus. The patients, often children and adolescents, should be followed carefully with neurological examinations, IQ tests and careful assessment of their development. If there is any deterioration of those parameters a shunt will be necessary.

It is interesting briefly to review the history of surgical treatment of hydrocephalus, as this common neurosurgical problem has only relatively recently been solved. Until early this century numerous remedies had been employed, including blood-letting, head-wrapping and repeated ventricular taps. In 1918, Walter Dandy introduced the technique of excising the choroid plexus to decrease the formation of CSF in patients with progressive hydrocephalus. In 1922, he described an operation of 3rd ventriculostomy, in which a hole was made in the thinned floor of the 3rd ventricle creating a fistula into the chiasmatic cisterns. Subsequently, the procedure was performed through the lamina terminalis. In 1939, Torkildsen introduced the ventriculocisternostomy to treat hydrocephalus caused by lesions obstructing the outflow from the 3rd ventricle. A thin rubber tube was inserted into the lateral ventricle through an occipital burr hole and passed subcutaneously into the cisterna magna.

All these procedures had significant limitations, risk or morbidity and substantial failure rates. The extracranial shunting procedures relied on the development of flow-directed valves allowing CSF to flow in one direction without reflux through the catheter. This type of valve was invented by an engineer, Holter, and was first used in 1952. Subsequently, numerous improvements and modifications have been made and at present there are a large variety of reliable shunt devices.

Operative procedure

The usual method of CSF diversion is a ventriculoperitoneal shunt, in which a catheter is placed into the lateral ventricle and is connected to a subcutaneous valve which is attached to a catheter threaded subcutaneously down to the abdomen and inserted into the peritoneal cavity. Alternative drainage sites such as the atrium, pleural cavity and ureter have now been largely abandoned, except in exceptional circumstances.

Technique of ventriculoperitoneal shunt (Fig. 3.6). The operation is performed under general anaesthesia and the shunt is usually inserted on the right side, so as to avoid interference with the dominant hemisphere. The head is turned to the left on the neurosurgical headrest. The head, neck, chest and abdomen are shaved, prepared with antiseptic solution and draped. It is absolutely essential to maintain the most strict sterile tech-

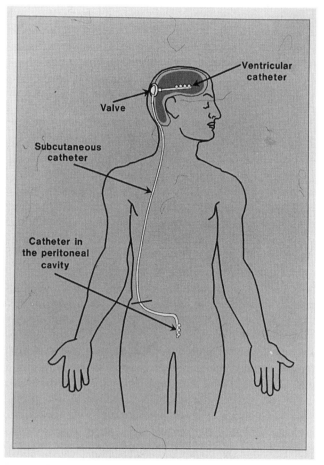

Fig. 3.6   Diagram of a ventriculoperitoneal shunt.

niques to avoid the serious complication of infection of the shunt. A small curvilinear incision is made in the parieto-occipital area and a small skin flap elevated. The peritoneal cavity is opened, either through a transverse rectus splitting incision in the right hypochondrium or through a midline incision. A burr hole is performed, the lateral ventricle cannulated and the ventricular catheter inserted into the lateral ventricle so that its tip lies in the frontal horn of the lateral ventricle, anterior to the choroid plexus. Insertion of the catheter in this way minimises the other major complication, shunt obstruction. As one of the major causes of obstruction of the ventricular catheter is blockage by the choroid plexus it is wise to place the perforations of the catheter into the frontal horn. The peritoneal catheter can be threaded subcutaneously between the abdominal and cranial wounds using one of many devices. Each catheter is joined to the valve which is then sutured in place. After checking that the system is functioning properly, the peritoneal catheter is placed within the peritoneal cavity.

There are numerous shunt systems and the type of shunt used, the particular clinical situation and the neurosurgeon's own preference results in many modifications of this basic system of implanting a ventriculoperitoneal shunt.

Postoperative care

The postoperative management is similar for any intracranial procedure. Initially the patient is nursed flat, to avoid rapid decompression of the ventricular system. Deterioration of neurological state or failure to improve will require an urgent CT scan to confirm that the catheter has been placed accurately into the ventricular system and to exclude the possibility of intracranial complications such as intracerebral haematoma.

Complications of ventriculoperitoneal shunt

The major possible complications are:

- Infection of the shunt
- Obstruction of the shunt
- Intracranial haemorrhage.

Shunt infection is a dreaded complication with possible disastrous consequences, particularly in patients who are shunt dependent. Avoidance of this complication is aided by:

- Meticulous sterile technique, including the use of a 'no touch' technique of the shunt and total avoidance of skin contact with the shunt
- Intra-operative prophylactic antibiotic medication.

Infection. The use of intra-operative prophylactic antibiotics during shunt placement is relatively well substantiated. Although the continuation of the antibiotics for 24–36 hours postoperatively has not been proven to be effective, it is a reasonable precaution. An infected shunt almost invariably needs to be removed and replaced by a new shunt, preferably in a different position and under appropriate antibiotic cover.

Obstruction. The shunt may fail to perform satisfactorily due to blockage of the ventricular catheter, malfunction or blockage of the valve or obstruction of the peritoneal catheter. The patient will usually present with recurrent symptoms of raised intracranial pressure and in some cases there may be an alarmingly rapid deterioration of neurological state. A useful clinical sign in the less acute case of shunt malfunction is failure of upgaze due to pressure of the distended 3rd ventricle on the superior colliculus. The diagnosis will usually be confirmed by CT scan. Compression of the valve is often helpful in determining the position of the obstruction. If the ventricular catheter is blocked the contents of the pump can be expressed but the valve will refill slowly. If the block lies in the valve or the peritoneal catheter the valve is usually not compressible.

The treatment of a malfunctioning shunt is by exploration and revision of the component that is not functioning adequately.

Intracranial haemorrhage. Intracranial haematomas may occur following the insertion of a ventriculoperitoneal shunt and may be either:

1. Intracerebral
2. Subdural.

The intracerebral haematoma will be due to the trauma of the passage of the ventricular catheter. Subdural haematomas are particularly likely to occur in patients with long-standing severe hydrocephalus. If there is a sudden decompression of the ventricular system the cortical mantle will fall away from the cranial vault, this may cause rupture of a bridging vein and the development of a subdural haematoma. Consequently, patients thought to be particularly at risk should initially be nursed lying flat and should be elevated gradually. Some neurosurgeons use shunts that incorporate an antisiphon device to decrease the possibility of a 'siphoning' effect causing further reduction of intracranial pressure.

Other CSF shunts

Also used sometimes are:

- Ventriculoatrial shunts
- Ventriculopleural shunts
- Lumboperitoneal shunts.

The ventriculoatrial shunt, in which the distal end is placed through the internal jugular vein into the right atrium, is occasionally necessary when there has been marked intraperitoneal sepsis or multiple abdominal operations. It will occasionally be necessary to place the shunt into the pleural cavity.

The lumboperitoneal shunt involves drainage of the CSF from the lumbar theca rather than the ventricle. This type of shunt can only be considered in patients with communicating hydrocephalus. A catheter is threaded percutaneously into the lumbar theca and then tunnelled subcutaneously to the anterior abdominal wall and placed into the peritoneal cavity. The technique has the theoretical advantage that the brain is not manipulated, but the disadvantage is that the shunts are not as reliable and are more difficult to assess if the patient develops symptoms resembling malfunction of the shunt.

NORMAL PRESSURE HYDROCEPHALUS

Normal pressure hydrocephalus was first described as a clinical entity by Hakim and Adams in 1965. They described a group of patients with symptoms of dementia, ataxia and incontinence, where the radiological studies showed hydrocephalus but the lumbar CSF pressure was normal.

Aetiology

The exact cause of the ventricular dilatation cannot be defined in every case. However, in a large percentage the communicating hydrocephalus may have resulted from obliteration of the subarachnoid pathways in the basal cisterns following an episode of meningitis or subarachnoid haemorrhage, either from rupture of an aneurysm, arteriovenous malformation or following trauma.

Although lumbar puncture pressure is, by definition, within the normal range, continuous monitoring of the intracranial pressure in these patients will frequently reveal abnormal wave formation, especially at night.

Clinical presentation

The classic clinical 'triad' consists of:

1. Dementia
2. Ataxia
3. Incontinence.

The syndrome is progressive and the disturbance of gait, which may be the first and most prominent symptom, is more of an apraxia than a true gait ataxia. Urinary incontinence is common but not universal. The dementia is similar to that seen in Alzheimer's disease, with profound loss of short-term memory. The patient does not usually complain of headaches.

Investigations

The CT scan will show dilated ventricles without significant cortical atrophy. The difficulty arises that normal pressure hydrocephalus may occur in patients with a CT scan appearance of cortical atrophy, but in these patients the degree of ventricular dilation should be more than would be expected just to compensate for the degree of atrophic change.

Other investigations, including isotope cisternography, neuropsychological assessment and CSF infusion studies, have been used. These investigations have a high failure rate in predicting which patients will benefit from a CSF shunt. Abnormal isotope cisternography, with prolonged ventricular retention of isotope and slight or delayed flow over the cerebral convexity, is associated with improvement following shunting in only a half to two-thirds of cases of normal pressure hydrocephalus. Improvement in symptoms after lumbar puncture and removal of CSF fluid may be a good prognostic sign but failure to improve does not exclude the diagnosis.

Continuous intracranial pressure monitoring is a useful technique as it will exclude patients with low intracranial pressure and make a definite diagnosis in those patients with intermittent waves of raised intracranial pressure, which occur particularly at night. However, some patients with intracranial pressure in the high normal range will also benefit from a CSF shunt.

Treatment

The major difficulty in the treatment of normal pressure hydrocephalus is in deciding which patient should be shunted. Dementia is a devastating disease with disastrous effects for the patient and profound social consequences for the patient's family and the general community. It is not surprising that the neurosurgeon is frequently asked to consider patients for a shunt where the diagnosis is far from certain. The slim chance that an operative procedure might be of some benefit is often considered worthwhile by the patient and their relatives. The following criteria can be used to assess those patients with the greatest chance of improvement following a shunt:

- A clinical presentation of the classic triad, particularly if the features of gait disturbance predominate
- The CT scan showing marked hydrocephalus with minimal cortical atrophy
- A clearly defined cause for the hydrocephalus, such as a past episode of subarachnoid haemorrhage, trauma or meningitis
- Abnormal pressure waves on continuous intracranial pressure monitoring.

Naturally, a patient who has all these positive criteria deserves a shunt and should make a good recovery following the operation. However, the usual situation is a patient who presents with only a few of these criteria and the neurosurgeon needs to make a careful assessment of whether a shunt is truly appropriate.

Operative procedure

The usual operation is a ventriculoperitoneal shunt but some surgeons prefer a lumboperitoneal shunt because there is no interference with an already impaired brain.

If the diagnosis has been correct and the shunt works satisfactorily, the patient can make a striking recovery with almost complete resolution of the symptoms.

BENIGN INTRACRANIAL HYPERTENSION

Benign intracranial hypertension, also known as pseudotumour cerebri, is, as its name implies, a disease of brain swelling which usually runs a benign, self-limiting course; the pathogenesis is poorly understood. The condition usually occurs in obese females.

Aetiology

The aetiology is generally poorly understood and the exact mechanisms of the raised pressure are not known. The condition is found typically in young, obese women, often with menstrual irregularities or taking an oral contraceptive pill and an endocrine disturbance has been suggested. However, careful endocrine studies have failed to show significant endocrine abnormalities. In a minority of patients a definite precipitating cause is found, these include:

- Hypoparathyroidism
- Vitamin A excess (used to treat acne)
- Pernicious anaemia
- Drug reaction — tetracycline, nalidixic acid, sulfamethoxazole, indomethacin, danazole, lithium carbonate, oral contraceptive steroids.

A similar condition results from venous sinus thrombosis. Prior to antibiotic therapy chronic mastoiditis was a cause of pseudotumour cerebri as a consequence of spread of inflammation to the sigmoid and lateral sinuses. This is now a relatively rare occurrence.

Presenting features

Most patients are obese females who present with:

- Headaches
- Visual disturbance.

The headaches have the features of raised intracranial pressure in that they are worse in the morning and exacerbated by straining, stooping and coughing.

The visual problems result from:

- Papilloedema
- Secondary optic atrophy
- Diplopia due to 6th cranial nerve palsy.

The papilloedema may be severe and the visual fields will show enlargement of the blind spot. Obscurations of vision may occur, particularly on standing or stooping, and the swelling of the optic discs may be so severe as to lead to visual failure and associated secondary optic atrophy.

An unusual but well recognised complication of benign intracranial hypertension is spontaneous CSF rhinnorhoea, usually associated with the empty sella syndrome (Ch. 8).

Investigations

The CT scan will show no cause for the papilloedema and the ventricles will often be smaller than usual.

Digital subtraction cerebral angiography may be performed to exclude thrombosis of a venous sinus as the cause.

If the CT scan shows no mass or lesion a lumbar puncture is usually performed; the pressure will be raised. CSF examination is normal in benign intracranial hypertension but biochemistry and cytological investigations should be performed to exclude underlying pathology.

If there is doubt as to the diagnosis continuous intracranial pressure monitoring is occasionally performed in order to assess the level of intracranial pressure.

Treatment

Benign intracranial hypertension is usually a self-limiting disease and most cases respond to simple conservative treatment. The usual measures undertaken are:

- Weight loss (the patients are usually obese)
- Cease any medication that may have led to the disease, e.g. oral contraceptives, tetracycline
- Diuretic therapy
- Acetazolamide (reduce CSF production).

Visual acuity, visual field examination (especially size of the blind spot) and fundal photography are essential to evaluate the progress of the disease. If there is no improvement with the above measures, treatment with glycerol or steroids may be tried. However, both of these medications will tend to increase obesity. Some clinicians recommend serial lumbar punctures but this is of limited value as the formation of CSF quickly replaces any that is withdrawn.

The major indications for surgical treatment are:

- Persistent severe papilloedema despite conservative measures
- Failing vision
- Intractable headaches despite conservative measures.

The surgical procedures that can be performed are:

- Optic nerve sheath decompression
- Lumboperitoneal shunt.

If the symptoms are primarily visual and headache is not a problem then optic nerve sheath decompression may be useful. In this procedure a small window of dura is excised from the optic nerve sheath to decompress the optic nerve head. If this procedure is not successful in improving papilloedema or reversing the failing vision, or if headaches are a major component of the disease, then a lumboperitoneal shunt can be performed. This operation is usually highly effective in reversing the symptoms and in improving the papilloedema.

FURTHER READING

Adams R D, Fisher C M, Hakim S, Ojemann R G, Sweet W H 1965 Symptomatic occult hydrocephalus with normal cerebrospinal fluid pressure: a treatable syndrome. New England Journal of Medicine 273: 117–126
Beks J W F, Bosch D A, Brock M 1976 Intracranial pressure III. Springer Verlag, Berlin
Black P McL 1980 Idiopathic normal pressure hydrocephalus. Journal of Neurosurgery 52: 371–377
Corbett J J, Savino P J, Thompson S, Kansu T, Schatz N J, Orr L S, Hopson D 1982 Visual loss in pseudotumour cerebri. Archives of Neurology 39: 461–474
Greer M 1968 Management of benign intracranial hypertension (pseudotumour cerebri). Clinical Neurosurgery 15: 161–174
Hakim S, Adams R D 1965 The special clinical problem of symptomatic hydrocephalus with normal cerebrospinal fluid pressure: Observations on cerebrospinal fluid hydrodynamics. Journal of Neurological Science 2: 307–372
Jefferson A, Clark J 1976 Treatment of benign intracranial hypertension by dehydrating agents with particular reference to measurement of the blind spot as a means for recording improvement. Journal of Neurology, Neurosurgery and Psychiatry 39: 627–639
Jennett B, Teasdale G 1981 Management of head injuries, Contemporary Neurology series. F A Davis, Philadelphia
Langfitt T W, Weinstein J D, Kassell N F, Simeone F A 1964 Transmission of intracranial pressure. I. Within the cranio-spinal axis. Journal of Neurosurgery 21: 989–997
Langfitt T W, Weinstein J D, Kassell N F, Gagliardi L J 1964 Transmission of intracranial pressure. II. Within the supratentorial space. Journal of Neurosurgery 21: 998–1005
Nulsen F E, Spitz E B 1952 Treatment of hydrocephalus by direct shunt from ventricle to jugular vein. Surgical Forum 2: 339–343
Shulman K, Marmarou A, Miller J D, Becker D P, Hochwald G M, Brock M 1980 Intracranial pressure IV. Springer Verlag, Berlin
Torkildsen A 1939 A new palliative operation in cases of inoperable occlusion of the sylvian aqueduct. Acta Chirurgica Scandinavica 82: 117–119

4. Head injuries

Head injuries are a major cause of morbidity and mortality in the community. Trauma is the third most common cause of death in the United States, exceeded only by cardiocerebral vascular disease and cancer. Trauma is the leading cause of death in youth and early middle age and the death is often associated with major head trauma. Head injury contributes significantly to the outcome in over half of trauma related deaths. There are approximately 2.5 deaths from head injury per 10 000 population in Australia and neurotrauma causes approximately 3.5% of all deaths. Road traffic accidents are responsible for about 65% of all fatal head injuries in Australia.

There is a wide spectrum of head injury from mild concussion to severe brain injury resulting in death. The management of the patient following a head injury requires the identification of the pathological processes that have occurred.

PATHOPHYSIOLOGY OF HEAD INJURY

Most head injuries result from blunt trauma, as distinct from a penetrating wound of the skull and brain caused by missiles or sharp objects. The pathological processes involved in a head injury are:

- Direct trauma
- Cerebral contusion
- Intracerebral shearing
- Cerebral swelling (oedema)
- Intracranial haemorrhage
- Hydrocephalus.

Direct trauma. Although penetrating injuries produce most of their damage by direct trauma to the brain this is not the case with blunt injuries, in which the energy from the impact has a more widespread effect.

Cerebral contusion. This may occur locally under the position of the impact although it usually occurs more severely at a distance from the area of impact as a result of a 'contra-coup' injury. As the brain is mobile within the cranial cavity the sudden acceleration/deceleration force will result in

59

the opposite 'poles' of the brain being jammed against the cranial vault. A sudden blow to the back of the head will cause the temporal lobes to slide across the floor of the middle cranial fossa and the frontal lobes across the floor of the anterior cranial fossa, causing contusion on the undersurface of those lobes and to the temporal and frontal poles of the brain as they strike the sphenoid ridge and frontal bones respectively. Cerebral contusion consists of lacerated haemorrhagic brain, and a 'burst temporal lobe' may result when the temporal pole has been severely injured.

Shearing forces. Intracerebral shearing forces occur as a result of the differential brain movement following blunt trauma, frequently in conjunction with a contra-coup type of injury. The rotational acceleration following injury will cause shear forces that result in petechial haemorrhages, (particularly in the upper brain stem, cerebrum and corpus callosum) and tearing of axons and myelin sheaths. The early pathological changes consist of retraction balls or microglial scars, and if the patient lives for a number of months before death then widespread degeneration of myelin will be apparent at postmortem.

Cerebral swelling. This occurs following trauma, either in a focal pattern around an intracerebral haematoma or diffusely throughout the cerebrum and/or cerebellum. The nature of the pathological processes are not clearly understood but involve a disturbance of vasomotor tone causing vasodilatation and cerebral oedema. In addition, cerebral contusion and petechial haemorrhages will contribute to the brain swelling.

Intracranial haemorrhage. Intracranial haemorrhage following trauma is discussed in more detail in Chapter 5 and may be:

- Intracerebral
- Subdural
- Extradural.

The intracranial haematoma or cerebral swelling may cause the types of cerebral herniation described in Chapter 3. The medial surface of the hemisphere may be pushed under the falx (subfalcine), the uncus and hippocampal gyrus of the temporal lobe may herniate through the tentorium causing pressure on the 3rd nerve and mid-brain (Fig. 4.1) or there may be a caudal displacement of the brain stem and/or cerebellum herniating into the foramen magnum.

Hydrocephalus. This occurs infrequently in the early stages after a head injury. It may be due to obstruction of the 4th ventricle by blood, swelling in the posterior fossa or as a result of a traumatic subarachnoid haemorrhage causing obstruction to the absorption of cerebrospinal fluid and resulting in a communicating hydrocephalus. This latter type of hydrocephalus is an uncommon, but important, cause of delayed neurological deterioration either in the weeks following the head injury or some years later (see Normal pressure hydrocephalus, Ch. 3).

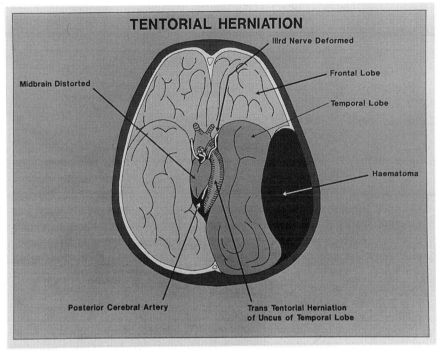

Fig. 4.1 Herniation of the uncus and hippocampal gyrus of the temporal lobe into the tentorial notch causing pressure on the 3rd nerve and mid-brain (Adapted from Jennett and Teasdale, 1981. Reproduced with permission).

Concussion

Concussion involves an instantaneous loss of consciousness as a result of trauma. The term 'concussion' was introduced by Paré and is derived from the Latin 'concutere' which means to shake. In 1941, Denny-Brown and Russell showed that concussion was produced by a blow on the cranium when it was free to move and subsequent studies showed that the acceleration/deceleration of the head resulted in shear strains, contra-coup injury, petechial and punctate haemorrhages throughout the brain stem, cerebral hemispheres and corpus callosum, and neuronal injury, the extent depending on the force of the impact. The term concussion is not strictly defined in respect to the severity of the injury. However, a minimum criterion is that the patient will have had a period of amnesia. The retrograde amnesia of most cerebral concussion is usually short-term, lasting less than 1 day. The initial retrograde amnesia may extend over a much longer period but it gradually shrinks down. A more reliable assessment of the severity of the head injury is the post-traumatic amnesia. If the amnesia following the head injury lasts more than 1 day then the concussion is regarded as being severe.

Associated injuries

Cranial nerves

The cranial nerves may be injured either as a result of direct trauma by the skull fracture, movement of the brain, or cerebral swelling.

The **olfactory nerves** are the most commonly affected and this may be as a result of either a fracture through the anterior cranial fossa, directly affecting the tracts, or tearing of the delicate nerve rootlets passing through the cribriform plate caused by the sudden brain movement, particularly from a blow to the back of the head.

8th nerve damage is often associated with a fracture of the petrous temporal bone. Deafness may be conductive, due to a haemotympanum, or sensorineural as a result of injury to the inner ear or to the nerve itself. Vertigo and nystagmus are due to vestibular nerve or end organ damage and usually resolve within a few months of the injury.

Facial paralysis is usually associated with a fracture through the petrous temporal bone, although this may only be evident on a high resolution CT scan using the bone 'window'. It may be either immediate, as a result of direct compression of the nerve, or delayed, due to bleeding and/or swelling around the nerve.

The **6th cranial** nerve has a long course from the brain stem to its entry into Dorello's canal and the nerve is easily damaged by torsion or herniation of the brain.

The **3rd nerve** may also be damaged by direct trauma or by brain herniation, the herniated uncus of the temporal lobe either impinging on the mid-brain or directly stretching the nerve.

The **optic nerve** is infrequently injured by direct trauma.

Skull fractures

Trauma may result in skull fractures which are classified as:

- Simple — a linear fracture of the vault
- Depressed — when the bone fragments are depressed beneath the vault
- Compound — when there is a direct communication with the external environment. This may result either from a laceration over the fracture or a fracture of the base of the skull which will be compound because there will be a direct connection outside the vault, usually via the air sinuses.

Scalp lacerations

The extent of the scalp laceration does not necessarily indicate the degree of trauma to the underlying brain.

Other injuries

The most common associated injuries are to the chest, skeletal and cardio-vascular systems.

INITIAL MANAGEMENT OF HEAD INJURY

The key aspects in the management of patients following head injury involve:

- Accurate clinical assessment of the neurological and other injuries
- Determination of the pathological process involved
- The concept that a change in the neurological signs indicates a progression or change in the pathological processes.

Immediate treatment at the site of the injury involves a rapid restoration and maintenance of an adequate airway, ventilation, essential circulatory resuscitation, first aid treatment of other injuries and the urgent transfer of the patient to hospital. It is essential to avoid hypoxia and hypotension as these will cause further brain injury.

Clinical assessment

It is fundamental to the management of the patient to know of changes in the neurological condition as soon as possible. It is essential to ascertain the type of accident that caused the head injury and the time injury occurred. An accurate assessment of the patient's initial neurological condition, albeit in non-medical terms, can be obtained from bystanders at the site of the accident or from the ambulance officers.

Neurological examination

An accurate neurological examination will help to determine the type and position of the pathological process and provide a baseline for comparison with subsequent examinations. Although a full neurological examination should be undertaken special emphasis should be given to the:

- Conscious state
- Pupillary size and reaction
- Focal neurological signs in the limbs.

The conscious state. If the patient will respond verbally an assessment should be made of the retrograde amnesia and post-traumatic amnesia.

There is a continuum of altered consciousness between those patients who are alert and respond appropriately to verbal command and those who are deeply unconscious. The first sign of a depressed conscious state is drowsiness, at which time the patient may be easily arousable and orientated in time, place and person. As the level of consciousness deteriorates the patient will become confused and more drowsy. The term 'coma' is generally restricted to patients who show no response to external stimuli, do not obey commands, are unable to utter comprehensible words, and do not open their eyes. However, the use of the words 'coma', 'semi-coma' or 'stuporose' should be avoided, as they convey different meanings to different observers. The assessment is more accurate and reproducible if either the exact nature of the response is described or, more simply, if the Glasgow coma scale is used.

The Glasgow coma scale (Table 4.1) gives a numerical value to the three most important parameters of the level of consciousness — opening of the eyes, best verbal response and best motor response. The exact response can be represented on a chart (Fig. 4.2) or the level of consciousness given as a numerical score — the sum of the three parameters of the Glasgow coma scale. A score of 8 or less indicates a severe injury.

Pupillary size and reaction. Careful evaluation of the pupil size and response to light is essential at the initial clinical assessment and during further observation. Raised intracranial pressure causing temporal lobe herniation will cause compression of the 3rd nerve, resulting in pupillary dilatation, which nearly always occurs initially on the side of the raised pressure. The pupil will at first remain reactive to light but subsequently will become sluggish and then fail to respond to light at all. As the intracranial pressure increases this same process commences on the contralateral side. A traumatic mydriasis will also result from direct trauma to the eye and the dilated pupil should not be confused with that due to a 3rd cranial nerve palsy.

Table 4.1 The Glasgow coma scale

Parameter	Response	Numerical Value
Eye opening	Spontaneous	4
	To speech	3
	To pain	2
	None	1
Best verbal response	Orientated	5
	Confused	4
	Inappropriate	3
	Incomprehensible sounds	2
	None	1
Best motor response to painful stimulus	Obeys commands	6
	Localise to pain	5
	Flexion to pain — withdrawal	4
	Flexion — abnormal	3
	Extension to pain	2
	None	1
	TOTAL	3–15

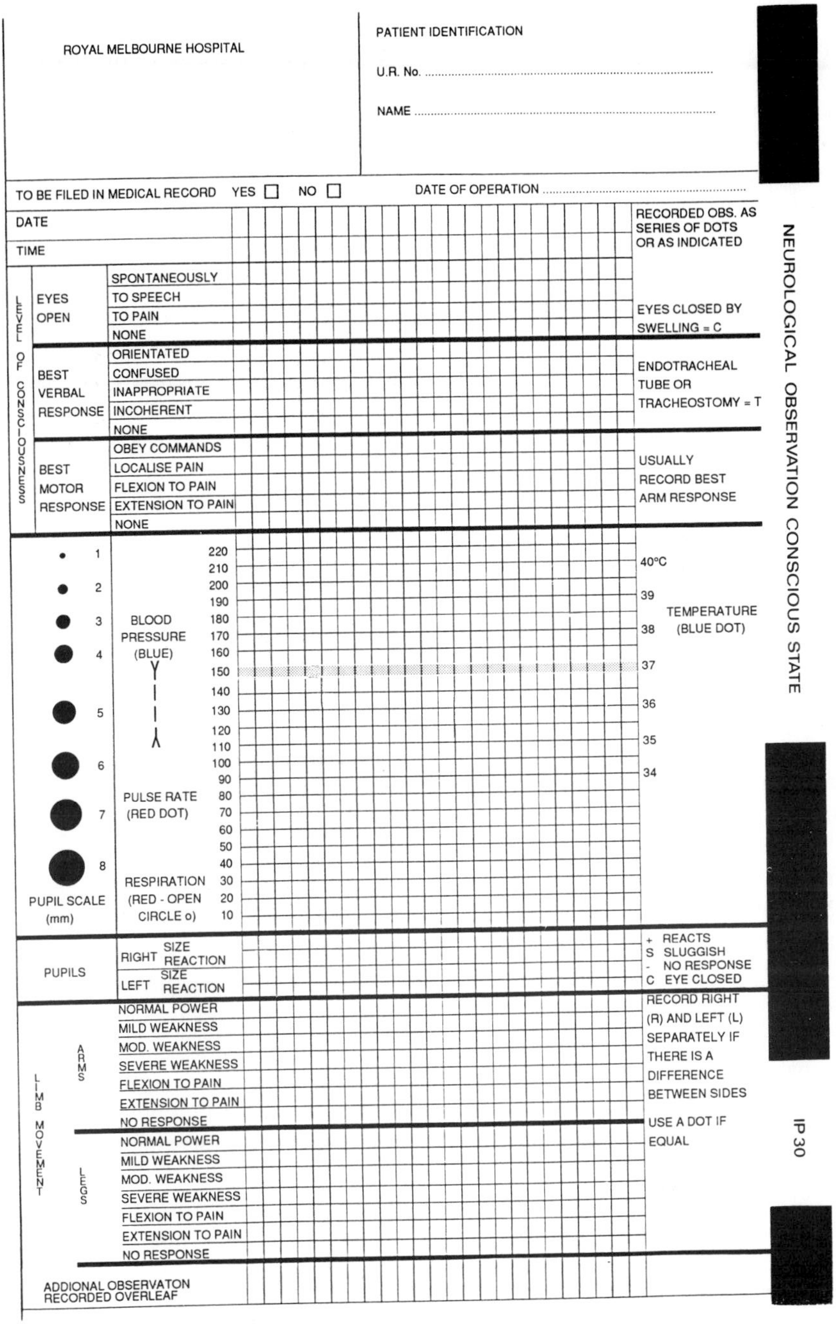

ROYAL MELBOURNE HOSPITAL

PATIENT IDENTIFICATION

U.R. No. ....

NAME ....

TO BE FILED IN MEDICAL RECORD   YES ☐   NO ☐   DATE OF OPERATION ....

NEUROLOGICAL OBSERVATION CONSCIOUS STATE

| DATE | | | RECORDED OBS. AS SERIES OF DOTS OR AS INDICATED |
| TIME | | | |

L E V E L O F C O N S C I O U S N E S S	EYES OPEN	SPONTANEOUSLY		EYES CLOSED BY SWELLING = C
		TO SPEECH		
		TO PAIN		
		NONE		
	BEST VERBAL RESPONSE	ORIENTATED		ENDOTRACHEAL TUBE OR TRACHEOSTOMY = T
		CONFUSED		
		INAPPROPRIATE		
		INCOHERENT		
		NONE		
	BEST MOTOR RESPONSE	OBEY COMMANDS		USUALLY RECORD BEST ARM RESPONSE
		LOCALISE PAIN		
		FLEXION TO PAIN		
		EXTENSION TO PAIN		
		NONE		

PUPIL SCALE (mm)

• 1
• 2
● 3
● 4
● 5
● 6
● 7
● 8

BLOOD PRESSURE (BLUE)
Y
|
|
λ

PULSE RATE (RED DOT)

RESPIRATION (RED - OPEN CIRCLE o)

220
210
200
190
180
170
160
150
140
130
120
110
100
90
80
70
60
50
40
30
20
10

40°C
39
38 TEMPERATURE (BLUE DOT)
37
36
35
34

PUPILS	RIGHT	SIZE		+ REACTS S SLUGGISH - NO RESPONSE C EYE CLOSED
		REACTION		
	LEFT	SIZE		
		REACTION		

L I M B M O V E M E N T	A R M S	NORMAL POWER		RECORD RIGHT (R) AND LEFT (L) SEPARATELY IF THERE IS A DIFFERENCE BETWEEN SIDES
		MILD WEAKNESS		
		MOD. WEAKNESS		
		SEVERE WEAKNESS		
		FLEXION TO PAIN		
		EXTENSION TO PAIN		
		NO RESPONSE		USE A DOT IF EQUAL
	L E G S	NORMAL POWER		
		MILD WEAKNESS		
		MOD. WEAKNESS		
		SEVERE WEAKNESS		
		FLEXION TO PAIN		
		EXTENSION TO PAIN		
		NO RESPONSE		

ADDIONAL OBSERVATON RECORDED OVERLEAF

IP 30

Fig. 4.2 The standard observation chart used at the Royal Melbourne Hospital and at many major trauma centres. The chart incorporates the Glasgow coma scale.

Disorders of ocular movement occur following head injury as a result of injury to an extra-ocular muscle or its nerve supply, or due to disturbance of the conjugate gaze centres and pathways. A destructive lesion of either a frontal or pontine gaze centre results in tonic overaction of the opposite frontal–pontine pathway for horizontal eye movement, causing ipsilateral deviation of the eyes with a frontal lobe lesion and contralateral gaze deviation with pontine lesions. The oculocephalic manoeuvre and caloric stimulation are important tests of functional activity of the brain stem reticular formation.

The oculocephalic response should only be performed after a cervical spine fracture has been excluded. The head is raised 30° and rotated from side to side in the horizontal plane. In the normal response the eyes maintain their position in space by moving opposite to the rotation of the head. The afferent impulses are from the cervical nerve roots and the semicircular canals.

Caloric testing should also be performed with the head elevated 30° so that the horizontal canal is positioned in the vertical plane. Irrigation with ice cold water causes ipsilateral tonic gaze deviation.

Skew deviation involves divergence of the eyes in the vertical plane and is a sign of a lesion within the brain stem.

Ocular bobbing occurs only after a very severe head injury resulting in pontine damage.

Focal neurological signs in the limbs. Neurological examination of the limbs will assess the tone, power and sensation. A hemiparesis will result from an injury of the corticospinal tract at any point from the motor cortex to the spinal cord. Following a severe brain injury the limbs may adopt an abnormal 'posturing' attitude. The decerebrate posture consists of the upper limbs adducted and internally rotated against the trunk, extended at the elbow and flexed at the wrist and fingers, with the lower limbs adducted, extended at the hip and knee with the feet plantar flexed. There is a continuum of severity of brain injury with the decerebrate posturing response being partial and unilateral and occurring only as a result of a painful stimulus to severe continuing bilateral decerebrate rigidity. The posture probably results from an upper brain stem injury. Less frequently, the upper limbs may be flexed, probably due to the injury predominantly involving the cerebral white matter and basal ganglia — corresponding to a posture of decortication.

Particular attention must be given to the patient's ventilation, blood pressure and pulse. At all times it is essential that care is taken to ensure the patient's ventilation is adequate. Respiratory problems may result either as a direct manifestation of the severity of the head injury or due to an associated chest injury. Cheyne–Stokes' breathing is due either to intrinsic brain stem damage or raised intracranial pressure causing pressure and distortion on the brain stem. Bradycardia and hypertension, the Cushing response, are also both indicative of brain stem compression due to raised intracranial pressure (Ch. 3).

Pyrexia frequently occurs following a head injury. A temperature lasting for more than 2 days is usually due to traumatic subarachnoid haemorrhage or may occur in patients with a severe brain stem injury.

General examination

Careful assessment must be made of any other injuries. Chest, skeletal, cardiovascular or intra-abdominal injury must be diagnosed and the appropriate management instituted. Hypotension or hypoxia may aggravate the brain injury, and, if severe, will themselves cause brain damage.

Radiological assessment

Following the clinical evaluation radiological assessment will be essential unless the injury has been minor. The CT scan will show the macroscopic intracranial injury and should be performed if:

- The patient is persistently drowsy or has a more seriously depressed conscious state
- There are lateralising neurological signs
- There is neurological deterioration
- There is CSF rhinorrhoea
- Associated injuries will entail prolonged ventilation so that ongoing neurological assessment is difficult.

The CT scan will clearly show the presence of intracerebral or extra-cerebral haematoma, as well as cerebral contusion, oedema and infarction. Small 'slit' ventricles and absence of the basal cisterns will indicate generalised brain swelling.

The indications for a skull X-ray have diminished since the introduction of the CT scan, especially as the bony vault can be assessed by the CT scan using the bone 'windows'. If a CT scan has not been performed, a skull X-ray is advisable if there has been any loss of consciousness or if the mechanism of injury is suggestive of an underlying fracture.

Cerebral angiography is indicated if a caroticocavernous fistula is suspected by the presence of a bruit over the orbit or by pulsating proptosis.

NB Radiological assessment of the cervical spine is essential in patients who have sustained a significant head injury, particularly if there are associated facial injuries.

FURTHER MANAGEMENT OF HEAD INJURY

Following the clinical and radiological assessment the subsequent management will depend on the intracranial pathology and the extent of any neurological injury.

Minor head injury

The patient would be assessed as described above. Any patient who has suffered a head injury must be observed for at least 4 hours. The following are the minimum criteria for obligatory admission to hospital:

- Loss of consciousness (post-traumatic amnesia) of greater than 10 minutes
- Persistent drowsiness
- Focal neurological deficits
- Skull fracture
- Persisting nausea or vomiting after 4 hours' observation
- If the patient does not have adequate care at home.

The further management of these patients will be careful observation; the neurological observations should be recorded on a chart displaying the features of the Glasgow coma scale. If there has been a period of significant loss of consciousness, or if the patient is drowsy, then the following measures should be instituted to minimise the development of cerebral swelling:

- Head of the bed elevated 20°
- Mild fluid restriction to 2–2.5 litres per day in an adult.

Should the patient's neurological state deteriorate an immediate CT scan is essential to re-evaluate the intracranial pathology; further treatment will depend on the outcome.

Severe head injury

The management of a patient following a severe head injury depends on the patient's neurological state and the intracranial pathology resulting from the trauma. In general, the following apply:

1. The patient has a clinical assessment and CT scan as described previously.
2. If the CT scan shows an intracranial haematoma causing shift of the underlying brain structures then this should be evacuated immediately.
3. If there is no surgical lesion, and following the operation, the management consists of:
   (a) careful observation using a chart with the Glasgow coma scale.
   (b) measures to decrease brain swelling, these include:
      (i) careful management of the airway to ensure adequate oxygenation and ventilation. Hypercapnia will cause cerebral vasodilation and so exacerbate brain swelling

(ii) elevation of the head of the bed 20°

(iii) fluid and electrolyte balance

Mild fluid restriction with an intake of between 1.5 and 2.0 litres per 24 hours is optimum for the average adult. Blood loss from other injuries should be replaced with colloid or blood and not with crystalloid solutions. Care should be taken to avoid over hydration, as this will increase cerebral oedema.

Following general injury there is retention of salt and water and excretion of potassium. The retention of water is usually greater than the retention of sodium, resulting in mild hyponatraemia. Following a severe head injury fluid and electrolyte abnormalities may occur for a variety of reasons. Severe hyponatraemia (sodium less than 130 mmol/l) may be due to excessive fluid intake or, occasionally, because of inappropriate excessive secretion of antidiuretic hormone. The urine is usually hypertonic with a high sodium level, probably as a result of suppression of aldosterone secretion occurring as a response to over hydration and expansion of the circulating volume. The term 'cerebral salt wasting', which has been applied to this syndrome, is usually inappropriate.

Serum sodium of less than 125 mmol/l may produce neurological impairment with depression of conscious state. The usual treatment is to restrict fluid intake to 800 ml per day or less.

Hypernatraemia is usually associated with hyperosmolality and often results from inadequate fluid intake. Other causes are diabetes insipidus, as a result of hypothalamic injury and excessive use of osmotic agents for control of intracranial pressure. Excessive administration of some feeding mixtures may lead to electrolyte abnormalities, particularly when complicated by diarrhoea.

(c) temperature control — pyrexia may be due to hypothalamic damage or traumatic subarachnoid haemorrhage. However, infection as a cause of the fever must be excluded. The most common sites of infection after a head injury are the respiratory and urinary tracts, particularly if a urinary catheter has been inserted. If the injury is compound, and especially if there has been a CSF leak, intracranial infection should be suspected. The temperature can usually be controlled using tepid sponges, and rectal paracetamol or aspirin. Chlorpromazine, to abolish the shivering response, should be administered if a cooling blanket is required. Every attempt should be made to control the temperature because hyperthermia can elevate the intracranial pressure, will increase brain and body metabolism and will predispose to seizure activity. Although hypothermia has been advocated in the management of a severe head injury no clearcut benefit has been demonstrated.

(d) nutrition — during the initial 2–3 days the fluid therapy will include 1.5–2 litres of 4–5% dextrose, providing 250–400 calories per day. Proper nutritional support should be commenced after 3–4 days. Feeding at this stage is best done by intragastric administration, usually by a nasogastric tube, unless this is precluded by other injuries. The nasogastric feeding should supply 2500–3000 calories per day with a calorie : nitrogen ratio of 180 : 1. The feeding should commence slowly, with dilute mixtures, and the stomach should be aspirated regularly to prevent regurgitation and pulmonary aspiration.

(e) routine care of the unconscious patient including bowel, bladder and pressure care.

More aggressive methods to control intracranial pressure are advisable if:

- The patient's neurological state continues to deteriorate and the CT scan shows evidence of cerebral swelling without an intracranial haematoma
- There is a posturing (decerebrate) response to stimuli
- The Glasgow coma score is less than 8.

In these patients an intracranial pressure monitor should be inserted to assess the intracranial pressure as accurately as possible. A catheter placed into the ventricle will give an accurate reading of the intracranial pressure and CSF can be drained to help in the control of the pressure. However, the disadvantages of an intraventricular catheter include difficulty of placement if the ventricles are small, possible injury to the brain during placement and infection resulting in ventriculitis following prolonged monitoring. A subdural catheter will also give an adequate measurement of the intracranial pressure but may be difficult to insert satisfactorily if the brain is swollen, and will tend to block. Extradural monitors are less accurate, although satisfactory recordings are obtainable with meticulous placement technique.

An intracranial pressure monitor will also be useful in patients requiring prolonged sedation and ventilation as a result of other injuries. Measurement of the intracranial pressure will provide another useful monitoring parameter and any sustained rise in the pressure will be an indication for careful reassessment and, if necessary, CT scan.

Following the insertion of the intracranial pressure monitor the patient will be transferred to the intensive care department. The techniques used to control intracranial pressure are as follows:

— Controlled ventilation, maintaining $Paco_2$ at 30 mmHg. Reduction of the $Paco_2$ will reduce cerebral vasodilatation and consequently decrease the intracranial pressure.
— If the pressure remains elevated despite hyperventilation CSF can be drained from a ventricular catheter if this has been inserted.

— Diuretic therapy utilising intermittent administration of mannitol or frusemide can be used if the preceding techniques have failed to control the intracranial pressure. Mannitol is an osmotic diuretic and may also exert its effect by increasing serum osmolality and drawing water out of the brain. The usual dose is 0.5–1.0 g/kg. The serum osmolality should not exceed 320 mOsM/kg.

— Barbiturate therapy can be considered if the intracranial pressure is resistant to treatment with the above techniques. Pentobarbitone (thiopentone), when given as a bolus dose (3–5 mg/kg) is frequently effective in temporarily reducing the intracranial pressure. There is probably little value in using barbiturate infusion at a dose to control burst suppression on EEG, although it has been postulated that this provides brain protection by reducing cerebral metabolism.

— Steroids. Although steroids dramatically reduce the oedema around cerebral tumours they have little effect in controlling the brain swelling following a head injury. Steroid medication is no longer considered advisable as there is no proven benefit for the patient and possible complications, such as gastrointestinal bleeding, poor wound healing and infection, may result from their administration.

Other techniques, such as hypothermia (to reduce cerebral metabolism and intracranial pressure) and hyperbaric oxygen, have been advocated in the past but have not been shown to have any proven benefit.

There is some controversy concerning the effectiveness of the more aggressive techniques to treat patients with severe head injuries. If a patient has suffered a profound brain injury and the neurological examination shows little or no remaining brain stem function then it is obvious that the aggressive techniques will provide no benefit and only delay the inevitable. Similarly, there are some patients who have suffered a severe head injury and whose intracranial pressure continues to rise despite all the above techniques. Other patients will have a fatal brain injury without any substantial rise in intracranial pressure, usually when the brain stem has been the primary site of injury. However, about 30% of patients who have suffered a severe brain injury will obtain substantial benefit from control of the intracranial pressure. Although clinical studies have not yet conclusively proved the value of intracranial pressure control in reducing morbidity following a brain injury, it is probable that a reduction in raised intracranial pressure will not only decrease the mortality but will improve the quality of the patient's outcome after a severe head injury.

Management of associated conditions

Scalp injury
A large scalp laceration may result in considerable blood loss. When the patient arrives in the emergency department 'spurting' arteries should be controlled with haemostatic clips prior to the application of a sterile bandage

to the head. The extent of the soft tissue scalp injury may not reflect the severity of the underlying brain injury. The principles of management are similar to those of soft tissue injury at other sites of the body and the wound should be closed without delay.

The hair should be shaved widely around the wound, which should be meticulously cleaned and debrided. The closure should be performed in two layers if possible, with careful apposition of the galea prior to closing the skin. The skin sutures should approximate the cut edges of the skin and care should be taken to avoid excessive tension which would cause skin necrosis and wound breakdown.

Straightforward, clean scalp lacerations can nearly always be closed with local anaesthetic infiltration. However, if the scalp wound has resulted in loss of soft tissue the wound may need to be extended to provide an extra 'flap' of healthy tissue so that the skin edges can be approximated without tension.

Skull fractures

Simple fracture. There is no specific management for a simple skull fracture that is undisplaced without an overlying skin injury. However, the presence of a fracture is an indication that the trauma was not trivial and it should provide a warning that a haematoma may develop beneath the fracture.

Compound fracture. A skull fracture may be compound either because of an overlying scalp laceration or if it involves an air sinus. The scalp wound should be debrided and closed as described above. A short course of prophylactic antibiotics should be administered to reduce the risk of infection.

Depressed skull fracture (Fig. 4.3). A skull vault fracture is considered to be significantly depressed if the inner table fragments are depressed by at least the thickness of the skull. About half the injuries are due to road trauma and most of the remainder are due to either objects falling on the head at work or to assault with a heavy, blunt instrument. A depressed fracture caused by a non-missile injury usually causes only focal brain damage, so that many patients never lose consciousness. If the underlying injured brain is an eloquent area the patient will exhibit focal neurological signs. Haemorrhage from the bony edges, the dura or underlying brain trauma may result in an intracranial haematoma which will cause progressive neurological deterioration. If the depressed fracture is compound and the dura has been lacerated there is a significantly increased risk of intracranial infection.

If the depressed skull fracture is compound, prophylactic antibiotics and tetanus prophylaxis should be administered and surgery, usually requiring a general anaesthetic, should be performed as soon as possible. A preoperative CT scan will not only show the position of the depressed skull fragments but also the presence of any underlying intracranial pathology (Fig. 4.4). At operation the scalp wound should be cleaned and debrided, as described previously, and the bone fragments elevated. If the dura has been penetrated, or if bone fragments and external foreign material have been driven down into the brain, this must be meticulously debrided and haemostasis obtained. It is desirable that the dura should be closed and this may require the use of a patch of pericranium or fascia lata from the thigh. If the wound and bone fragments are heavily contaminated, and particularly

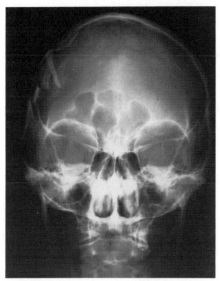

Fig. 4.3 Depressed skull fracture.

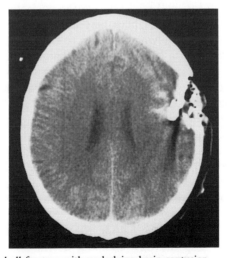

Fig. 4.4 Depressed skull fracture with underlying brain contusion.

if there has been some delay in surgery, the bone should not be replaced and a reconstructive cranioplasty may be necessary later.

If the depressed fracture is closed there is no urgency in elevating the bone fragments, provided there is no underlying intracranial complication. There is controversy over whether a depressed fragment might lead to epilepsy due to continued pressure on the brain. In general, the depressed fragments should be elevated if:

- Careful studies using the bone 'windows' on the CT scan show that the dura might have been penetrated
- There is significant brain compression
- The fracture is compound
- Cosmetic considerations such as a frontal fracture in a young child.

The risk of epilepsy following a depressed fracture is 15% for the whole group, but the risk ranges from 3–70% depending upon other associated intracranial pathology resulting from the injury. Prophylactic anticonvulsant medication should be continued for one year if the dura has been penetrated.

Cerebrospinal fluid rhinorrhoea

A fracture involving the base of the anterior cranial fossa may cause tearing of the basal dura resulting in a fistula into the frontal, ethmoid or sphenoid sinuses (Fig. 4.5). This type of fistulous connection should also be suspected if the patient suffers from an episode of meningitis or if the radiological investigations show a fracture in the appropriate site. An intracranial aerocele is proof of a fistulous connection. CSF rhinorrhoea may also occur as a result of a fistula through the tegmen tympani into the cavity of the middle ear, and may leak via the eustachian tube.

The diagnosis of CSF rhinorrhoea may be difficult. In the early stages following a head injury involving fractures to the facial bones, CSF needs to be differentiated from a bloody nasal discharge. Allergic rhinitis is the major differential diagnosis in patients presenting weeks or months after a head injury. Testing for sugar in the nasal discharge may help to identify the fluid as being CSF. CSF isotope scans using technetium-99 injected through the lumbar theca are only likely to be positive if there is a large leak. High resolution CT scanning following the administration of intracisternal contrast may help to identify the position of the hole.

The major concern of a dural fistula is the risk of intracranial infection, particularly bacterial meningitis. A CSF leak may not become apparent for a few days after the head injury, but as the brain swelling decreases the dural tear becomes unplugged. Alternatively, CSF leakage may cease due to a brain hernia 'plugging' the hole in the dura and bone. Although the brain hernia might stop the CSF escaping it will not provide protection against future intracranial infection, as the dural defect will remain.

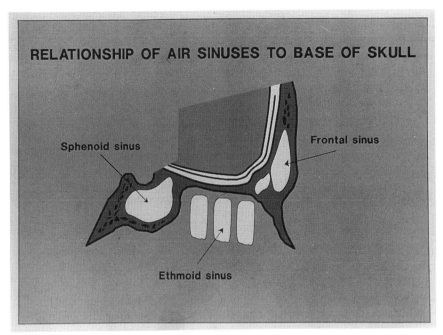

Fig. 4.5 Relationship of base of skull to air sinuses.

There is controversy concerning the indications for an anterior cranial fossa exploration and dural repair, but there is general agreement that surgery should be performed if:

- Cerebrospinal fluid leakage continues for more than 5 days, indicating the fistula is not trivial
- There is an intracranial aerocele
- There has been an episode of meningitis in a patient with a fracture of the anterior cranial fossa.

Patients with a possible dural fistula should be placed on prophylactic antibiotic medication. In general, penicillin is recommended as *Pneumococcus* is the most common organism; amoxycillin is appropriate in children due to the risk of haemophilus infection. Broad spectrum antibiotics may lead to the development of resistant organisms and should be avoided. Nasal swabs may indicate the need for more individualised antibiotic prophylaxis.

It is best to delay surgery for 2 or 3 weeks, until the initial brain swelling has resolved. Early surgery, using a craniofacial type of exposure, has been advocated by some neurosurgeons if there are associated major facial and anterior vault fractures. However, early surgery may result in further damage to an already swollen frontal lobe during the retraction necessary to obtain adequate exposure of the dural tear.

The operative procedure involves a frontal craniotomy with repair of the dural defect using either pericranium or fascia lata taken from the thigh.

Cerebrospinal fluid otorrhoea

CSF otorrhoea may occur as a result of a base of skull fracture involving the petrous temporal bone. Unlike fractures of the anterior cranial fossa the leakage nearly always settles and the fistula does not usually provide a route of infection, unless there is evidence of chronic middle ear infection. Occasionally, a persistent leak may require surgical exploration and repair.

Cranial nerve injuries

Injuries to the cranial nerves occurring directly as a result of the trauma are not helped by surgery. Steroid medication is appropriate for patients with a delayed facial nerve palsy following fracture of the petrous temporal bone. Some otologists recommend surgical decompression of the facial nerve when the palsy is delayed but, as the facial function nearly always recovers, operative intervention is usually not justified.

Post-traumatic epilepsy

The indications for prophylactic medication following head injury are discussed in Chapter 21.

MISSILE INJURIES

Although most literature on missile injuries is related to warfare, these injuries are unfortunately becoming more common in civilian conflict, particularly as a result of the increased availability of firearms. In general the cranial injury is directly proportional to the velocity of the missile. The 'high velocity' injury is defined as resulting from a missile travelling faster than the speed of sound (1050 ft/sec), and modern rifle bullets have a muzzle velocity greater than 3000 ft/sec.

The pathological processes involve scalp injury, depressed skull fracture, intracranial haemorrhage and the intracranial pathological sequelae resulting from a 'closed' head injury, including cerebral contusion, haemorrhage, swelling and raised intracranial pressure. The pattern of injury will depend on the velocity of the weapon and the trajectory of the missile through the bone and brain. A high velocity wound may result in a rapid increase of intracranial pressure of more than 3000 mmHg due to the temporary cavity about the missile, which might be 50 times as large as the missile itself. The high intracranial pressure resulting from the cavitation may result in death from failure of the respiratory and cardiac centres in the brain stem.

Management

Rapid transport of the patient to hospital and urgent treatment is of paramount importance. The early definitive treatment resulting from prompt transport and the introduction of antibiotics were the major factors in lowering mortality from head wounds in the Korean and Vietnam wars.

The management of the patient after transfer to hospital is essentially the same as described for severe head injuries previously. Antibiotics should be administered immediately, in large intravenous doses because of the risk of infection; penicillin and chloramphenicol were the most commonly used during the Vietnam conflict. After neurological assessment, a CT scan should be performed to ascertain the position of the intracranial haematomas, depressed bone fragments and metal fragments.

Surgery is not appropriate if the patient is brain dead with no evidence of brain stem reflexes. Patients with less severe injuries should have urgent surgical intervention, particularly as early exploration reduces the risk of subsequent infection.

The operation is performed under general anaesthetic and intravenous diuretic therapy is administered to reduce intracranial pressure. A large scalp flap is designed, with excision and debridement of the entry and exit wounds. Meticulous care is taken to remove any accessible bone or metallic fragments. Haematoma and necrotic brain debris are excised. A water-tight dural closure should be performed and the scalp should be closed in the two layers (galea and skin). Following surgery, a repeat CT scan will identify any further retained bone or metallic fragments. Accessible fragments should be removed, but isolated deep or inaccessible bone or metallic fragments are probably best left as further neurological damage may occur during an attempt at excision of these particles. In civilian practice, infection is unlikely if exploration has taken place within 2 hours of the injury. In general it is thought that retained metallic fragments have less potential for infection than other debris.

Postoperative management is similar to that described for severe head injury, with particular attention to controlling intracranial pressure. Prophylactic antibiotics and anticonvulsant medication are administered.

REHABILITATION

Some form of rehabilitation is essential following any significant head injury. If the injury has been relatively minor then the necessary rehabilitation may involve only advice and reassurance to the patient and family. However, rehabilitation following a severe head injury will usually involve a team of paramedical personnel, including physiotherapists, occupational therapists, speech therapists and social workers.

The major groups of disabilities resulting from a head injury are:

- Impairment of motor function — hemiparesis, quadriparesis, ataxia, poor coordination
- Speech disturbances — dysphasia, dysarthria
- Impairment of special senses — vision, hearing

- Cognitive disturbance — memory impairment, intellectual disability, personality change.

The general aims of the rehabilitation process are:

- In the initial period, to prevent complications such as contractures of the limbs and provide counselling for the family
- To maximise the neurological recovery by restoring old skills and teaching new skills. This is usually undertaken in a rehabilitation unit
- Retraining for future employment, if necessary and if possible.

The rehabilitation process should commence as soon as possible after the head injury and should initially concentrate on preventing complications. Limb contractures and pressure sores are avoided by frequent patient turning, physiotherapy and the use of splints. As the neurological state improves the patient's rehabilitation will normally be undertaken in a rehabilitation unit. Orthotic devices will assist hemiplegic patients to walk and, if they can follow simple instructions, most are able to relearn the activities of daily living.

The speech therapist may provide valuable assistance for patients with dysarthria and swallowing difficulties. Formal speech therapy probably does little to improve global aphasia but it does offer important psychological support for the patient with a severe communication disorder.

Damage to the non-dominant hemisphere results in perceptual disturbances, particularly relating to visual spatial tasks. Although the perceptual problems may resolve with time and rehabilitation, the problems associated with cognitive disturbances and alteration of personality may persist. Family counselling and support is essential to help the relatives understand and cope with these long-term disabilities.

FURTHER READING

Becker D P, Miller J D, Ward J D, Greenberg R P, Young H F, Sakalas R 1977 The outcome from severe head injury with early diagnosis and intensive management. Journal of Neurosurgery 47: 491–502
Cushing H 1908 Surgery of the head. In: Kean W W (ed) Surgery — Principles and Practice. W B Saunders, Philadelphia, vol 3: 217–276
Cushing H 1918 Notes on penetrating wounds of the brain. British Medical Journal 1: 22–226
Blackwood W, Corsellis J A N (eds) 1976 Greenfield's neuropathology. Edward Arnold, London
Gurdjian E S, Thomas R S 1964 Surgical management of a patient with head injury. Clinical Neurosurgery 12: 56–74
Holbourn A H S 1943 Mechanisms of brain injuries. The Lancet ii: 438–441
Jamieson K G, Yelland J D 1975 Surgical repair of anterior fossa because of rhinorrhoea, aerocele or meningitis. Journal of Neurosurgery 39: 328–331
Jefferson A, Reilly G 1972 Fractures of the floor of the anterior cranial fossa. The selection of patients for dural repair. British Journal of Surgery 59: 585–592
Jennett B, Miller J D 1972 Infection after depressed fracture of the skull. Implications for management of non-missile injuries. Journal of Neurosurgery 36: 333–339

Jennett B, Miller J D, Braakman R 1974 Epilepsy after non-missile depressed skull fracture. Journal of Neurosurgery 41: 208–216

Jennett B, Teasdale G 1981 Management of head injuries, Contemporary Neurology series. F A Davis, Philadelphia

Johnston I H, Johnston J A, Jennett B 1970 Intracranial pressure changes following head injury. The Lancet ii: 433–436

Langfitt T W 1978 Measuring the outcome from head injuries. Journal of Neurosurgery 48: 673–678

Plum F, Posner J B 1972 The diagnosis of stupor and coma, 2nd edn. F A Davis, Philadelphia

Russell W R, Schiller F 1949 Crushing injuries of the skull: Clinical and experimental observations. Journal of Neurology, Neurosurgery and Psychiatry 12: 52–60

Teasdale G, Jennett B 1974 Assessment of coma impaired consciousness. The Lancet ii: 81–84

Walsh F B, Hoyt W F 1969 Clinical neuro-ophthalmology. Williams & Wilkins, Baltimore, Vol 3.

5. Traumatic intracranial haematomas

Intracranial haematoma formation following head injury is the major cause of fatal injuries in which death may have been potentially avoidable and in which many survivors are unnecessarily disabled following head injury due to a delay in the evacuation of the haematoma. The incidence of intracranial haematomas and the type of haematoma varies widely depending on the different admission policies. In general hospitals that receive an unselected series of patients, the incidence varies between 1–5% of all head injuries, while the incidence will be much higher in specialist neurosurgical centres.

Classification of traumatic intracranial haematomas

The general classification depends on the relationship of the haematoma to the dura and brain. Haematomas can be:

- Extradural
- Subdural
- Intracerebral.

However, many haematomas occupy more than one of the intracranial sites (Table 5.1).

EXTRADURAL HAEMATOMA

Extradural haematomas are more likely to occur in the younger age group as the dura is able to strip more readily off the underlying bone. In patients under 20 years of age, extradural haematomas account for about two-thirds of all traumatic intracranial haematomas, but represent less than 5% of haematomas in patients over the age of 50. Although an extradural haematoma may occur in the presence of a severe head injury and coexist with a severe primary brain injury, the important feature of an extradural haematoma is that it may occur when the injury to the underlying brain is either trivial or negligible.

Table 5.1 Position of traumatic intracerebral haematomas

Series	Extradural only (%)	Extradural and intradural (%)	Subdural only (%)	Subdural and intracerebral (%)	Intracerebral only (%
International Collaborative Study Glasgow, Rotterdam, Groningen, Los Angeles	16	7	22	34	20
Brisbane Jamieson & Yelland	13	11	34	36	6
Melbourne Royal Melbourne Hospital	14	8	29	31	18

Distribution of extradural haematomas

The most common sites for extradural haematoma are the temporal region followed by the frontal area. Posterior fossa and parasagittal extradural haematomas are relatively uncommon. The relative proportions in a consecutive series of 100 cases from the Royal Melbourne Hospital are shown in Figure 5.1. In most cases the haemorrhage is from a torn middle meningeal artery or its branches but haematomas may also develop from haemorrhage from extradural veins, the superior sagittal sinus, transverse sinus or posterior meningeal artery, the last two being responsible for the posterior fossa extradural haematomas. A fracture overlies the haematoma in nearly all (95%) of adults and most (75%) children.

Clinical presentation

As previously mentioned, an extradural haematoma may occur as a result of a severe head injury and the haematoma will then become manifest as a further deterioration of the neurological state, particularly with lateralising features involving a 3rd nerve palsy (dilatation of the pupil) and progressive hemiparesis.

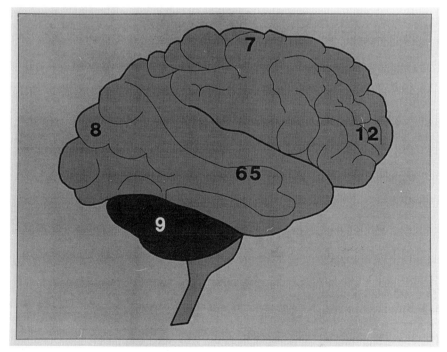

Fig. 5.1 Frequency of sites of extradural haematomas in Royal Melbourne Hospital series of 100 consecutive cases.

More frequently the extradural haematoma occurs following a head injury that has resulted in only a transient loss of consciousness and in approximately one-quarter of cases there has been no initial loss of consciousness. In these patients the most important symptoms are:

- Headache
- Deteriorating conscious state
- Focal neurological signs (dilating pupil, hemiparesis)
- Change in vital signs (hypertension, bradycardia).

Headache. This is the outstanding initial symptom in patients who have not lost consciousness or who have regained consciousness. The headache increases in severity and is followed by vomiting.

Deteriorating conscious state. This is the most important neurological sign, particularly when it develops after a 'lucid' interval. It is essential that the drowsiness that occurs in a patient following a head injury is not misinterpreted just as the patient wishing to sleep. It is well to remember the nursery rhyme:

Its raining, its pouring,
The old man is snoring,
He bumped his head and went to bed,
And didn't get up in the morning.

This is a classic description of an extradural haematoma leading to drowsiness and death.

Focal neurological signs. These will depend upon the position of the haematoma. In general, a temporal haematoma will produce a progressive contralateral spastic hemiparesis and an ipsilateral dilated pupil. Further progression will result in bilateral spastic limbs, a decerebrate posture and bilaterally dilated pupils (Ch. 4, Fig. 4.1). Occasionally the hemiparesis may initially be ipsilateral, due to compression of the contralateral crus cerebri of the tentorial edge, but it is rare for the opposite pupil to be involved first.

The change in vital signs. The change in vital signs shows the classic Cushing response to a rise in intracranial pressure — bradycardia accompanied by an increase in blood pressure. Disturbances in respiration will develop into a Cheyne–Stokes pattern of breathing.

Extradural haematomas occurring at other than the temporal position show modifications of this clinical presentation. Frontal haematomas show evidence of lateralising signs late in their evolution, the predominant features being a deterioration of consciousness and pupil abnormalities. In the posterior fossa the vital signs tend to be affected early, followed by a change in conscious state. The pupils and limbs may not be affected until the patient becomes deeply unconscious. Haematomas in the posterior fossa may cause sudden respiratory failure.

Radiological investigations

The CT scan will show the typical hyperdense (white) biconvex haematoma (Fig. 5.2) with compression of the underlying brain and distortion of the lateral ventricle.

Treatment

The treatment of extradural haematoma is urgent craniotomy with evacuation of the clot.

As soon as an extradural haematoma is suspected clinically the patient should have an urgent CT scan. In some cases the rate of neurological deterioration may be so rapid that there is not sufficient time for a CT scan and the patient should be transferred immediately to the operating theatre. Infusion of mannitol (25% solution, 1 g/kg) or frusemide (20 mg intravenously) may temporarily reduce the intracranial pressure during the transfer to the operating theatre. If unconscious, the patient should be intubated and hyperventilated during the transfer. **It is essential that there should be no delay in evacuating the haematoma. An extradural haematoma is a surgical emergency which will result in death if not removed promptly.**

Operation for extradural haematoma

The type of operation performed will depend on the circumstances in which the patient is being treated.

1. If a CT scan has been performed and the position of the haematoma is known, the skin flap will be lifted directly over the haematoma.

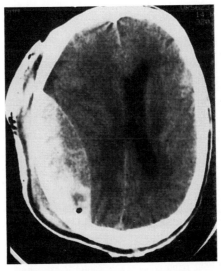

Fig. 5.2 Extradural haematoma with the typical hyperdense biconvex appearance.

2. If the patient's neurological state is stable or only slowly progressive and if the surgeon is trained in neurosurgical operations, a formal craniotomy can be performed over the site of the haematoma.
3. A craniectomy, rather than a craniotomy, should be performed:
   (a) if the surgeon is inexperienced
   (b) if craniotomy instruments are not available
   (c) if the rate of neurological deterioration has been so rapid that time has not permitted a CT scan to be performed, exploratory burr holes should be inserted first in the temporal region and then in the frontal and parietal areas (Fig. 5.3). When the haematoma is identified the burr hole incision should be extended and the bone over the region of the haematoma should be rapidly removed. If the haematoma is not found on the first side that is explored burr holes should be performed in the same order on the other side. The following are guidelines for the position of the haematoma if a CT scan has not been performed:
      (i) it underlies the fracture (that may have been seen on the skull X-ray)
      (ii) it underlies a boggy swelling on the skull
      (iii) it is on the same side as the pupil that dilated first
      (iv) in 85% of cases it is on the contralateral side to the hemiparesis.

Following removal of the bone of the vault by craniotomy or craniectomy it is easy to evacuate the haematoma. The original source of the haematoma, usually the bleeding middle meningeal artery in the temporal haematoma, is controlled by diathermy or with a haemostatic clip. The haematoma will have stripped away the dura from the inner table of the vault, often resulting in considerable oozing from the dural surface. The dura should be

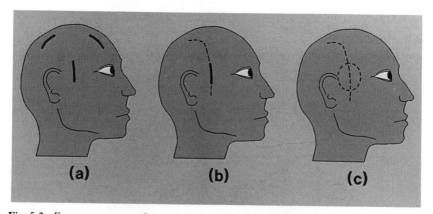

Fig. 5.3 Emergency surgery for suspected extradural haematoma. (A) Position of exploratory burr holes. (B) If haematoma found in the temporal position the skin wound is extended. (C) Further bone removed to enable complete evacuation of haematoma and haemostasis.

opened, if a CT scan has not previously been performed, to exclude the coexistence of a subdural haematoma. It should then be closed in a water-tight fashion. It is usually advisable to insert a closed system, low pressure extradural drain to evacuate any blood that may continue to ooze.

The postoperative care is similar to that for any other intracranial procedure. If the neurological state fails to improve following the evacuation of the haematoma, or if there is further deterioration, another CT scan should be performed to exclude recurrence of the haematoma formation.

Prognosis. If the initial head injury has resulted in only a transient loss of consciousness, the patient should make a full recovery following removal of the extradural haematoma, provided the haematoma has been evacuated early enough to prevent permanent neurological disability. The damage caused by an extradural haematoma is potentially reversible, provided the haematoma is evacuated before pressure from the blood clot has caused secondary intracranial pathological effects.

SUBDURAL HAEMATOMA

Subdural haematomas have been classified into acute, subacute and chronic, depending on the time they become clinically evident following injury:

- Acute subdural haematoma — less than 3 days.
- Subacute subdural haematoma — 4–21 days.
- Chronic subdural haematoma — more than 21 days.

The CT scan enables a further classification depending on the density of the haematoma relative to the adjacent brain. An acute subdural haematoma is hyperdense (white) and a chronic subdural haematoma is hypodense. Between the end of the 1st week and the 3rd week the subdural haematoma will be isodense with the adjacent brain.

Acute subdural haematoma

The acute subdural haematoma frequently results from severe trauma to the head and commonly arises from cortical lacerations. Occasionally, an acute subdural haematoma will result from a less severe trauma caused by rupture of a bridging vein or focal tear of a cortical artery. Cases of spontaneous acute subdural haematoma have been reported and in these patients it is essential to exclude a ruptured aneurysm or bleeding diathesis as a cause. Acute subdural haematomas are bilateral in approximately one-third of cases, in comparison with less than 3% of extradural haematomas.

An acute subdural haematoma usually presents in the context of a patient with a severe head injury whose neurological state is either failing to improve or deteriorating. The features of deteriorating neurological state — decrease in conscious state and/or increase in lateralising signs should raise the possibility of a subdural haematoma.

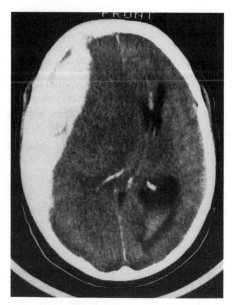

Fig. 5.4   Acute subdural haematoma causing marked shift of the lateral ventricle.

The CT scan will show the characteristic hyperdense haematoma, which is concave towards the brain, with compression of the underlying brain and distortion of the lateral ventricles (Fig. 5.4). Over 80% of patients with acute subdural haematomas have a fracture of either the cranial vault or the base of skull, which may be evident on the bone 'windows' of the CT scan.

It may be possible to evacuate an acute subdural haematoma through burr holes. If the haematoma is liquid the blood can be washed out with gentle irrigation. However if bleeding persists a craniotomy will be required for haemostasis. If the haematoma has become solidified a craniotomy will be necessary to evacuate the clot.

Chronic subdural haematoma in the adult

In 1863, Virchow first proposed chronic inflammation of the meninges as being the cause of a chronic subdural haematoma. In 1914, Trotter suggested trauma as the aetiological factor and in 1932 Gardner, and later Zollinger and Gross, proposed that an osmotic gradient occurred from the breakdown of haemoglobin. However, it was subsequently shown that the osmolarity of the haematoma did not change with time and so this theory was abandoned.

Chronic subdural haematoma can be divided into two major groups. The first involves patients having suffered a significant, and often severe head injury. However, in approximately one-third of patients there is no definite history of preceding head trauma. The aetiology of the subdural haematoma in this non-traumatic group is probably related to rupture of a fragile bridging vein in a relatively atrophic 'mobile' brain. In this group the majority of patients are over 50 years of age. Shrinkage of the brain resulting from atrophy allows the brain to become more mobile and increases the space traversed by the veins bridging between the cortex and the vault. A relatively trivial injury may result in movement of the brain, like a walnut inside its shell, with tearing of the bridging vein.

Clinical presentation

The presence of a chronic subdural haematoma should be considered if the neurological state of a patient being treated in hospital for a significant head injury begins to deteriorate. Alternatively, the patient may present without the history of a significant head injury in one of three characteristic ways:

1. Raised intracranial pressure without significant localising signs. The patient presents with headache, vomiting and drowsiness and the absence of focal neurological signs raising the differential diagnosis of a cerebral neoplasm or chronic subdural haematoma.
2. Fluctuating drowsiness. The predominant characteristic is a decline in the level of consciousness and the patient may abruptly become deeply unconscious.
3. A progressive dementia, which may be misdiagnosed as Alzheimer's disease. However, the course of the dementia is usually more rapid and progressive. Focal neurological signs may develop, particularly a hemiparesis with an extensor plantar response. In up to 20% of cases the hemiparesis may be ipsilateral to the side of the haematoma due to shift of the brain causing the contralateral crus cerebri to be compressed by the tentorial edge.

A chronic subdural haematoma will be diagnosed on the CT scan as a hypodense, extracerebral collection causing compression of the underlying brain (Fig. 5.5). In 25% of cases the haematoma is bilateral (Fig. 5.6)

Operation

The chronic subdural haematoma can be drained through burr holes. No attempt should be made to excise the membrane of the haematoma. As these haematomas may be multiloculated it is advisable to insert more than one burr hole and to visualise the underlying brain at each site. The haematoma fluid should be washed out completely and after the operation it is usually advisable to place a subdural catheter for further drainage in a closed drain system.

Following the operation the patient is nursed flat, or even with the head down initially, to encourage the brain to expand into the haematoma space. Careful attention should be given to the fluid intake and serum electrolytes.

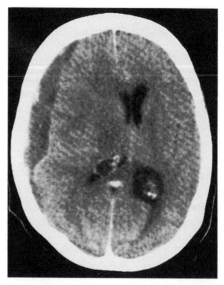

Fig. 5.5 Chronic subdural haematoma. The fluid is hypodense compared with the adjacent brain.

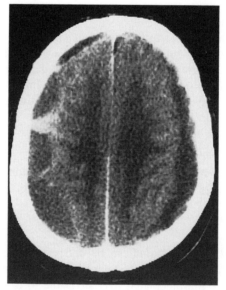

Fig. 5.6 Bilateral chronic subdural haematoma. The collection on the left is not as hypodense, indicating that it is more recent than the haematoma fluid on the right. It also has a hyperdense area, indicating more recent haemorrhage.

The normal daily fluid requirements are given (3 litres/day in adults) provided there is no clinical or radiological evidence of brain swelling. The patient should be slightly more hydrated after this type of operation than other intracranial procedures, in an attempt to encourage the brain to swell into the previous haematoma space. However, hyponatraemia is a common occurrence, both prior to and following surgery, and if the serum sodium decreases to less than 130 mmol/l the fluid intake should be reduced.

Subdural haematomas in infancy

The infantile chronic subdural haematoma, or effusion, is a distinct clinical entity. Birth trauma is a frequent cause but in many cases a past history is inadequate to establish the nature of the injury with certainty. Chronic subdural haematomas occur in 10% of 'battered children' and the violent shaking of an infant may be sufficient to lacerate bridging cerebral veins without evidence of external trauma. Subdural bleeding in infants occurs bilaterally in 85% of cases and is usually over the dorsolateral surfaces of the frontal and parietal lobes.

The earliest finding in infants with chronic subdural haematomas is excessive cranial enlargement as the sutures are unfused. The symptoms are non-specific and usually involve listlessness, irritability and failure to thrive.

The diagnosis will be confirmed by CT scan. Treatment initially involves aspiration of the fluid but if, after 2 or 3 weeks, repeated taps have failed to reduce the volume significantly, a shunt may be inserted to drain the fluid from the subdural space to the peritoneal cavity.

INTRACEREBRAL HAEMATOMA

Intracerebral haematomas occur either as a result of a penetrating injury (such as a missile injury), a depressed skull fracture or following a severe head injury. Intracerebral haematoma is frequently associated with subdural haematoma.

The size of the haematoma varies considerably and multiple haematomas are frequently seen on the CT scan following a severe head injury. The contra-coup injury described in Chapter 4 may be responsible for a 'burst' temporal lobe which results in a large temporal haematoma associated with subdural blood.

An intracerebral haematoma should be suspected in any patient with a severe head injury or in a patient whose neurological state is deteriorating.

The CT scan will show the size and position of the haematomas (Fig. 5.7).

A large intracerebral haematoma should be evacuated, unless the patient's neurological state is improving. Small intracerebral haematomas, particularly if multiple, are not removed but the clinician must be aware that they may expand and require subsequent evacuation.

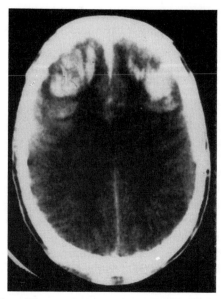

Fig. 5.7 Traumatic frontal intracerebral haematomas resulting from contra-coup injury.

FURTHER READING

Gardner W J 1932 Traumatic subdural haematoma with particular reference to the latent interval. Archives of Neurology and Psychiatry 27: 847–855

Hooper R S 1959 Observations on extradural haemorrhage. British Journal of Surgery 47: 71–87

Jamieson K G, Yelland J D 1968 Extradural haematoma. Report of 167 cases. Journal of Neurosurgery 29: 13–23

Jamieson K G, Yelland J D 1972 Traumatic intracerebral haematoma. Report of 63 surgically treated cases. Journal of Neurosurgery 37: 528–532

Jennett B, Teasdale G 1981, Intracranial haematoma. In: Jennett B, Teasdale G (eds) Management of head injuries. Contemporary Neurology Series. F A Davis, Philadelphia

Jennett B, Murray A, Carlin J et al 1979 Head injuries in three neurosurgical units, Scottish Head Injury Management Study. British Medical Journal 2: 955–958

Reilly P J, Adams J H, Graham D I et al 1975 Patients with head injury who talk and die. Lancet ii: 375–381

Teasdale G, Galbraith S 1981 Acute traumatic intracranial haematomas. In: Progress in neurological surgery 10. Karger, Basel

Trotter W 1914–1915 Chronic subdural haemorrhage of traumatic origin and its relation to pachymeningitis haemorrhagica interna. British Journal of Surgery 2: 271–291

Weir B K A 1971 The osmolarity of subdural haematoma fluids. Journal of Neurosurgery 34: 528–533

6. Brain tumours

Brain tumours are responsible for approximately 2% of all cancer deaths. Central nervous system tumours comprise the most common group of solid tumours in young patients, accounting for 20% of all paediatric neoplasms. The overall incidence of brain tumours is 4–5/100 000 population per year. A study by the United States Department of Health in 1966 showed the incidence to be 2/100 000 per year at two years old and 1/100 000 during the teenage years. The incidence increases after the 4th decade of life to reach a maximum of 13/100 000 per year in the 7th decade.

Classification

The general brain tumour classification is related to the cell of origin, and is shown in Table 6.1.

Table 6.2 shows the approximate distribution of the more common brain tumours.

This chapter will discuss the tumours derived from the neuroectoderm and metastatic tumours. The following chapters will describe the benign brain tumours and pituitary cells.

Aetiology

Epidemiology studies have not indicated any particular factor (viral, chemical or traumatic) that would cause brain tumours in humans, although a range of cerebral tumours can be induced in animals experimentally. There is no genetic predisposition but chromosome 22 abnormalities have been noted in meningiomas. Von Recklinghausen's disease is inherited as an autosomal dominant pattern and these patients have increased risk of gliomas, meningioma and spinal and cerebral schwannomas, as well as peripheral nerve schwannomas, plexiform neurofibroma and cutaneous neurofibromas.

There is no specific evidence linking central nervous system tumours to environmental carcinogens although many chemicals, especially ethyl and methyl nitrosourea and anthracene derivatives, show carcinogenic activity in animals and produce central nervous system tumours.

Table 6.1   General classification of brain tumours

Neuroepithelial tumours
  Gliomas
    Astrocytoma (including glioblastomas)
    Oligodendrocytoma
    Ependymoma
    Choroid plexus tumour
  Pineal tumours
  Neuronal tumours
    Ganglioglioma
    Gangliocytoma
    Neuroblastoma
  Medulloblastoma

Nerve sheath tumour — acoustic neuroma

Meningeal tumours
  Meningioma

Pituitary tumours

Germ cell tumours
  Germinoma
  Teratoma

Lymphomas

Tumour-like malformations
  Craniopharyngioma
  Epidermoid tumour
  Dermoid tumour
  Colloid cyst

Metastatic tumours

Local extensions from regional tumours
  e.g. glomus jugular (i.e. jugulare) carcinoma of ethmoid

Table 6.2   Incidence of common cerebral tumours (%)

Neuroepithelial		52
Astrocytoma	44	
(all grades including glioblastoma)		
Ependymoma	3	
Oligodendroglioma	2	
Medulloblastoma	3	
Metastatic		15
Meningioma		15
Pituitary		8
Acoustic neuroma		8

Viral induction of brain tumours has been used in animal models but there is no firm evidence for viral aetiology in humans. A human polyoma JC virus injected into primates produces tumours similar to human astrocytomas after an 18 month incubation period. This type of 'slow virus' effect may account for some of the problems of isolating viruses from human tumours.

There is growing evidence that oncogenes are involved in cellular transformation to malignancy. However, it is difficult to assign a direct role because transformation (spontaneous or induced) is a multistep process requiring both initiation and promotion. Exactly how oncogenes implement the transformation process is not completely known, although some are known to be involved with two key cellular functions, phosphorylation and cellular proliferation. Epidermal growth factor receptor amplification has been reported, as well as rearrangement of the epidermal growth factor receptor gene in patients with glioblastoma. It is possible that the induction of epidermal growth factor receptor expression may accompany the malignant transformation of human brain cells of glial origin.

Although immunosuppression is known to increase markedly the risk of primary lymphoma of the brain, particularly in transplant recipients, there is not the corresponding increased incidence of gliomas.

At present there is considerable conjecture regarding the role of other possible aetiological agents, including trauma, electromagnetic radiation and organic solvents but, as yet, there is no convincing evidence to implicate these as being involved with the development of brain tumours in humans.

GLIOMA

Neuroectodermal tumours arise from cells derived from neuroectodermal origin. Gliomas comprise the majority of cerebral tumours and arise from the neuroglial cells. There are four distinct types of glial cells; astrocytes, oligodendroglia, ependymal cells and neuroglial precursors. Each of these gives rise to tumours with different biological and anatomical characteristics. The neuroepithelial origin of microglia is in question.

ASTROCYTOMA

The most common gliomas arise from the astrocyte cells which comprise the vast majority of intraparenchymal cells of the brain. Their function appears to be as a supporting tissue for the neurons. The tumours arising from astrocytes range from the relatively benign to the highly malignant. The term 'malignant' for brain tumours differs from its usage for systemic tumours. Intrinsic brain tumours very rarely metastasise (except for medulloblastoma and ependymoma) and 'malignant' refers to aggressive biological characteristics and a poor prognosis.

Classification

There are many classification systems of brain tumours in general and gliomas in particular. The period of systematic classification of tumours began in 1846, when Virchow described the neuroglia and related it to brain tumours. Although Virchow created the term 'glioma', these tumours had already been described under other names. In 1926, Bailey and Cushing described a histogenetic classification system which compared the predominant cell in the tumour with the embryonal development of the neuroglia. The comparison with stages of cytogenesis was probably more of a working hypothesis than an oncological theory for the origin of the tumour cells. The theory that gliomas originate from proliferation of cells of varying degrees of maturity lying dormant in the brain is not generally accepted except in the case of medulloblastoma, which may arise from a primitive layer in the cerebellar cortex.

A valuable prognostic system of subclassification of astrocytoma was described by Kernohan, in 1949. Astrocytomas were graded from 1 to 4, with Grade 4 being the most malignant and Grade 1 cytologically, but not necessarily biologically, benign. Ringertz simplified the four grade classification of Kernohan into a three tiered system; the comparison between the two is shown in Figure 6.1. The glioblastoma multiforme, equivalent to the Kernohan Grade 3 and 4 tumours, is the most common adult cerebral tumour, accounting for approximately half of all gliomas. The low grade gliomas — the astrocytoma, or Grade 1 or 2 Kernohan astrocytoma, account for only 10–15% of astrocytomas.

Pathology

Macroscopic changes

An astrocytoma may arise in any part of the brain, although it usually occurs in the cerebrum in adults and the cerebellum in children.

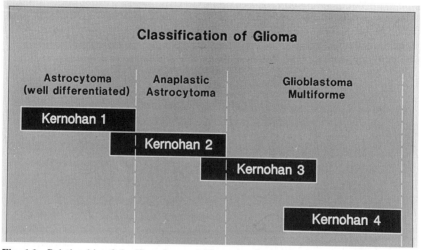

Fig. 6.1 Relationship of the Kernohan and 'three tiered' classification system for astrocytomas.

A low grade tumour in the cerebral hemispheres invades diffusely into the brain. The tumour does not have a capsule and there is no distinct tumour margin. The low grade gliomas are usually relatively avascular with a firm fibrous or rubbery consistency. Fine deposits of calcium are present in 15% of astrocytomas. Occasionally, a low grade astrocytoma may invade diffusely throughout the cerebral hemisphere. In contrast, the macroscopic appearance of a high grade tumour, the glioblastoma multiforme, is characterised by a highly vascular tumour margin with necrosis in the centre of the tumour. Although, in certain areas, the margin of the tumour may seem to be macroscopically well defined from the surrounding brain, there are microscopic nests of tumour cells extending well out into the brain.

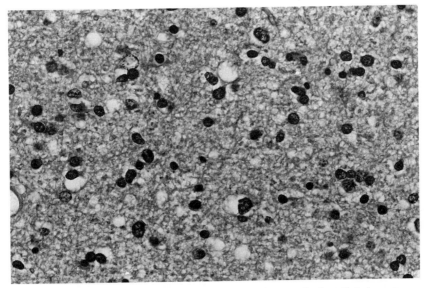

Fig. 6.2 Low grade astrocytoma. There is only a slight increase in the cellularity and mild nuclear atypia. There is a disturbed architecture with formation of triplets and quadruplets of astrocytes (haematoxylin and eosin, ×40).

Microscopic changes

The histological appearance of the tumour varies with the tumour grade. The Kernohan Grade 1 astrocytoma is characterised by an increased cellularity, composed entirely of astrocytes (Fig. 6.2). The Grade 2 astrocytoma shows mild to moderate nuclear pleomorphism but no mitotic figures. In the Grade 3 astrocytoma 50–75% of the astrocytes have a normal appearance but mitotic figures are frequent, there is increased vascularity, as evidenced by endothelial and adventitial cell proliferation, and necrosis is present in the tumour. In the Grade 4 astrocytoma very few astrocytes appear normal.

There is marked cellular pleomorphism, extensive endothelial and adventitial cell proliferation and numerous mitotic figures with extensive necrosis (Fig. 6.3). The major histological features of glioblastoma multiforme, using the three tiered system described above, are endothelial proliferation and necrosis. The anaplastic astrocytoma is characterised by nuclear pleomorphism and mitoses, which are absent in the astrocytoma.

Clinical presentation

The presenting features can be classified under:

- Raised intracranial pressure
- Focal neurological signs
- Epilepsy.

The duration of the symptoms and the progression and evolution of the clinical presentation will depend on the grade of the tumour — that is its rate of growth. A patient presenting with a low grade astrocytoma (Grade 1) may have a history of seizures extending over many years, antedating the development of progressive neurological signs and raised intracranial pressure. The tumour may evolve histologically into the more malignant anaplastic astrocytoma or glioblastoma multiforme. Patients with the higher grade tumours present with a shorter history and glioblastoma multiforme is characterised by a short illness of weeks or a few months.

Raised intracranial pressure

Raised intracranial pressure is due to the tumour mass, surrounding cerebral oedema and hydrocephalus due to blockage of the CSF pathways. The features of raised intracranial pressure are described in detail in Chapter 3. The major symptoms are **headache, nausea and vomiting, and drowsiness**.

Headache is the most common symptom in patients with cerebral astrocytoma and occurs in nearly three-quarters of patients; vomiting occurs in about one-third. The headaches are usually gradually progressive and although frequently worse on the side of the tumour, they may be bitemporal and diffuse. Characteristically, the headache is worse on waking and improves during the day. Nausea and vomiting occur as the intracranial pressure increases and the patient frequently indicates that vomiting may temporarily relieve the severe headache. Drowsiness, that is, a deterioration of conscious state, is the most important symptom and sign of raised intracranial pressure. The extent of impairment of conscious state will be related to the severity of raised intracranial pressure. An alert patient with severely raised intracranial pressure may rapidly deteriorate and become deeply unconscious when there is only a very small further rise in the pressure within the cranial cavity.

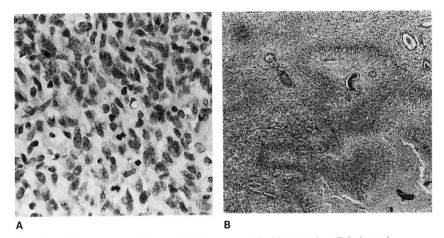

Fig. 6.3 Glioblastoma multiforme. (A) There is a marked increase in cellularity and variation in nuclear size shape and staining density with frequent mitotic figures (haematoxylin and eosin, ×40). (B) Low power view of the same tumour showing pallisaded necrosis typical of glioblastoma multiforme.

Focal neurological deficits

Focal neurological deficits are common in patients presenting with cerebral gliomas; the nature of the deficit will depend on the position of the tumour.

Patients presenting with tumours involving the frontal lobes frequently have pseudopsychiatric problems, personality change and mood disturbance. These changes are particularly characteristic of the 'butterfly glioma', so-called because it involves both frontal lobes by spreading across the corpus callosum, giving it a characteristic macroscopic (Fig. 6.4) and CT scan appearance. This type of tumour may also occur posteriorly, with spread across the splenium of the corpus callosum into both parieto-occipital lobes.

Limb paresis results from interference with the pyramidal tracts, either at a cortical or a subcortical level, and occurs in just under 50% of patients. **Field defects** associated with tumours of the temporal, occipital and parietal lobes are common, but may be evident only on careful testing. **Dysphasia**, either expressive or receptive, is a particularly distressing symptom occurring in patients with tumours involving the relevant areas of the dominant hemisphere.

The particular characteristics of posterior fossa and brain stem gliomas will be discussed in the following section on paediatric tumours.

Epileptic seizures

Seizures are the most frequent initial symptom in patients with cerebral astrocytoma and occur in between 50 and 75% of all patients. Tumours adjacent to the cortex are more likely to be associated with epilepsy than

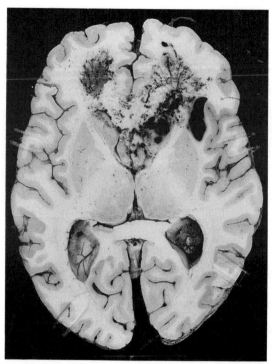

Fig. 6.4 'Butterfly glioma'. Glioblastoma multiforme of corpus callosum spreading into both frontal lobes.

those deep to the cortex and tumours involving the occipital lobe are less likely to cause epilepsy than those which are more anteriorly placed. Astrocytomas may produce either generalised or focal seizures; the focal characteristics will depend on the position within the brain and the cortical structures involved.

Investigations

Computer tomography. A CT scan of the brain is the essential radiological investigation; an accurate diagnosis can be made in nearly all tumours. Low grade gliomas show decreased density on the CT scan; this does not enhance with contrast and there is little or no surrounding oedema. Calcification may be present (Fig. 6.5). High grade gliomas are usually large and enhance vividly following intravenous injection of contrast material (Figs. 6.6 and 6.7). The enhancement is often patchy and non-uniform and frequently occurs in a broad, irregular rim around a central area of lower density. Although tumour cysts may occur in the high grade tumours, the central area of low density surrounded by the contrast enhancement is usually due to tumour necrosis. High grade tumours are surrounded by marked

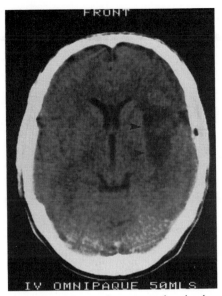

Fig. 6.5 Low grade astrocytoma. CT scan shows non-enhancing low density lesion with little or no mass effect.

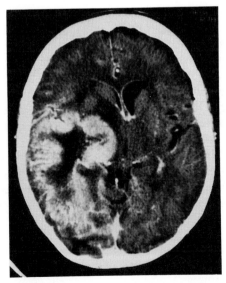

Fig 6.6 Glioblastoma multiforme. CT shows a large tumour with contrast enhancement particularly at the margins surrounding a necrotic centre. There is marked surrounding oedema with compression of the ventricles.

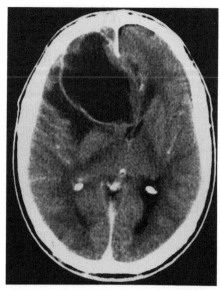

Fig. 6.7 Cystic anaplastic astrocytoma. There is a contrast enhancing margin, surrounding cerebral oedema and shift of the lateral ventricles.

cerebral oedema and there is frequently considerable distortion of the lateral ventricles. Compression of the lateral ventricle in one hemisphere, with pressure extending across the midline, may result in an obstructive hydrocephalus involving the opposite lateral ventricle.

Although the CT scan is the most important radiological investigation, other radiological studies may provide useful information.

Magnetic resonance imaging. When used with gadolinium contrast enhancement, MRI improves the visualisation of the low grade astrocytomas and improves the anatomical localisation of the tumour (Fig. 6.8).

Cerebral angiography. This was the standard study in most patients with astrocytomas prior to the introduction of computer tomography. It provides helpful information on the vascular supply of the tumour but is now only rarely indicated.

Plain X-rays. Plain X-rays of the skull do not need to be performed as a routine. The most common abnormality is erosion of the sella turcica due to long-standing raised intracranial pressure. Radiologically visible calcification is present in about 8% of patients with astrocyte derived gliomas.

Management

Following the presumptive diagnosis of a glioma the management involves:

- Surgery
- Radiotherapy
- Other adjuvant treatments.

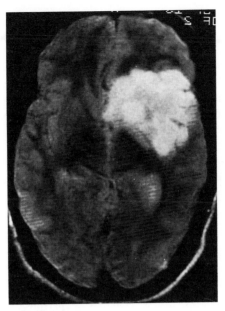

Fig. 6.8   MRI of low grade glioma.

Surgery

Surgery is performed with three principle aims:

- To make a definite diagnosis
- Tumour reduction to alleviate the symptoms of raised intracranial pressure
- Reduction of tumour mass as a precursor to adjuvant treatments.

The patient is started on glucocorticoid steroid therapy (e.g. dexamethasone) when presenting with clinical features of raised intracranial pressure with the aim of decreasing the cerebral oedema prior to surgery.

The type of operation performed will largely be determined by the position of the tumour and by the patient's clinical presentation. In general, the tumour is excised as radically as possible, provided the surgery will not result in any disabling neurological deficit. Craniotomy is performed in the position that provides the best access to the tumour. If the tumour has not grown to involve the cortical surface, a small incision is made in a non-eloquent gyrus or sulcus and the subcortical brain is divided down to the tumour mass. The tumour is excised, often with the aid of an ultrasonic aspirator. Occasionally, the tumour may involve one of the 'poles' of the hemisphere and the excision may entail a partial lobectomy. Although a craniotomy with radical tumour excision will alleviate the symptoms of raised intracranial pressure, for oncological reasons there is controversy as to whether it is valid as a cytoreductive procedure. Most high grade gliomas weigh approximately 100 g at the time of diagnosis and consist of 10^{11} cells. A radical tumour excision is able to excise the macroscopic tumour but cannot remove the tumour cells that are infiltrating deep into the adjacent, often vital, areas of normal or oedematous brain. Consequently, a radical excision is unlikely to achieve more than a 90–95% reduction in tumour cell numbers, resulting in 10^{10} cells remaining. Whether the 1–2 logs of tumour cell reduction are a significant reduction in tumour burden prior to adjuvant therapy aimed at improving the effectiveness of subsequent treatment, is still not resolved.

Alternatively, a biopsy, which can be performed most accurately using stereotactic methods, may be undertaken to obtain the definite histological diagnosis, without macroscopic tumour excision, if:

- The tumour is small and deep seated
- The tumour is diffuse, without major features of raised intracranial pressure, and macroscopic resection is not feasible
- The tumour involves highly eloquent areas (e.g. speech centre) without pronounced features of raised intracranial pressure.

Stereotactic biopsy involves localisation of the tumour with a stereotactic frame applied to the head of the patient using the CT scan. The three dimensional coordinates of the tumour are ascertained. The surgeon chooses the point of entry and the desired path through the brain and a computer program determines the necessary angles for the biopsy probe and the depth to the tumour (Fig. 6.9).

Postoperative care. The postoperative management of astrocytoma involves the routine care of a patient following a craniotomy. Careful neurological observations are performed, as prompt intervention is essential if the patient's neurological state deteriorates as a result of either increasing cerebral oedema or postoperative haemorrhage. A postoperative haematoma may occur in the region of the tumour excision or may be extracerebral, either subdural or extradural. A CT scan should be performed urgently if there is neurological deterioration, to determine the exact pathology. Occasionally, postoperative deterioration may be so rapid as to require urgent re-exploration of the craniotomy without prior radiological assessment.

In the initial postoperative period it is essential to avoid over hydration of the patient so as not to precipitate the cerebral oedema. The patient is nursed with the head of the bed elevated 20°, so as to promote venous return and reduce intracranial venous pressure. Steroid medication is usually required in the initial postoperative period and is gradually decreased over the following days. The steroids may need to be re-instituted during the course of radiotherapy.

The patient is usually mobilised as soon as possible, if necessary with the help of a physiotherapist.

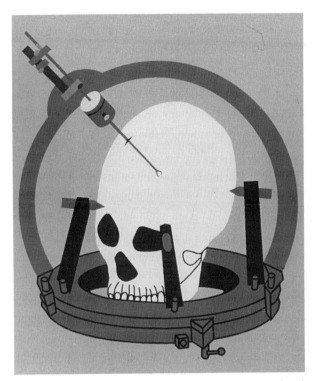

Fig. 6.9 Schematic diagram of stereotactic biopsy of cerebral tumour using the Brown–Roberts–Wells (BRW) system.

Radiation therapy

Postoperative radiation therapy is generally an effective adjunct to surgery in the treatment of higher grade gliomas. It has been shown to double the median survival for high grade gliomas to 37 weeks.

Radiation treatment is planned to optimise the homogeneity of the radiation dose throughout the tumour volume selected and to minimise high dose regions in normal brain transited by the radiation beam. The size of the daily radiation fraction is related to the incidence of complications and a maximum daily dose is usually between 180 and 200 rads. The total radiation dose varies depending on the tumour type, location and size of field, but for gliomas it is usually between 4500 and 6000 rads (4.5–6 Gy). Opinion varies regarding the tissue volume that should be treated for malignant glioma but there is no convincing evidence for the superiority of whole brain irradiation over radiation to the tumour area and a 'generous volume' of surrounding brain. The selection of the proper radiation dose for gliomas is as controversial as selection of the appropriate brain volume to be treated. Although increasing the radiation dosage from 5000 to 6000 rads does slightly improve survival, the higher dose of radiation therapy significantly increases the risk of brain necrosis.

Prognosis

At present there is no satisfactory treatment for the malignant cerebral glioma — the anaplastic astrocytoma and glioblastoma multiforme. The median survival following surgery is approximately 17 weeks and when radiation therapy is used as an adjuvant the median survival is approximately 37 weeks. Chemotherapy for high grade gliomas has been disappointing and the best results with surgery, radiation therapy and chemotherapy consistently show a median survival time of less than 1 year.

The role of surgery, radiation therapy and other adjuvant therapies in low grade gliomas is even less certain than for the high grade glioma. The low grade tumour may remain relatively quiescent for some years before it either continues to grow slowly or changes to a more anaplastic tumour with resulting debilitating neurological deterioration. In general, the same principles for surgical excision apply for low grade gliomas as for high grade tumours. However, patients having a radical excision of a tumour have been shown to have a higher 5 year survival (50%) than those with a subtotal excision (less than 20%). Radiation therapy has been shown to improve the survival in some groups of patients with low grade tumours. In general, other adjuvant therapies are not used for the treatment of low grade gliomas.

Other adjuvant therapies

Many different adjuvant therapies have been investigated for the treatment of glioma. These include the use of new chemotherapeutic agents, new methods of administering cytotoxic chemicals, immunotherapy, hyperthermia, new techniques of radiotherapy and photoradiation therapy.

The lack of effectiveness of the present treatment of gliomas is related to the biology of the tumour. The most common position for tumour recurrence following conventional treatment is locally, in the tumour bed, indicating that treatment has failed in local control. Although light microscopy shows high grade gliomas to have a relatively well defined border with the adjacent brain, special staining techniques, including monoclonal antibodies, show malignant cells extending well out into the surrounding brain. It is the failure to control the growth of these cells that is largely responsible for the local tumour recurrence. As indicated previously, a good surgical resection with 90% of the tumour excised would still result in 10^{10} cells being present. Effective radiotherapy will result in 1 log (90%) or at the most 2 logs (99%) of cell kill and it is unlikely that subsequent chemotherapy would reduce remaining tumour cells by more than 90%. Consequently, the effect of cytoreductive surgery, radiotherapy and chemotherapy would result in approximately 10^8 cells remaining; the immune system is unlikely to be able to cope with a tumour burden of more than 10^5 cells. It follows that, for any extra treatment to be effective, whether surgery or adjuvant therapy, it must provide at least 1 log of cell kill.

Chemotherapy. Conventional chemotherapy has been disappointing. Many of the chemotherapy agents that are active in vitro, or in other systemic tumours, have reduced activity in malignant brain tumours, either by exerting an inherently limited cytotoxic potential on brain tumour cells or by the inability of the chemotherapeutic agent to reach the cells that are responsible for the tumour recurrence. A study of brain tumour cell kinetics of high grade gliomas shows only a small proportion of the cells (5–10%) in an active growth phase; this has serious consequences for any cell cycle-specific cytotoxic agent. The most commonly used single agent cytotoxic regime involves administration of nitrosourea compounds. The high lipid solubility and low ionisation of these agents ensures a relatively effective penetration of the cytotoxic compound into the tumour. Combination therapy, utilising many different cytotoxic compounds, has been used in various trials but none of the combinations has been shown to be more beneficial than the use of the single nitrosourea.

It has been postulated that a reason for the lack of effectiveness of chemotherapy is the inability of the cytotoxic compound to reach the tumour cells which are invading the normal adjacent brain. This has resulted in new techniques of delivering the cytotoxic agent. High dose chemotherapy with bone marrow rescue has largely been abandoned because of its high morbidity and lack of effectiveness. Techniques of disrupting the blood–brain barrier have been used before chemotherapy infusion to improve the delivery of chemotherapeutic agents to tumour cells within the environment of a normal blood–brain barrier. This has resulted in substantially increased neurotoxicity to the normal brain without significantly improving survival. Intracarotid chemotherapy suffers from serious limitations — the perfusion of the tumour mass is less than expected because most tumours are not supplied entirely by one carotid artery and 'streaming' of the cytotoxic agent results in very high doses of chemotherapy to small areas, with relative hypoperfusion in other regions. Complications such as serious retinal damage and neurotoxicity have further reduced the attractiveness of this technique.

Radiotherapy. Improvements to enhance the effect of radiotherapy have included the use of radiosensitisers, such as metronidazole and misonidazole, which increase the radiosensitivity of hypoxic tumour cells without a corresponding increase in the sensitivity of euoxic cells. However, the clinical trials have shown only a marginal advantage. The use of interstitial brachytherapy, involving stereotactic implanted radioactive sources into the tumour, has the advantage of applying a high dose of radiotherapy to the tumour while sparing the surrounding brain. However, the clinical trials performed so far have resulted in a high incidence of radionecrosis to the surrounding brain and improvements in the technique will need to be devised before this method would become acceptable.

Hyperthermia. This has inherent basic limitations as, although cell death occurs at approximately 42°C, damage to the surrounding brain occurs at 45°C, so there is a very narrow therapeutic index. In addition, there is a marked tolerance of tumour cells to hyperthermia and the treatment has not been effective.

Immunotherapy. The possibilities for immunotherapy as an adjuvant treatment have been investigated for many years. Investigations have included the use of active immunotherapy techniques and, more recently, the application of adoptive immunotherapy. This technique involves stimulating peripheral blood lymphocytes in vitro with human recombinant interleukin-2 to produce lymphokinine activated killer cells (LAK cells) which can be administered in conjunction with interleukin-2. However, the LAK cells do not cross the blood–brain barrier and so need to be injected in close proximity to the tumour cells. Recent studies using this technique have been disappointing.

Photoradiation therapy. This is a technique that offers special advantages as an adjuvant therapy of malignant brain tumours since it has been shown to be an effective method of controlling local tumours. The technique involves the selective uptake of sensitiser into the brain tumours, followed by open or intra-operative irradiation of the sensitised tumour cells with light of an appropriate wavelength to activate the sensitiser and selectively destroy the tumour cells. Clinical studies using this method have shown a favourable trend, although formal phase III studies have not been undertaken.

OLIGODENDROGLIOMA

Oligodendrogliomas are responsible for approximately 4% of all gliomas and occur throughout the adult age group with a maximum incidence in the 5th decade. The tumour is rare in children.

Pathology

Nearly all oligodendrogliomas occur above the tentorium, most are located in the cerebral hemispheres and about half of these are in the frontal lobes. Oligodendrogliomas may project into either the 3rd or lateral ventricles.

Oligodendrogliomas have the same spectrum of histological appearance as astrocytomas, ranging from the very slow growing, benign tumour to the more rapidly growing, malignant variety with abundant mitotic figures, endothelial proliferation and foci of necrosis. Calcium deposits are found by histological examination in up to 90% of oligodendrogliomas. Unlike the astrocyte group, most oligodendrogliomas are well differentiated.

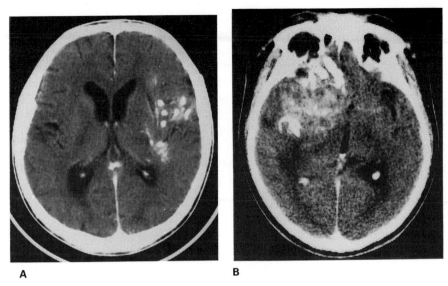

A   **B**

Fig. 6.10 Oligodendrogliomas. (A) Non-enhancing low grade calcified tumour. (B) contrast enhancing high grade oligodendroglioma.

Clinical presentation

The presenting features are essentially the same as for the astrocyte group but, as these tumours are more likely to be slow growing, epilepsy is common, occurring in 80% of patients and seen as an initial symptom in 50%. The features of raised intracranial pressure and focal neurological deficits are each present in approximately one-third of patients.

As for astrocyte tumours, MRI with contrast may be beneficial but other investigations are usually unnecessary.

Radiological investigation

CT scanning is the fundamental investigation. It will confirm the diagnosis of an intracranial tumour and in many cases the diagnosis of oligodendroglioma will be highly probable. Calcification will be present in 90% of cases and over half show contrast enhancement (Fig. 6.10).

Treatment and results

Treatment involves:

- Surgical resection
- Radiotherapy
- Other adjuvant treatments.

The standard treatment for oligodendroglioma has been an aggressive re-section of the tumour followed by radiation therapy, although there is some disagreement regarding the effectiveness of radiotherapy for these lesions. Chemotherapy is sometimes advocated for the higher grade tumours.

The survival of patients depends on the degree of histological malignancy. Five year survival rates are between 30 and 50% with a small number of patients living for many years (up to 5% for 20 years). However, most tu-mours with histological features of oligodendroglioma also have a component of astrocyte derived cells, usually anaplastic astrocytoma, and the tumour behaves biologically and clinically as an anaplastic astrocytoma rather than an oligodendroglioma.

RECURRENT CEREBRAL GLIOMA

As discussed earlier, most high grade cerebral gliomas will recur within one year of the initial treatment with surgery and radiotherapy. Low grade tumours may recur either as a continuing progression of the slow growth or, alternatively, the histological characteristics may alter and the tumour may become more anaplastic and rapidly growing.

The clinical presentation of a recurrent tumour will be evidenced by either a progression of the focal neurological signs or the signs of an increase in the intracranial pressure. The diagnosis will be confirmed by CT scan in most cases. The major differential diagnosis is postradiotherapy radiation necrosis, which may develop as early as 4 months or as late as 9 years after radiotherapy. The radiological investigations usually show an avascular mass and the diagnosis may be suspected from the dose of radiotherapy that has been administered. However, there may be considerable difficulty in differ-entiating necrosis from recurrent glioma, and sometimes an operation is required both for definitive diagnosis and to remove the mass.

The initial deterioration following a diagnosis of recurrent glioma can usually be temporarily halted by the use of steroid medication. The major decision is whether further surgery and other adjuvant therapy should be undertaken. In general, a further operation involving debulking of the tumour would be considered if:

- The patient is <65 years old
- There has been a symptom-free interval of one year or more since the first operation
- Debilitating irreversible neurological signs are absent
- The tumour is in an accessible position and repeat surgery would not result in additional morbidity.

Adjuvant therapies

Adjuvant therapies have little benefit for patients with recurrent tumour and, considering the morbidity involved, are not usually indicated.

EPENDYMOMA

Ependymomas are glial neoplasms arising from the ependyma and constitute approximately 5% of all gliomas. Approximately two-thirds of ependymomas occur in the infratentorial compartment and most of these present in children, adolescents and young adults. The supratentorial ependymomas occur mostly in adults.

Pathology

The tumour arises from the ependyma of the ventricle and, although predominantly intraventricular, the tumour often invades into the adjacent cerebellum, brain stem or cerebral hemisphere. The 4th ventricular tumours usually arise from the floor or lateral recess of the 4th ventricle and they may extend into the subarachnoid space to encase the medulla or upper cervical spinal cord. Alternatively, the tumour may grow laterally through the foramen of Luschka and into the cerebellopontine angle.

The tumours are nodular, soft and pale. Calcification is common, especially in supratentorial ependymomas.

There are numerous histological classification systems of ependymomas and the World Health Organization classification divides these tumours into myxopapillary, papillary and subependymoma types of non-anaplastic ependymoma and anaplastic ependymoma.

The myxopapillary variety occur in the cauda equina and are discussed in the chapter on spinal cord tumours (Ch. 15).

In an adult the subependymoma may be encountered as an incidental autopsy finding — a discrete nodular mass based in the brain's ventricular surface, particularly the floor or lateral recess of the 4th ventricle or the septum pellucidum — or it may be large enough to present clinically. It is usually heavily calcified and is composed of cells with astrocytic as well as ependymal features.

The papillary and anaplastic varieties of ependymoma are responsible for the majority of clinically symptomatic ependymomas. The cellularity and architecture of the ependymomas vary but a diagnostic feature is the presence of rosettes, and most ependymomas contain areas in which perivascular pseudorosettes are conspicuously developed. In these formations the blood vessel is surrounded by an eosinophil halo composed of the radiating tapering processes of the cells. Blepharoplasts frequently occur in ependymomas but may be difficult to visualise. These are tiny intracytoplasmic spherical or rod-shaped structures which represent the basal bodies of cilia, and are most frequently encountered in the apical portion of cells that form ependymal rosettes.

Clinical presentation

Posterior fossa ependymomas

Details will be discussed in the section on paediatric tumours, page 125.

The patients present with features of raised intracranial pressure due to hydrocephalus as a result of obstruction of the 4th ventricle, ataxia due to cerebellar involvement and occasionally features of brain stem pressure or infiltration.

Supratentorial tumours

Virtually all patients with supratentorial ependymomas present with features of raised intracranial pressure, often due to hydrocephalus as a result of obstruction of the CSF pathways. Ataxia is common and focal neurological deficits may occur due to involvement of the underlying cerebral hemisphere.

Radiological investigation

The CT scan will show a tumour that arises in the ventricle and enhances after administration of intravenous contrast. Calcification is common in the tumours arising from the lateral ventricles (Fig. 6.11). There is frequently associated hydrocephalus. In the posterior fossa differentiation from a medulloblastoma may be difficult.

Treatment

The treatment of ependymomas is initially surgical, with an attempt to perform a radical macroscopic resection of the tumour. The supratentorial

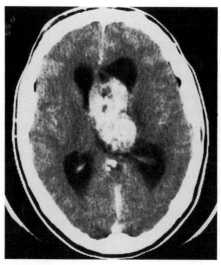

Fig. 6.11 Calcified contrast enhancing ependymoma involving lateral ventricles.

tumours are often very large and may extend throughout the lateral and 3rd ventricles, but the associated hydrocephalus makes the excision of the intraventricular portion feasible. However, the tumour may arise from the ventricular wall in the region of the basal ganglia and blend imperceptibly with the underlying cerebral structures so that a complete excision is not possible. The 4th ventricular tumours can be excised from the ventricle but the microscopic infiltration into the underlying brain stem cannot be removed surgically. Postoperative radiation therapy is advisable and, as these tumours may spread through the CSF pathways, sometimes whole neuraxis radiation is recommended.

The prognosis is related to the degree of anaplasia of the tumour and for intratentorial tumours varies from 15 to 50% 5 year survival. The prognosis for the supratentorial tumours is better, particularly in adults.

PINEAL TUMOURS

Tumours arising in the region of the pineal gland are mostly not of pineal origin, but are generally called 'pineal', as they have a similar clinical presentation.

The tumours are relatively uncommon, accounting for 0.5% of all intracranial tumours. However, they occur more frequently in Japan and China, where the incidence is up to 5%. Most tumours have their clinical appearance between 10 and 30 years of age.

Classification

Classification of pineal region tumours in decreasing frequency

- Germinoma
- Teratoma
- Pineocytoma
- Pineoblastoma
- Miscellaneous — glioma
                  — cyst.

The germinoma is the most common pineal region tumour and is similar in histological appearance to germinoma of the gonads and mediastinum; it occurs predominantly in males. The teratoma is less common and, like the germinoma, also arises from displaced embryonic tissue. The other tumour types are rare.

Clinical presentation

Patients with pineal tumours present with:

- Raised intracranial pressure

- Neurological signs due to focal compression
- Endocrine disturbance.

Raised intracranial pressure. The features of raised intracranial pressure, such as headaches, drowsiness and papilloedema, are due to hydrocephalus, which is a result of the tumour occluding the aqueduct of Sylvius.

Focal compression. Compression of the efferent cerebellar pathways in the superior cerebellar peduncle results in limb ataxia and distortion of the quadrigeminal plate, produces limitation of upgaze, convergence paresis with impairment of reaction of pupils to light and accommodation (Parinaud's syndrome) and may result in convergence–retraction nystagmus on upgaze (Koerber–Salius–Elschnig syndrome).

Endocrine disturbance. Endocrine disturbances are uncommon but include precocious puberty in 10% of patients, almost invariably male, and diabetes insipidus in 10%.

Radiological investigations

CT scan and MRI will show a pineal region tumour and will often suggest the correct pathological diagnosis (Fig. 6.12). On CT scan, before contrast, a germinoma will be a hyperdense lesion in the region of the pineal gland infiltrating into the surrounding tissue and there will be uniform vivid enhancement following intravenous contrast. Calcification is uncommon.

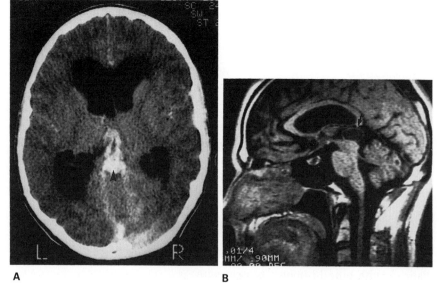

A   **B**

Fig. 6.12   (A) Pineal region germinoma causing obstructive hydrocephalus. (B) pineal cyst.

Management

This consists of surgery and radiotherapy.

A ventriculoperitoneal shunt is frequently required as the hydrocephalus is often severe.

There is controversy over whether the definitive treatment should be an attempt at surgical excision or radiotherapy. As most of the tumours are germinomas, and these tumours are very radiosensitive, a course of radiotherapy is usually given as the initial treatment. If serial CT scans show the tumour has failed to respond to the radiotherapy then surgery may be necessary. Alternatively, if the features on the initial CT and MR scans are atypical, and the lesion does not resemble a germinoma, exploration of the tumour and surgical excision may be appropriate as the initial procedure.

The preferred surgical approach is usually by a posterior fossa craniotomy, above the cerebellum and below the tentorium cerebelli. Alternative supratentorial surgical exposures include approaching the tumour through the corpus callosum or by retracting the occipital lobe.

METASTATIC TUMOURS

Metastatic tumours are responsible for approximately 15% of brain tumours in clinical series but up to 30% of brain tumours reported by pathologists. Approximately 30% of deaths are due to cancer and 1 in 5 of these have intracranial metastatic deposits at autopsy. The metastatic tumours most commonly originate from:

- Carcinoma of the lung
- Carcinoma of the breast
- Metastatic melanoma
- Carcinoma of the kidney
- Gastrointestinal carcinoma.

In 15% a primary origin is never found.

Most metastatic tumours are multiple and one-third are solitary. In about half of these systemic spread is not apparent. The incidence of tumours in the cerebrum relative to the cerebellum is 8 to 1, and most occur in the distribution of the middle cerebral artery. The size of the tumours may vary considerably if the deposits are multiple. Metastatic tumours are often surrounded by intense cerebral oedema.

Clinical presentation

The interval between the diagnosis of the primary cancer and cerebral metastases varies considerably. In general, secondary tumours from carcinoma of the lung present relatively soon after the initial diagnosis, with a median interval of 5 months. Although cerebral metastases may present within a few months of the initial diagnosis of malignant melanoma or carcinoma of the breast, some patients may live many years (up to 15 years) before an intracranial tumour appears.

The presenting features are similar to those described for other intracranial tumours:

- Raised intracranial pressure
- Focal neurological signs
- Epileptic seizures.

Headache and vomiting, indicative of raised intracranial pressure, occur in most patients and the presenting history is usually short, often only a few weeks or months. The increased intracranial pressure will be caused by either the tumour mass and surrounding oedema or, in posterior fossa tumours, obstructive hydrocephalus.

The pattern of focal neurological signs will depend on the position of the tumour deposits and the patient may present with a progressive hemiparesis or speech disturbance with supratentorial tumours or gait ataxia with cerebellar tumours.

Epileptic seizures occur in approximately 25% of patients and may be either focal or generalised.

Occasionally, metastases, especially melanoma or choriocarcinoma, present following an intracerebral haemorrhage.

Radiological investigations

The CT scan will diagnose the metastatic tumour and will show whether the deposits are solitary or multiple (Fig. 6.13). Most metastatic tumours are relatively isodense on the unenhanced CT scan and they enhance vividly after intravenous contrast material. Tumours that may be hyperdense prior to contrast are melanoma, choriocarcinoma, mucoid adenocarcinoma (e.g. from the gastrointestinal tract) and 50% of lymphomas. There is usually considerable surrounding cerebral oedema with distortion of the ventricular system.

MRI following gadolinium contrast will demonstrate small metastatic tumours often not visible on the CT scan (Fig. 6.14).

Treatment

Steroid medication (e.g. dexamethasone) will control cerebral oedema and should be commenced immediately if there is raised intracranial pressure.

Surgery to remove the metastasis is indicated if:

- There is a solitary metastasis in a surgically accessible position
- There is no systemic spread.

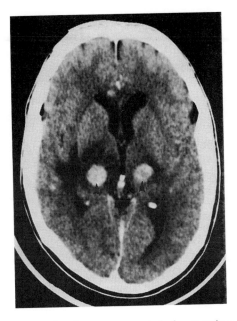

Fig. 6.13 Multiple contrast enhancing tumours typical of metastatic melanoma.

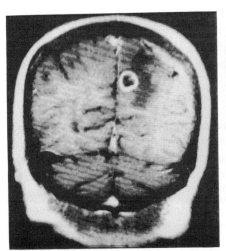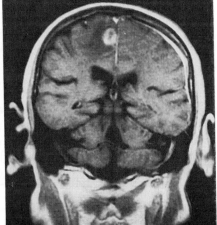

Fig. 6.14 MRI following gadolinium shows multiple small metastatic tumours.

Removal of a solitary secondary is preferable only if the primary site of origin has been, or will be, controlled. However, excision of a single metastasis will provide excellent symptomatic relief and consequently may be indicated even if the primary site cannot be treated satisfactorily. Surgery is, of course, mandatory if the diagnosis is uncertain.

Radiotherapy, together with steroid medication to control cerebral oedema, is used to treat patients with multiple cerebral metastases and may be advisable following the excision of a single metastasis. The treatment, up to 4500 rads, is usually given in a 2 week course.

Anticonvulsant medication is given both to patients who have suffered epileptic seizures and as a prophylactic measure.

Prognosis

About 30% of patients with solitary metastatic deposits from carcinoma of the lung or melanoma and 50% of patients with carcinoma of the breast survive one year following surgical excision. In those patients where the source of the metastatic tumour is undetermined, about 50% survive one year.

Leptomeningeal metastases

Meningeal carcinomatosis is widespread, multifocal sealing of the leptomeninges by systemic cancer. The clinical presentation includes:

- Hydrocephalus, causing headaches and vomiting
- Cranial nerve abnormalities due to direct invasion by the tumour
- Spinal root involvement due to local infiltration.

The CT scan findings may be subtle but frequently show excessive enhancement of the meninges. Lumbar puncture can be performed if there is no evidence of raised intracranial pressure. Malignant cells may be seen in the CSF, the protein concentration is increased and the glucose reduced.

PARANASAL SINUS TUMOURS

Tumours of the paranasal sinuses may spread directly to involve the brain. These uncommon tumours most frequently arise from the ethmoid or maxillary sinuses, less frequently from the sphenoid sinus and rarely from the frontal sinus. The tumours invade through the floor of the anterior cranial fossa in the region of the cribriform plate and may extend through the dura into the frontal lobe (Fig. 6.15). The tumours are usually squamous cell carcinoma and less frequently adenocarcinoma or adenoid cystic adenocarcinoma. The esthesioneuroblastoma is a rare nasal tumour arising from the olfactory epithelium that may invade through the cribriform plate.

The patients usually present with a blood stained or purulent nasal dis-

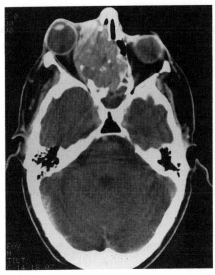

Fig. 6.15   Carcinoma of the ethmoid extending through the cribriform plate into the anterior cranial fossa.

charge and pain in the involved region. Cerebrospinal fluid rhinorrhoea may occur if the dura has been breached.

Surgical excision using a craniofacial resection may be the only method of controlling these tumours and, if the tumour has spread into the orbit, an adequate resection may involve orbital exenteration.

CHORDOMAS

Chordomas are rare tumours arising from notochord cell nests. They may arise throughout the craniospinal axis but occur predominantly at the ends of the axial skeleton in:

- The basi-occipital region
- The sacrococcygeal region.

The intracranial chordoma presents as a skull base tumour. It infiltrates and erodes the sphenoid and basi-occiput and may spread into the petrous bones, the paranasal sinuses, the sella turcica and the cavernous sinuses. The tumour will compress and distort the adjacent brain and engulf the cranial nerves and arteries.

These tumours do not have histological features of malignancy and only rarely metastasise. However, it is not usually possible to excise the cranial tumours completely; most patients die within 10 years of initial presentation.

Spinal chordomas occur predominantly in the sacrococcygeal region, although they may also arise in the cervical area. Like the cranial tumours, spinal chordomas invade and destroy the bone and compress the adjacent neural structures. Remote metastases occasionally occur. Patients with spinal chordomas present with back pain, radicular pain and slowly progressive lumbosacral nerve root involvement resulting in sphincter difficulties and sensory and motor disturbances in the legs.

Histological appearance

The tumours consist of notochord cells and mucoid stroma. Many of the cells may be coarsely vacuolated and some will contain a single large vacuole giving a 'signet ring' appearance. The characteristic histological appearance are physaliphorous (bubble-bearing) cells containing multiple vacuoles.

Clinical presentation

The majority of intracranial chordomas arise between 20 and 60 years of age. The clinical features result from the widespread tumour extension and include:

- Raised intracranial pressure, causing headaches and vomiting
- Multiple cranial nerve palsies, often unilateral
- Nasopharyngeal obstruction.

The radiological appearances are of a destructive lesion at the base of the skull or in the vertebral bodies (Fig. 6.16).

Treatment

It is rarely possible to excise all the tumour. Postoperative radiotherapy is usually administered but is of doubtful value.

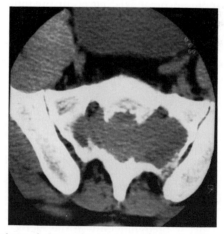

Fig. 6.16 Sacral chordoma. A destructive tumour extending into the vertebral canal.

PAEDIATRIC TUMOURS

Intracranial tumours are the most common form of solid tumour in childhood, with 40% of the tumours occurring above the tentorium cerebelli. The most common supratentorial tumours are astrocytomas, followed by anaplastic astrocytomas and glioblastoma multiforme. Craniopharyngioma occur more commonly in children than adults and are situated in the suprasellar region; this tumour is described in Chapter 8. Other, less common, supratentorial tumours include primitive neuroectodermal tumours, ependymomas, ganglioglioma and pineal region tumours.

POSTERIOR FOSSA TUMOURS

Sixty per cent of paediatric brain tumours occur in the posterior fossa. The relative incidence of the tumours is:

1. Cerebellar astrocytoma 30%
2. Medulloblastoma   30%
3. Ependymoma   20%
4. Brain stem glioma   10%
5. Miscellaneous   10%
   a. choroid plexus papilloma
   b. haemangioblastoma
   c. epidermoid, dermoid
   d. chordoma.

Clinical presentation

The presenting clinical features of posterior fossa neoplasms in children are related to:

- Raised intracranial pressure
- Focal neurological signs.

Raised intracranial pressure. This is the most common presenting feature. It is due to hydrocephalus caused by obstruction of the 4th ventricle and is manifest by headaches, vomiting, diplopia and papilloedema.

The headaches begin insidiously, gradually becoming more severe and frequent; they are worst in the early morning. There is usually no specific headache localisation. Vomiting is frequently associated with the headaches and may temporarily relieve the headache. Raised intracranial pressure may result in a strabismus causing diplopia due to stretching of one or both of the 6th (abducens) cranial nerves. This is a so-called 'false localising sign'. Papilloedema is usually present at the time of diagnosis. In infants, an expanding head size is an additional sign of raised intracranial pressure.

Focal neurological signs. These are due to the tumour invading or compressing the cerebellum (nuclei and tracts), the brain stem and cranial nerves. Truncal and gait ataxia results particularly from midline cerebellar involvement. Horizontal gaze paretic nystagmus often occurs, with tumours around the 4th ventricle. Upbeat vertical nystagmus is indicative of brain stem involvement.

Disturbances of bulbar function, such as difficulty in swallowing with nasal regurgitation of fluid, dysarthria and impaired palatal and pharyngeal reflexes, result from brain stem involvement. In addition, compression or tumour invasion of the pyramidal tracts may result in hemiparesis and, if the ascending sensory pathways are involved, sensory disturbance will occur in the trunk and limbs.

The tumour may directly envelop the lower cranial nerves — glosso-pharyngeal, vagal, spinal accessory and hypoglossal, as well as the 7th cranial nerve.

Neck stiffness and head tilt may occur in children with posterior fossa neoplasms, and may be due to herniation of a cerebellar tonsil or tumour tissue resulting in dural irritation.

Investigations

CT scan and MRI have replaced the need for the previous radiological investigations that included radio-isotope brain scanning, air ventriculography and posterior fossa angiography. The CT scan will show the presence of a posterior fossa tumour, its position and whether it arises primarily in the brain stem, 4th ventricle or from the cerebellum (Figs. 6.17, 6.18 and 6.19).

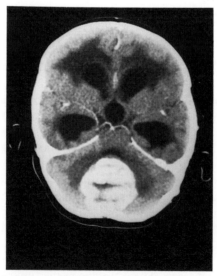

Fig. 6.17 Contrast enhancing medulloblastoma arising from the vermis causing obstructive hydrocephalus.

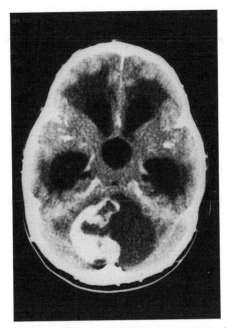

Fig. 6.18 Cystic cerebellar astrocytoma causing obstructive hydrocephalus. There is a contrast enhancing nodule in a large cyst.

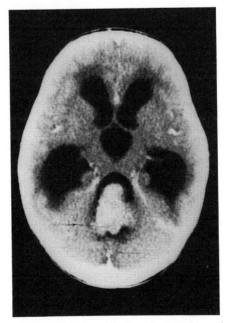

Fig. 6.19 Contrast enhancing ependymoma in the 4th ventricle causing obstructive hydrocephalus.

Management

The treatment of posterior fossa tumours involves:

- Surgery
- Radiotherapy
- Chemotherapy.

A preliminary CSF shunt may need to be performed in a child with severely raised intracranial pressure due to hydrocephalus. The CSF diversion can be achieved by either an external drain or a ventriculoperitoneal shunt. An external drain is a temporary measure only, because of the risk of infection. A ventriculoperitoneal shunt provides immediate and controlled relief of intracranial hypertension and the subsequent posterior fossa operation can be performed as a planned elective procedure, rather than an urgent operation in suboptimal conditions. A criticism of a preoperative ventriculoperitoneal shunt is that it might promote the metastatic spread of tumour. A filtering chamber in the shunt system may lessen this risk but this predisposes to shunt malfunction.

Steroid medication to control local oedema is commenced preoperatively. The operation is performed in either the sitting or prone position through a vertical midline incision. A posterior fossa craniotomy is performed, usually with excision of the bone down to and around the foramen magnum. Tumour excision is aided by the use of magnifying loupes and illumination with a fibre-optic headlight, or by the use of an operating microscope.

Postoperative care involves careful monitoring of the neurological signs. Postoperative haemorrhage or oedema may result in rapid deterioration of the neurological state, and in respiratory arrest. An urgent CT scan may indicate the cause and site of the problem but the deterioration may be so rapid that the wound may need to be reopened without the benefit of prior scanning.

If a ventriculoperitoneal shunt has not been inserted prior to tumour removal an exacerbation of the obstructive hydrocephalus may occur if the tumour excision has failed to relieve the CSF obstruction. Disturbances of bulbar and lower cranial nerve function may cause difficulty in swallowing. Nasogastric feeding may be necessary until the protective mechanisms return, and great care should be taken to avoid aspiration.

Medulloblastoma

The medulloblastoma is a malignant tumour usually arising in the midline from the cerebellar vermis, although it may occur more laterally in a cerebellar hemisphere in older patients. The tumour expands to invade the adjacent cerebellum and large tumours completely fill the 4th ventricle (see Fig. 6.17).

The tumours arise from the external granular layer of the fetal cerebellum (Obersteiner's layer). Histologically, the medulloblastoma is highly cellular, with numerous mitoses. True rosettes do not occur but the cells are seen in concentric patterns around homogeneous material or blood vessels (pseudorosettes).

Presenting features. The presenting features are related to hydrocephalus and cerebellar dysfunction. Truncal ataxia is typically present in children with medulloblastoma but cranial nerve deficits, except for a 6th nerve palsy, are uncommon in the early stages.

Surgery. At surgery the cerebellar vermis is split in the midline and it is usually possible to obtain a gross macroscopic excision of the tumour with complete removal from the 4th ventricle.

Radiation therapy. Medulloblastoma is relatively radiosensitive and radiation therapy is recommended to the entire neuraxis because of the tendency of the tumour to seed along the CSF pathways. Adjuvant chemotherapy is sometimes recommended and numerous protocols using a variety of chemotherapeutic agents have been investigated. There is no uniformity of opinion as to which drugs or routes of administration are the most effective and whether chemotherapy should be administered as part of the initial treatment plan or only used at the time of recurrence of the tumour.

Prognosis. Although the combination of radical surgery and irradiation has improved the prognosis, the 5 year survival rate is approximately 40%.

Cerebellar astrocytoma

The cerebellar astrocytoma is frequently a benign, slowly growing cystic tumour which is the most favourable of all the intracranial paediatric neoplasms. The tumours may arise in either the hemisphere or vermis and frequently consist of a large tumour cyst with a relatively small solid component in the wall of the cyst (see Fig. 6.18). Less frequently the tumour may be entirely solid with little or no cystic component. Histologically, the solid portion of the tumour is usually a Grade 1 or 2 astrocytoma.

Presenting features. The clinical presenting features are similar to those of a medulloblastoma, but as the tumours may be located more laterally the presenting features are accompanied by ipsilateral cerebellar disturbance. The duration of symptoms is variable but tends to be longer than with medulloblastoma, averaging 6–12 months.

Surgery. A complete surgical excision is usually possible and it is only necessary to excise the solid component from the cystic tumour.

Radiation therapy. Postoperative radiation therapy is not usually indicated if an excision has been possible. The prognosis is the most favourable of all intracranial childhood tumours with a cure rate in excess of 75%.

Ependymoma

The ependymoma of the 4th ventricle arises from the floor of the 4th ventricle and is attached to, and may infiltrate the underlying brain stem (see Fig. 6.19).

Pathological features. The pathological features and histology are described earlier in the chapter, see page 111.

Presenting features. The presenting features are similar to those described for a medulloblastoma, although the initial symptoms and signs are usually due to hydrocephalus. Involvement of the dorsal brain stem results in unilateral or bilateral facial weakness.

Surgery. The surgical excision of the ependymoma involves splitting the inferior vermis to obtain access to the fourth ventricle. It is usually possible to perform a gross macroscopic excision of the tumour from the ventricle and adjacent cerebellum but, as the tumour often originates from the floor of the fourth ventricle, total excision is rarely possible.

Radiation therapy. Postoperative radiation therapy is usually administered to the posterior fossa and, as the tumour seeds along the CSF pathways, entire neural axis irradiation is often recommended, particularly in the higher grade ependymoma.

There is no definite advantage from adjuvant chemotherapy, although it may be used at the time of tumour recurrence.

Brain stem glioma

The brain stem glioma arises predominantly in the pons, less frequently in the medulla but may infiltrate extensively throughout the brain stem. The tumour infiltrates between the normal structures with a histological appearance varying from the relatively benign astrocytoma to anaplastic astrocytoma and glioblastoma multiforme. Over 50% of brain stem gliomas examined at autopsy will have the microscopic features of glioblastoma multiforme.

Clinical presentation. The clinical presentation characteristically includes progressive multiple bilateral cranial nerve palsies with involvement of pyramidal tracts and ataxia. Facial weakness and 6th cranial nerve palsy are common and an internuclear ophthalmoplegia is indicative of an intrinsic brain stem lesion. The child's personality often changes — they become apathetic. Raised intracranial pressure is less common than with other paediatric posterior fossa neoplasms, as obstruction of the 4th ventricle or aqueduct of Sylvius occurs late in the illness.

The CT scan appearance is of an expanded brain stem. Magnetic resonance imaging has considerably improved the accuracy of the diagnosis (Fig. 6.20).

Surgery. Surgical treatment is not usually indicated, although either an open or a stereotactic biopsy may be performed if there is any doubt of the diagnosis.

Radiation therapy. Palliative radiation therapy is the only treatment but tumour usually causes death within 18 months of diagnosis.

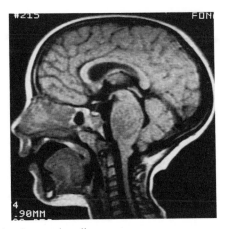

Fig. 6.20 MR scan showing pontine gliomas.

FURTHER READING

Apuzzo M J, Jepson J H, Luxton G, Little P M 1984 Ionising and non-ionising radiation treatment of cerebral malignant gliomas: specialised approaches. Clinical Neurosurgery 31: 470–496

Bailey P, Cushing H 1971 A classification of tumours of the glioma group on a histogenetic basis with a correlated study of prognosis. J B Lippincott, Philadelphia, 1926. Reprinted Argosy Antiquarian, New York

Burger P C, Vogel F S 1982 Surgical pathology of the nervous system and its coverings, 2nd edn. John Wiley, New York

Dohrmann G J, Farwell J R, Flannery J I 1976 Ependymomas and ependymoblastomas in children. Journal of Neurosurgery 45: 273–283

Higginbotham N L, Phillips R J, Farr H W 1979 Chordoma: thirty five year study at the Memorial Hospital. Cancer 29: 1841–1850

Kaye A H, Morstyn G, Apuzzo M J 1988 Photoradiation therapy and its potential in the management of neurological tumours. Journal of Neurosurgery 69: 1–14

Kernohan J W, Maybon R F, Svein H J, Adson A W 1949 A simplified classification of gliomas. Mayo Clinic Proceedings 24: 71–75

Kornblith P L, Walker M 1988 Chemotherapy of gliomas. Journal of Neurosurgery 68: 1–17

Liebel S A, Sheline G E 1987 Radiation therapy for neoplasms of the brain. Review article. Journal of Neurosurgery 66: 1–22

Rich T A, Schiller A, Suit H D, Mankin H J 1985 Clinical and pathologic review of 48 cases of chordoma. Cancer 56: 182–187

Ringertz N 1950 Grading of gliomas. Acta Pathologica Microbiologica Scandinavica 27: 51–64

Wold L F, Laws E R Jr 1983 Cranial chordomas in children and young adults. Journal of Neurosurgery 59: 1043–1047

Zulch K J 1986 Brain tumours, their biology and pathology, 3rd edn. Springer Verlag, Berlin

7. Benign brain tumours

The benign brain tumours may be intimately associated with, and surrounded by, the adjacent brain, but the tumour cells do **not** invade the underlying brain. This is in contradistinction to the gliomas, which are intrinsic brain tumours actively invading the adjacent brain. This chapter will discuss the more common benign brain tumours — meningioma and acoustic neuroma — and give a brief description of the less common tumours — haemangioblastoma, epidermoid and dermoid, and colloid cysts.

MENINGIOMA

Meningiomas are the most common of the benign brain tumours and constitute about 15% of all intracranial tumours, being about one-third of the number of gliomas. Although they may occur at any age, they reach their peak incidence in middle-age, are very uncommon in children and occur more frequently in women than men.

The term meningioma was introduced by Harvey Cushing in 1922, although the tumour had been described in the late eighteenth century. The tumour arises from the arachnoid layer of the meninges, principally the arachnoid villi and granulations.

Aetiology

As for other brain tumours, no definite aetiological factor has been identified. However, the possibility that head trauma predisposes to the development of meningioma has been the subject of controversy for many years. Although epidemiological studies do not support trauma as an aetiological factor, there have been cases reporting the development of meningiomas at the site of substantial meningeal trauma.

Position of meningiomas (Fig. 7.1)

The most common location is in the parasagittal region arising either from the wall of the superior sagittal sinus (parasagittal) or from the falx (falcine). Less frequently the tumours may arise from the convexity of the cranial

129

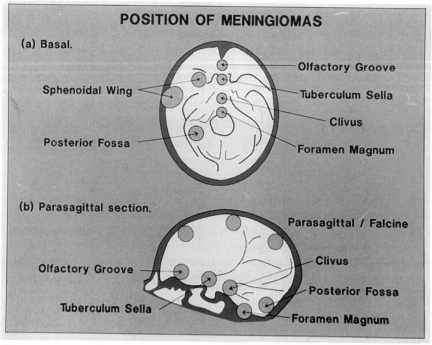

Fig. 7.1 Typical positions of intracranial meningiomas.

vault, where they are particularly concentrated in the region of the coronal suture. Sphenoidal ridge meningiomas are divided into those that arise from the inner part of the lesser wing of sphenoid and the adjacent anterior clinoid process, and those arising from the outer sphenoidal ridge, comprising the greater wing of the sphenoid and the adjacent pterion (the junction of the temporal, parietal and frontal bones). Less frequently, the tumours may arise from the olfactory groove, tuberculum sella (suprasellar) or posterior fossa (Table 7.1)

Meningiomas usually occur as a single intracranial tumour but multiple intracranial meningiomas may present in von Recklinghausen's disease.

Table 7.1 Position of intracranial meningiomas (%)

Parasagittal and falx	25
Convexity	20
Sphenoidal wing	20
Olfactory groove	12
Suprasellar	12
Posterior fossa	9
Ventricle	1.5
Optic sheath	0.5

Pathology

Unlike gliomas, where the classification system is based on the histological appearance of the tumour, meningiomas are usually classified according to their position of origin rather than their histology. The reason for this is that the biological activity of the tumour, the presenting features, the treatment and prognosis are all related more to the site of the tumour than the histology.

The major histological types are:

— Syncytial or endotheliomatous — sheets of cells with varying amounts of stroma.
— The transitional type characterised by whorls of cells which may undergo hyalin degeneration with subsequent deposition of calcium salts. These calcified concentric **psammoma bodies** form the characteristic feature of many transitional meningiomas but they may also be present in the syncytial or fibroblastic types.
— The fibroblastic type contains abundant reticulin and collagen fibres.
— Angioblastic meningiomas are much less common and their characteristic feature is the predominance of vascular channels separated by sheets of cells. Histologically, these tumours resemble cerebellar haemangioblastomas.
— Malignant meningiomas occur infrequently. The indications of malignancy include cellular pleomorphism, increased numbers of mitotic figures and local invasion of brain.

Clinical presentation

Meningiomas present with features of:

- Raised intracranial pressure
- Focal neurological signs
- Epilepsy.

The position of the tumour will determine the features of the clinical presentation. The tumours grow slowly and there is frequently a long history, often of many years, of symptoms prior to the diagnosis.

Parasagittal tumours (Fig. 7.2)

These tumours most often arise in the middle third of the vault and the patient may present with focal epilepsy and paresis, usually affecting the opposite leg and foot as the motor cortex on the medial aspect of the posterior frontal lobe is affected. Tumours arising anteriorly are often bilateral and patients present with features of raised intracranial pressure. As these tumours involve the frontal lobes, pseudopsychiatric symptoms, as well as

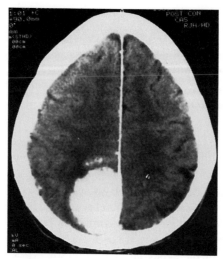

Fig. 7.2 Parasagittal meningioma.

impairment of memory, intelligence and personality, may occur. Urinary incontinence is occasionally a symptom of a large frontal tumour, especially if it is bilateral. Tumours arising from the posterior falx may affect the parieto-occipital region and produce a homonymous hemianopia. If the tumour lies above the calcarine fissure the inferior quadrant is more affected; when the tumour is below the fissure the upper quadrant is predominantly affected.

Convexity tumours (Fig. 7.3)

Convexity tumours may grow to a large size if situated in front of the coronal suture. They present with raised intracranial pressure. More posterior tumours will cause focal neurological symptoms and focal epilepsy.

Sphenoidal ridge tumours

Tumours arising from the **inner sphenoidal ridge** cause compression of the adjacent optic nerve and patients may present with a history of uni-ocular visual failure. If the tumour is large enough to cause raised intracranial pressure papilloedema will develop in the contralateral eye. The presenting features of primary optic atrophy in one eye and papilloedema in the other is known as the Foster Kennedy syndrome, and was described in 1911. Inner sphenoidal ridge tumours may also cause compression of the olfactory tract resulting in anosmia.

Patients with tumours involving the **outer sphenoidal ridge** present with features of raised intracranial pressure, often severe papilloedema with relatively inconspicuous localising symptoms or signs. Tumours in this region occur as a thin sheet, and are known as 'en plaque'. They may cause an excessive bony reaction resulting in proptosis (Fig. 7.4).

Olfactory groove tumours (Fig. 7.5)

Olfactory groove meningiomas cause anosmia, initially unilateral and later bilateral. The presenting features may include symptoms of raised intracranial pressure, failing vision either from chronic papilloedema or direct optic nerve and field defects from chiasm compression. These tumours may

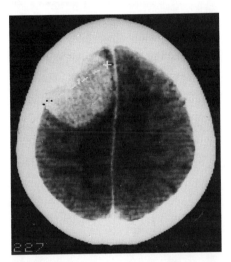

Fig. 7.3 Convexity meningioma.

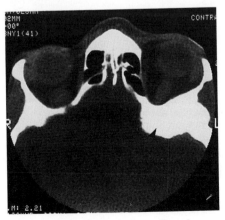

Fig. 7.4 Hyperostosis of the sphenoidal ring causing unilateral proptosis due to a sphenoidal ring meningioma.

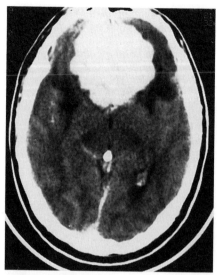

Fig. 7.5 Olfactory groove meningioma.

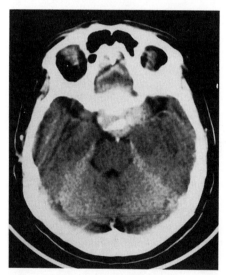

Fig. 7.6 Tuberculum sella meningioma.

also present with the Foster Kennedy syndrome and the intellectual and psychiatric problems caused by frontal lobe compression described for inner spheroidal ridge meningiomas.

Suprasellar tumours (Fig. 7.6)

Suprasellar meningiomas arising from the tuberculum sella will cause visual failure and a bitemporal hemianopia, but the lack of endocrine disturbance

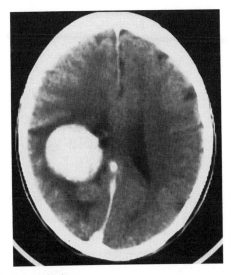

Fig. 7.7   Intraventricular meningioma.

will distinguish the clinical presentation of this tumour from that of a pituitary tumour.

Ventricular tumours (Fig. 7.7)

Tumours arising in the lateral ventricle present with symptoms of raised intracranial pressure extending over several years and associated with a mild global disturbance of function of one hemisphere and frequently a homonymous hemianopia.

Posterior fossa (Fig. 7.8)

Posterior fossa tumours may arise from the cerebellar convexity or from the cerebellopontine angle or clivus. The cerebellopontine angle tumours simulate an acoustic neuroma with symptoms involving the acoustic nerve, trigeminal nerve and facial nerve, ataxia due to cerebellar involvement and raised intracranial pressure, often due to hydrocephalus caused by obstruction of the 4th ventricle.

Radiological investigations

The CT scan appearance shows a tumour of slightly increased density prior to contrast; it enhances vividly and uniformly following intravenous contrast. Hyperostosis of the cranial vault may be a focal process at the site of the tumour attachment or, as seen with en plaque meningioma, a more diffuse sclerosis. These bone changes may also be seen on plain skull X-ray.

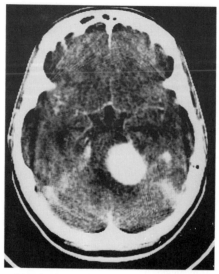

Fig. 7.8 Meningioma arising in the cerebellopontine angle and from the tentorial edge.

Magnetic resonance imaging will demonstrate meningiomas following the intravenous injection of gadolinium contrast (Fig. 7.9). Cerebral angiography is no longer necessary as a diagnostic investigation but may be useful pre-operatively to ascertain the position of the cerebral vessels. It will demonstrate external carotid artery supply to the tumour with a characteristic tumour blush, differentiating it from a glioma or metastatic tumour (Fig. 7.10). Angiography also allows pre-operative embolisation of the tumour, if necessary.

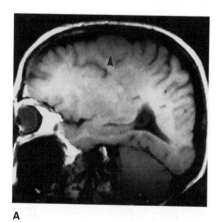
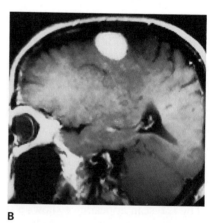

A   B

Fig. 7.9 MRI of parasagittal meningioma. The meningioma may be isodense on the plain T1 and T2 scans (A) but will enhance vividly after i.v. gadolinium (B).

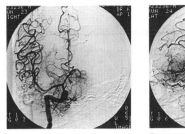 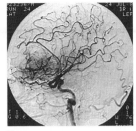 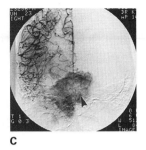

A   **B**   **C**

Fig. 7.10 Cerebral angiogram of olfactory groove meningioma showing displacement of anterior cerebral arteries (A & B) and the characteristic tumour blush, usually due to the external carotid artery supply (C).

Preoperative management

Meningiomas are frequently surrounded by severe cerebral oedema and patients should be treated with high dose steroids (dexamethasone) prior to surgery if possible. Pre-operative embolisation of the tumour vasculature may be considered advisable in some anterior basal and sphenoidal wing tumours where the major vascular supply is not readily accessible in the early stages of the operation.

Treatment

The treatment of meningiomas is total surgical excision, including obliteration of the dural attachment. Although this objective is usually possible there are some situations where complete excision is not possible because of the position of the tumour. Tumours arising from the clivus, in front of the brain stem or those situated within the cavernous sinus, are notoriously difficult to excise without causing devastating morbidity.

Radiation therapy is not generally advised for tumours that have been incompletely excised as meningiomas are radioresistant.

Postoperative management

The postoperative care of patients following excision of a meningioma involves the routine management of patients following a craniotomy but with particular attention to the minimisation of cerebral oedema. Steroid therapy is continued initially and gradually tapered. Care is taken to avoid excessive hydration and the patient is nursed with the head of the bed elevated to promote venous return. Neurological deterioration requires urgent assessment and a CT scan will determine the pathological cause, either postoperative haemorrhage or cerebral oedema.

Tumour recurrence

The risk of tumour recurrence depends on the extent of tumour excision. When the tumour and its dural origins are completely excised, the risk of recurrence is remote. The most common source of recurrence is from a tumour that has invaded a venous sinus and which was not resected (e.g. superior sagittal sinus or cavernous sinus). Recurrence is more common if the tumour has histological features of malignancy.

ACOUSTIC NEUROMA

Acoustic schwannomas arise from the 8th cranial nerve and account for 8% of intracranial tumours. Schwannomas occur less frequently on the 5th cranial nerve and rarely involve other cranial nerves. The acoustic schwannoma takes origin from the vestibular component of the 8th cranial nerve near the internal auditory meatus, at the transition zone where the Schwann cells replace the oligodendroglia.

Macroscopically, the acoustic schwannoma is lobulated with a capsule that separates it from the surrounding neural structures. Small tumours occupy the porus of the internal auditory canal and, as the tumour grows, the 8th nerve is destroyed and the adjacent cranial nerves become stretched around the tumour. The 7th nerve is typically displaced on the ventral and anterior surface of the tumour and the trigeminal nerve is carried upwards and forwards by the upper pole. The 6th nerve lies ventral and usually medial to the major mass and the lower cranial nerves are displaced around the inferior pole of the tumour. As the tumour grows medially it compresses and displaces the cerebellum and distorts the brain stem. Large tumours will result in obstruction of the 4th ventricle and hydrocephalus.

Clinical presentation

The presenting features will depend on the size of the tumour at the time of diagnosis. The earlier symptoms are associated with 8th nerve involvement. Tinnitus and unilateral partial or complete sensorineural hearing loss are the earliest features. Episodes of vertigo may occur but these may be difficult to distinguish from Menière's disease. Although the tumour causes compression of the facial nerve, the growth of the tumour is so slow that facial paresis is not evident until the tumour is large. At that stage 5th nerve compression may be evident, with diminished facial sensation and a depressed corneal reflex. Cerebellar involvement will result in ataxia and compression of the pyramidal tracts from a very large tumour causing brain stem compression will cause a contralateral hemiparesis. If a large tumour has caused obstructive hydrocephalus the patient will also present with features of raised intracranial pressure.

Radiological investigations

The CT scan will show an enhancing tumour in the cerebellopontine angle (Fig. 7.11). The internal auditory meatus will be widened indicating that the tumour has arisen from the 8th cranial nerve (Fig. 7.12). While there is no difficulty in diagnosing a tumour large enough to be evident on the CT scan, very small acoustic neuromas, which are predominantly within the internal auditory canal, may be more difficult to diagnose. These tumours may be seen on high quality CT scan but are particularly evident using MRI, especially following gadolinium contrast (Fig. 7.13).

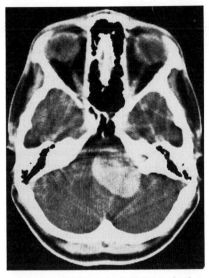

Fig. 7.11 Acoustic neuroma. A contrast enhancing tumour in the cerebellopontine angle arising from the 8th cranial nerve in the internal auditory canal.

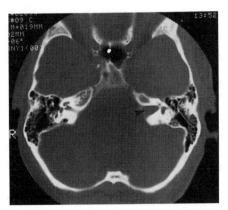

Fig. 7.12 Widened internal auditory meatus, indicative of an acoustic neuroma.

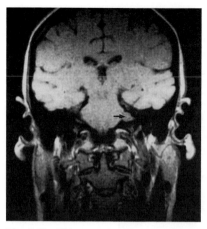 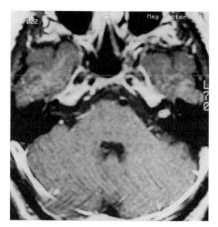

Fig. 7.13   MR scans showing small acoustic neuroma.

Other investigations

Pure tone audiometry, both by air and bone conduction is an essential part of the investigation of a patient with an acoustic neuroma. Other special auditory tests have been developed, including the use of brain stem auditory evoked response tests (which is particularly sensitive for changes in the retrocochlear auditory system) and are helpful in diagnosing a small intracanalicular tumour.

Vestibular function is impaired early in patients with acoustic neuromas and nystagmus is a frequent neurological finding. The Hallpike caloric test is carried out with the patient supine on a couch and the head raised to 30°C above horizontal, bringing the horizontal canals into the vertical plane with the position of maximum sensitivity to thermal stimuli. Warm and cool water is irrigated and the nystagmus reaction observed. The caloric response on the side of the acoustic nerve tumour is depressed or absent.

Differential diagnosis

The major differential diagnoses for a cerebellopontine angle tumour in decreasing frequency are:

- Meningioma
- Metastatic tumour
- Exophytic brain stem glioma
- Epidermoid tumour.

Treatment

The total excision of a large acoustic neuroma remains one of the major operative challenges in what Cushing has described as 'the gloomy corner of neurologic surgery'.

The aim of the operation is complete resection of the tumour while sparing the adjacent neural structures. If the patient presents with a large tumour causing severe hydrocephalus and raised intracranial pressure, a preliminary ventriculoperitoneal shunt or ventricular drain may be considered. Steroid administration prior to surgery is advisable if the tumour is large. The patient is usually positioned on their side, with the head flexed in the three-point headrest, although some surgeons prefer the patient to be in the sitting position. The operation is performed through a unilateral retrosigmoid craniotomy. After opening the dura, removal of CSF from either the cisterna magna or lateral cisterns provides exposure for exploration of the cerebellopontine angle. The central 'core' of a large tumour is debulked, often with the aid of the ultrasonic aspirator or CO_2 laser. The capsule of the tumour is then gently peeled away from the cerebellum, brain stem and cranial nerves. If the schwannoma is large the 8th nerve is so intimately incorporated into the tumour capsule that its functional preservation is impossible. The posterior rim of the internal auditory meatus is drilled away, allowing access to the internal auditory canal, so that a complete excision of the tumour is possible. Excision of large acoustic neuromas may be technically difficult and tedious, as the adjacent vital neurological structures, the brain stem and cranial nerves, are often adherent to the capsule. It may be possible to preserve the acoustic section of the 8th cranial nerve if the tumour is small.

Alternative surgical procedures include a translabyrinthine operation. However, this approach provides only restricted access for large tumours, making total excision difficult, and this method cannot preserve the hearing when the tumour is small.

Postoperative care

The postoperative management is similar to that indicated for the posterior fossa tumours in the previous chapter. Any neurological deterioration must be investigated urgently. A postoperative haemorrhage in this region may be rapidly fatal.

Postoperative swallowing difficulties may occur if there has been injury to the lower cranial nerves or brain stem. Great care should be taken to avoid aspiration and nasogastric feeding may be necessary. Facial paralysis will occur if the 7th nerve is not intact at the end of the operation and may result even if the nerve is in continuity due to neuropraxia of the nerve. A tarsorrhaphy may be necessary to prevent corneal ulceration and will be essential if there is a facial palsy and corneal sensation is diminished due to 5th nerve damage.

The cosmetic appearance of a permanent facial paralysis can be improved by a number of procedures including:

- Nerve anastomoses, such as a hypoglossal–facial anastomosis
- Cross facial nerve grafts
- Facial slings.

HAEMANGIOBLASTOMA

Haemangioblastomas are uncommon intracranial tumours accounting for 1–2% of all brain tumours and approximately 10% of posterior fossa tumours.

The haemangioblastoma arises from proliferation of endothelial cells. The tumour usually occurs in young adults, although it may occur at any age. It usually occurs in the posterior fossa and often produces a large cyst. Although haemangioblastoma may occur as a component of Lindau's disease, which includes multiple haemangioblastomas, haemangioblastomas of the retina (von Hippel tumour), renal tumour, renal cyst, pancreatic cyst and tubular adenomata of the epididymis, the majority of patients with the cerebellar tumour do not have Lindau's disease. Incomplete forms of the syndrome may occur and cerebellar haemangioblastomas occur in about 20% of patients with retinal haemangioblastoma.

Clinical presentation

The tumour presents as a slowly growing posterior fossa mass with features of raised intracranial pressure and cerebellar involvement. Occasionally the patient may be polycythaemic due to increased circulating erythropoetin.

Radiological investigations

The CT scan shows a cerebellar tumour which may involve the vermis and hemispheres and which shows vivid enhancement following intravenous contrast (Fig. 7.14). There is usually a low density cyst surrounding the tumour nodule, although haemangioblastomas may sometimes be solid. If considered necessary, vertebral angiography will confirm the highly vascular mass.

Total surgical excision through a posterior fossa craniotomy is nearly always possible. Great care must be taken not to enter the highly vascular tumour during the dissection and excision.

COLLOID CYST OF THE THIRD VENTRICLE

The colloid cyst of the 3rd ventricle is situated in the anterior part of the ventricle and is applied to the roof just behind the foramen of Munro.

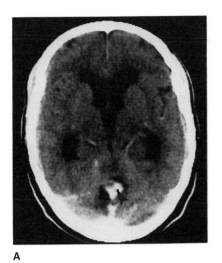
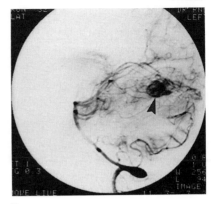

A   B

Fig. 7.14 Haemangioblastoma in the vermis of the cerebellum. (A) A vividly enhancing tumour nodule in the wall of a cyst. (B) Vertebral angiogram shows small tumour nidus.

Several possibilities as to the origin of the tumour have been proposed, including the paraphysis, choroid plexus epithelium, ependyma or a diverticulum of the diencephalon.

The cyst consists of a thin, outer fibrous capsule lined by a layer of epithelium; the contents consist of mucoid material, epithelial debris and mucin. The cyst may be very small and asymptomatic, as was the case with Harvey Cushing, where a 1 cm colloid cyst was found at postmortem. As the tumour grows it will cause bilateral obstruction to the foramen of Munro causing raised intracranial pressure from hydrocephalus. The headaches may fluctuate, being aggravated by stooping and relieved by standing upright. Episodes of abrupt, sudden leg weakness causing the patient to fall may occur without a change in conscious state. Alternatively, an abrupt loss of consciousness may occur and, although this is is usually transient, might be fatal.

Radiological investigations

The usual CT scan picture is a high density, rounded tumour in the anterior 3rd ventricle which enhances following intravenous contrast (Fig. 7.15), although isodense, hypodense and non-enhancing tumours have been reported. Magnetic resonance imaging helps to define the position of these tumours (Fig. 7.15).

Treatment

Surgical excision is performed through a craniotomy with a small incision in the anterior corpus callosum giving access to the lateral ventricle. The

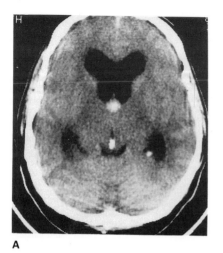
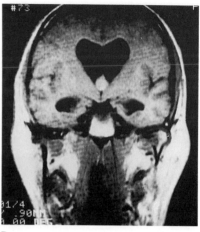

A   B

Fig. 7.15 Colloid cyst of the 3rd ventricle. (A) CT scan shows hyperdense tumour before contrast. (B) MRI.

tumour is seen expanding the foramen of Munro and, using the operating microscope, a complete excision is usually possible. Great care must be taken during the operation to preserve the venous structures, including the septal veins, thalamostriate vein and internal cerebral veins. Damage to the columns of the fornix will result in severe postoperative memory disturbance.

EPIDERMOID AND DERMOID CYSTS

Epidermoid and dermoid cysts arise from epithelial cells embryologically misplaced intracranially, particularly into the meninges and ventricles and, less frequently, into the parenchyma of the brain. Rarely, the cells can be implanted as a result of trauma such as a lumbar puncture, which can implant skin into the spinal canal causing an epidermoid cyst.

Epidermoid cysts make up about 1% of brain tumours, although their incidence is higher in Japan, where the incidence of dermoid cysts is much less.

Epidermoid tumours are found principally in the arachnoid spaces, cisterns or in the diploë of the bone. The most frequent localisations are the cerebellopontine angle, the suprasellar and parasellar regions, the lateral or 4th ventricles and the quadrigeminal cistern.

Dermoid tumours occur mostly in the posterior fossa as a midline lesion and a fistula may connect the dermoid with the skin.

Histology

The epidermoid cyst contains desquamated epithelium surrounded by keratin-producing squamous epithelium. The dermoid cyst includes dermal elements such as hair follicles, sebaceous glands and sometimes sweat glands.

Clinical presentation

The cysts usually present following a long history of symptoms related to their position. Cranial nerve abnormalities such as trigeminal neuralgia and hemifacial spasm may occur with cerebellopontine angle epidermoid tumours and the suprasellar cyst will produce visual impairment with optic atrophy and often a bitemporal hemianopia. Leakage of epidermoid cyst contents may result in a chemical meningitis and in patients with posterior fossa dermoid cysts, bacterial meningitis may occur through the dermal sinus connecting the cyst with the skin.

Radiological investigations

The CT scan of an epidermoid cyst is characterised by a low density lesion that does not enhance. The dermoid cyst will also have areas which are even less dense than CSF, indicating the presence of fat (Fig. 7.16).

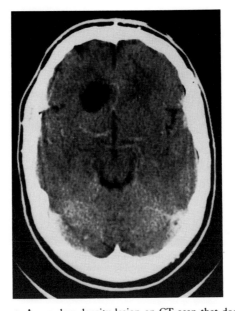

Fig. 7.16 Dermoid cyst. A very low density lesion on CT scan that does not enhance.

Treatment

The treatment is operative, with resection of the cyst. Complete excision may be prevented by the cyst wall being densely adherent to major vessels and important neural structures.

FURTHER READING

Cushing H, Eisenhardt L 1938 Meningiomas: their classification, regional behaviour, life history and surgical end results. Charles C Thomas, Springfield
Cushing H 1917 Tumours of the nervus acusticus and the syndrome of the cerebellopontine angle. W B Saunders, Philadelphia
Di Tullio M V, Rand R W 1978 The Rand-Kurze suboccipital transmeatal operation. In: Rand R W (ed) Microneurosurgery. C V Mosby, St Louis, ch 13, pp 206–232
Kennedy F 1911 Retrobulbar neuritis as an exact diagnostic sign of certain tumours and abscesses in the frontal lobes. American Journal of Medical Science 142: 355–368
King T T 1982 The translabyrinthine operation for removal of acoustic nerve tumours. In: Schmidek H H, Sweet W H (eds) Operative surgical techniques: indications, methods and results. Grune and Stratton, New York, ch 42, pp 609–636
Little J R, McCarty C S 1974 Colloid cysts of the third ventricle. Journal of Neurosurgery 39: 230–235
Rand R W, Kurze T 1965 Facial nerve preservation by posterior fossa transmeatal microdissection in total removal of acoustic neuromas. Journal of Neurology, Neurosurgery and Psychiatry 28: 311–316
Russell D S, Rubenstein L J 1977 Pathology of tumours of the nervous system, 4th edn. Williams & Wilkins, Baltimore
Zulch K J 1986 Brain tumours, their biology and pathology, 3rd edn. Springer Verlag, Berlin

8. Pituitary tumours

Pituitary adenomas account for 8–10% of all intracranial tumours.

In 1886, Pierre Marie first made the connection between acromegaly and pituitary adenomas. Patients may present with signs of either endocrine disturbance or with compression on the adjacent neural structures, especially the optic pathways.

CLASSIFICATION

Historically, three main types of pituitary adenomas were defined by their cytoplasmic staining characteristics; chromophobic, acidophilic and basophilic, the implication being that these tumours were either hormonally inactive, secreted growth hormone or produced adrenocorticotrophic hormone (ACTH), respectively.

The development of immunoperoxidase techniques and electron microscopy has provided a more refined classification of pituitary adenomas based on the specific hormone that is produced. This classification is shown in Table 8.1.

PATHOLOGY

Pituitary adenomas arise from the anterior lobe (adenohypophysis) of the pituitary gland which develops from Rathke's pouch, an ectodermal diver-

Table 8.1 Classification of pituitary adenomas

Hormone secreted	Percentage of tumours
Prolactin	40
Growth hormone	20
Null cell (no hormone)	20
ACTH	15
Prolactin and growth hormone	5
FSH/LH	1–2
TSH	1
Acidophil stem cell (no hormone)	1–2

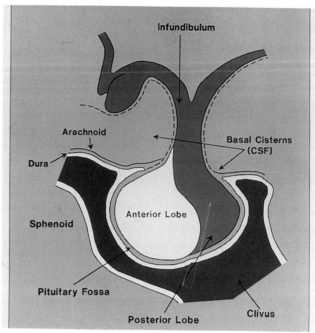

Fig. 8.1   Pituitary gland.

ticulum arising from the roof of the stomodeum, immediately in front of the buccopharyngeal membrane. The posterior lobe (neurohypophysis/pars nervosa) arises from the infundibulum developing from the floor of the diencephalon (Fig. 8.1).

The tumour arises within the pituitary fossa. If it is less than 10 mm in diameter it is known as a 'microadenoma'. The tumour may grow locally within the sella and cause erosion and remodelling of the floor of the sella and posterior clinoid processes (macroadenoma). The tumour usually spreads superiorly into the suprasellar cisterns, where it may cause compression of the optic pathways, particularly the optic chiasm. Further growth superiorly causes compression of the hypothalamus and, if large enough, obstruction of the 3rd ventricle, resulting in hydrocephalus (Figs. 8.2 and 8.3).

The tumour may also grow laterally out of the sella into the cavernous sinus. Occasionally the lateral extension may be sufficient to cause disturbance of the cranial nerves in the cavernous sinus but it is rare for the tumour to penetrate further laterally, into the temporal lobe.

The tumour may infrequently extend inferiorly through the floor of the pituitary fossa into the sphenoid sinus, resulting in CSF rhinorrhoea.

The localisation of microadenomas within the pituitary fossa corresponds somewhat with the regional distribution of the normal adenohypophyseal

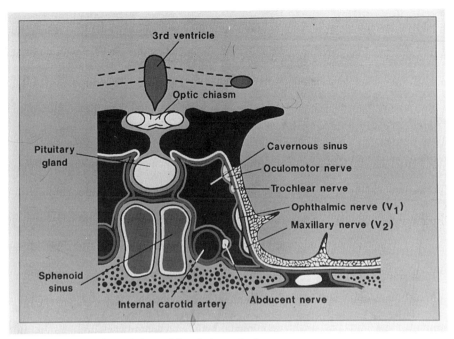

Fig. 8.2 Anatomical relations of the pituitary gland.

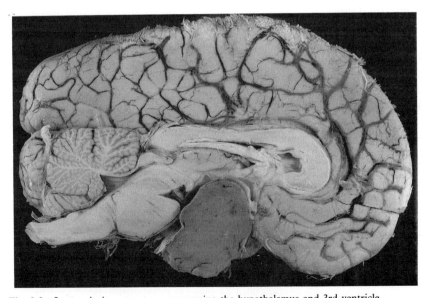

Fig. 8.3 Large pituitary tumour compressing the hypothalamus and 3rd ventricle.

cells. Prolactin and growth hormone secreting microadenomas tend to occur laterally, whereas most adenomas secreting ACTH occur in the central zone.

The pituitary hormones are synthesised in the rough endoplasmic reticulum and are packaged in the golgi apparatus. After packaging they can be visualised by either electron microscopy or immunoperoxidase staining as secretory granules within the cytoplasm. The hormone is released from the cell by exocytosis, following fusion of the granule with the cell membrane which usually occurs at the vascular pole of the cell. Adenomas may either be densely or sparsely granulated and this will determine their staining properties (Figure 8.4).

Multiple endocrine neoplasia type I (Werner's syndrome) is an autosomal dominant disorder representing the inherited occurrence of both benign and malignant neoplasms involving the pituitary gland, parathyroid gland and pancreas.

Functional types of pituitary adenoma

Prolactin cell adenoma

Prolactin is a 23 500-Da polypeptide hormone produced by the prolactin secreting cells (lactotrophs) situated predominantly in the posterolateral hypophysis and constituting 15–20% of adenohypophyseal cells. The best known physiological functions of prolactin are stimulation of breast growth and promotion of lactation. Its role in the male is poorly understood but it is important in spermatogenesis.

Unlike the secretion of other pituitary hormones which is controlled primarily by a hypothalamic releasing hormone, prolactin secretion is primarily under the influence of an inhibitory agent, 'prolactin inhibiting factor'.

Prolactinomas are the most frequently occurring pituitary adenoma. The majority present as microadenomas in young females with symptoms of hypersecretion causing amenorrhoea and galactorrhoea; impotence may be the only symptom in males. This explains the much greater surgical frequency of prolactinomas in women, and why these tumours may grow to a large size in males and elderly females.

Three-quarters of prolactin secreting tumours are chromophobic by light microscopy, the rest being either weakly acidophilic or composed of a mixture of cells. The serum levels of prolactin will be elevated and levels exceeding 1000 ng/ml are suggestive of an invasive prolactinoma. A minor elevation of serum prolactin is not necessarily diagnostic of a prolactin secreting adenoma, as any lesion of the hypothalamus, pituitary or pituitary stalk which interferes with the production or release of prolactin inhibiting factor may cause some increase in the serum prolactin.

Growth hormone cell adenoma

Growth hormone is a single chain 21 000-Da polypeptide produced by cells situated principally in the lateral part of the gland. Growth hormone aden-

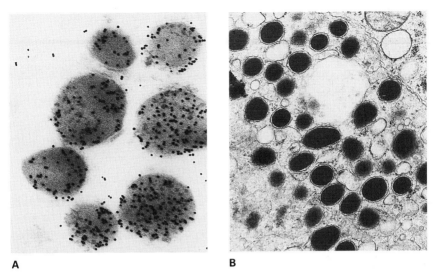

A   B

Fig. 8.4 (A) Membrane bound electron dense granules of growth hormone synthesised in the endoplasmic reticulum and packaged by the golgi apparatus ($\times$ 20 000). (B) Immunogold labelling of granules with antiserum against growth hormone ($\times$ 75 000).

omas represent approximately 15–20% of pituitary adenomas. Under light microscopy the features are either acidophil or chromophobe, depending on the extent of the cytoplasmic granules. The adenomas may be composed of either densely or sparsely granulated cells, occurring with approximately equal frequency; about 10% of tumours show a mixture of both cell types (Fig. 8.4).

Hyperprolactinaemia occurs quite frequently in growth hormone producing adenomas and may result either from an adenoma producing both hormones or from a growth hormone producing adenoma being of sufficient size to interfere with the release of prolactin inhibiting factor, thereby elevating the serum prolactin secondarily.

ACTH (corticotrophic) adenomas

ACTH is a single chain polypeptide which stimulates the adrenal cortex and promotes secretion of cortisol and related steroids. Adenomas producing ACTH are the cause of Cushing's disease. The adenomas are densely granulated with basophilic cytoplasm.

ACTH producing tumours constitute approximately 15% of adenomas, over 80% of which are microadenomas. About 15–20% of adenohypophyseal cells are corticotrophs, located in the central component of the anterior lobe of the pituitary gland, and it is not surprising that most microadenomas are located centrally rather than laterally, as occurs with the other hormone producing microadenomas.

Gonadotroph cell adenomas

Follicle stimulating hormone (FSH) and luteinising (LH) cells represent approximately 10% of the normal pituitary cells and are scattered throughout the adenohypophysis. Adenomas resulting from these cells are very uncommon and most are functionally silent.

Thyrotroph cell adenoma

Thyroid stimulating hormone (TSH) producing tumours are rare.

Null cell adenomas

Twenty to thirty per cent of pituitary adenomas have no clinical or biological evidence of hyperfunction. Mild hyperprolactinaemia may occur secondary to distortion of the pituitary stalk. Most (75%) of null cell adenomas are chromophobic, with few or no cytoplasmic granules. Approximately 20% of null cell tumours show marked accumulation of mitochondria and are called 'oncocytomas'.

Clinically, null cell adenomas are aggressive and, as they are hormonally silent, may grow to a large size, so that patients present with visual disturbance.

About 10% of pituitary adenomas are invasive, with extensive penetration of the pituitary capsule, dural sinuses, and surrounding bone. Most invasive pituitary adenomas are sparsely granulated or chromophobic and are either hormonally inactive or prolactin producing.

Metastasising pituitary carcinoma, either extracranially or throughout the CSF pathway, is extremely rare.

CLINICAL PRESENTATION (Table 8.2)

The presenting features are due to:

- The size of the tumour
- Endocrine disturbance.

Headache occurs principally in patients with acromegaly and is uncommon in other types of pituitary tumour.

Visual failure

Careful assessment of the visual fields, the visual acuity and the optic fundi are essential.

Suprasellar extension of the pituitary tumour causes compression of the optic chiasm resulting in a bitemporal hemianopia. The bitemporal hemianopia initially involves the upper quadrants, before extending to the

Table 8.2   Clinical manifestations of pituitary tumours

'Mass' effects
  Headaches (especially acromegaly)
  Superior extension
    Chiasmal syndrome (impaired visual acuity and fields)
    Hypothalamic syndrome (disturbance in thirst, appetite, satiety, sleep, and
    temperature regulation; diabetes insipidus — uncommon; inappropriate ADH
    syndrome — uncommon)
    Obstructive hydrocephalus
  Lateral extension
    Cranial III, IV, VI, diplopia
    Cranial V, facial pain
    Temporal lobe dysfunction
  Inferior extension
    Nasopharyngeal mass
    CSF rhinorrhoea

'Endocrine' effects
  Hyperpituitism
    GH — gigantism/acromegaly
    PRL — hyperprolactinaemic syndrome
    ACTH — Cushing's disease
    TSH — thyrotoxicosis
  Hypopituitism
    GH — child: shortness of stature, hypoglycaemia
    PRL — adult female: failure of postpartum lactation
    ACTH — hypocortisolism (Addison's)
    TSH — hypothyroidism
    LH/FSH — hypogonadism

Acute deterioration
  Pituitary apoplexy

GH = growth hormone; PRL = prolactin; TSH = thyroid stimulating hormone; LH = luteinising hormone; FSH = follicle stimulating hormone; ACTH = adrenocorticotrophic hormone.

lower quadrants of the visual field. If the chiasm is prefixed, that is placed more anteriorly than usual, a homonymous hemianopia may occur due to compression of the optic tract. Bilateral central scotomas result from the tumour pressing on the posterior part of the chiasm where the macular fibres decussate. Primary optic atrophy will be evident in patients with long-standing compression of the chiasm.

Ocular palsies occur in about 10% of patients and are due to invasion of the cavernous sinus. The 3rd nerve is the most frequently affected, followed by the 6th and 4th cranial nerves. Facial pain results from compression of the trigeminal nerve, usually the ophthalmic division, as a result of cavernous sinus invasion.

Endocrine abnormalities

Endocrine disturbance is due either to hypopituitism or excess secretion of a particular pituitary hormone.

Hypopituitarism

Hypopituitarism results from failure of the hormones secreted by the adenohypophysis and it gives rise to the clinical features first described by Simmonds in 1914. Pituitary gland failure does not occur if the tumour is a microadenoma, but may be clinically evident in the larger tumours. The endocrine secretions are not equally depressed but there is a selective failure and the order of susceptibility is as follows: growth hormone, gonadotrophin, corticotrophin, thyroid stimulating hormone.

Gonadotrophic deficiency prior to puberty retards the development of secondary sex characteristics, adult men have poor beard growth, women suffer from amenorrhoea and both sexes have loss of libido and deficient pubic and axillary hair. The biochemical abnormality is manifest by a low oestrogen and androgen production with reduced urinary 17-keto steroids.

Hypopituitarism initially results in vague symptoms, including lack of energy, undue fatiguability, muscle weakness and anorexia and, when prolonged and severe, it will cause low blood pressure. Clinical hypothyroidism is manifest by physical and mental sluggishness and a preference for warmth. When the hypopituitism is severe, episodic confusion occurs and the patient will become drowsy. It is essential to recognise the features of severe pituitary insufficiency as an endocrine crisis can be precipitated by minor stressful events occurring during hospital investigation or as a result of an intercurrent infection.

Pituitary apoplexy results from spontaneous haemorrhage into a pituitary tumour. It is characterised by sudden, severe headache followed by transient or more prolonged loss of consciousness with features of neck stiffness, vomiting and photophobia. The condition is similar to subarachnoid haemorrhage resulting from a ruptured aneurysm, but is often associated with paralysis of one or more of the ocular muscles (usually bilateral) and acute visual deterioration. An acute endocrine crisis may be precipitated by the apoplexy (Fig. 8.5).

Prolactinoma

The prolactin secreting tumour may be a microadenoma or macroadenoma within the pituitary fossa. The patients are usually women who present with infertility associated with amenorrhoea and galactorrhoea, although the tumour may occasionally cause infertility in men. Large prolactinomas occur in the elderly and in males, and these can cause endocrine disturbance associated with hypopituitism and visual failure.

Acromegaly

Acromegaly results from a growth hormone secreting pituitary adenoma which, as described previously, consists of cells that stain either as acido-

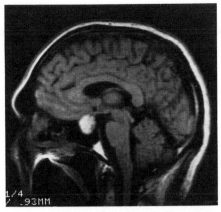

Fig. 8.5 MR scan showing recent haemorrhage into pituitary tumour.

phils, chromophobes or both. The onset of acromegaly is slow and insidious, usually during the third and fourth decades of life, with both sexes being affected equally. The clinical features (Table 8.3) include bone and soft tissue changes that are evident as an enlarged supraciliary ridge, enlarged frontal sinuses and increased mandibular size, which will cause the chin to project (prognathism) (Fig. 8.6). The hands and feet enlarge, the skin becomes coarse and greasy and sweats profusely. The voice becomes hoarse and gruff and thoracic kyphosis occurs as a result of osteoporosis.

Other problems associated with acromegaly include hypertension, cardiac hypertrophy and diabetes. Headache is often severe in patients with pituitary tumours causing acromegaly and patients complain of lack of energy, physical weakness and lassitude.

Suprasellar extension of the tumour occurs in about 15% of cases and may result in compression of the optic pathways.

A pituitary adenoma with excessive growth hormone secretion occasionally presents in childhood and results in giantism.

Cushing's disease

Cushing's disease is due to ACTH producing pituitary adenomas. Over 80% of the tumours are microadenomas and the remainder are either macroadenomas involving the whole of the sella or with extrasellar extension.

The onset is insidious and the disease may affect children or adults. Severe obesity occurs, the skin is tense and painful and purple striae appear around the trunk. Fat is deposited, particularly on the face (moon face), neck, cervicodorsal junction (buffalo hump) and trunk. The skin becomes a purple colour due to vasodilatation and stasis. Spontaneous bruising is common. The skin is greasy, acne is common and facial hair excessive. Pa-

Table 8.3 Clinical manifestations of growth hormone-producing pituitary tumours

Endocrine effects
    Excess GH on tissue growth and intermediary metabolism
        Skin and subcutaneous tissue overgrowth
        Skeletal overgrowth
        Visceromegaly
        Increased BMR, heat intolerance, hyperhydrosis
        Carbohydrate intolerance
        Diabetes mellitus
    Associated pituitary dysfunction
        Owing to pituitary compression or destruction
        Hypopituitism
    Associated thyroid dysfunction
        Goitre
        Thyrotoxicosis — toxic nodular goitre, Graves' disease
    Associated multiple endocrine neoplasia type 1
        Associated multiple endocrine neoplasia type 1
        Primary hyperparathyroidism
        Tumours of the endocrine pancreas syndromes

Neurological
    Related to tumour mass effects
    Related to GH hypersecretion
        Acroparaesthesias
        Entrapment neuropathies
        Peripheral neuropathy
        Myopathy

Ophthalmological
    Related to tumour mass effects
    Related to GH hypersecretion
        Glaucoma
        Exophthalmos

Laryngeal
    Voice changes
    Cord fixation

Sleep disorders

Skeletal
    Acral changes
    Arthropathy

Cardiovascular
    Hypertension
    Cardiomegaly
    Congestive heart failure
    Conduction defects and arrhythmias

Dermatological
    Acral changes
    Hyperhydrosis
    Acne
    Hypertrichosis
    Hyperpigmentation
    Acanthosis nigricans

tients complain of excessive fatigue and weakness. There is wasting and flaccidity of the muscles. Osteoporosis predisposes to spontaneous fractures.

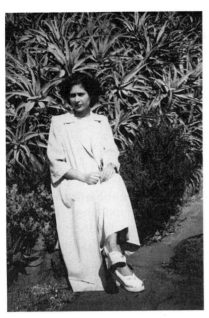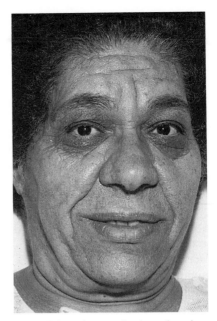

Fig. 8.6   58 year old female with acromegaly. On the left is a photograph taken when she was 25 years old.

Glucose tolerance is impaired, the serum potassium is low and vascular hypertension occurs. If untreated, 50% of cases are fatal in 5 years.

Cushing's syndrome, that is an excessive cortisol production, is due to an ACTH producing pituitary adenoma (Cushing's disease) in 90% of cases. Other causes of Cushing's syndrome are an adrenal adenoma or carcinoma, an ectopic source of ACTH production such as from an oat cell carcinoma of the lung or aberrant adrenocortical tissue occurring outside the adrenal gland.

Nelson–Salassa syndrome. This consists of an ACTH producing pituitary adenoma in a patient who has undergone bilateral or subtotal adrenalectomy. Before the development of CT scanning and transphenoidal microsurgery, patients with Cushing's disease often underwent total adrenalectomy when pneumoencephlography had failed to reveal a pituitary tumour. However, accelerated growth of an existing adenoma is induced by the loss of normal corticosteroid feedback. Unlike the adenomas of Cushing's disease, about half the patients with Nelson's syndrome have macroadenomas. Patients have marked cutaneous hyperpigmentation due to secretion of either beta melanocyte stimulating hormone and/or beta lipotropin.

Laboratory investigations

Radioimmunoassay will help identify the hormone being secreted.

Serum prolactin level in patients with prolactinomas will vary from just above the upper limit of normal to values greater than 10 000 ng/ml (normal 0–23 ng/ml in females; 0–20 ng/ml in males). The levels may show considerable variation in a particular patient and prolactin levels greater than 200 ng/ml are almost always indicative of a pituitary tumour. As mentioned previously, hyperprolactinaemia may be associated with other pituitary tumours and has been noted in some patients with acromegaly. Null cell tumours may be associated with mild hyperprolactinaemia due to distortion of the pituitary stalk or impingement on the hypothalamus.

Serum growth hormone is measured by radioimmunoassay, the normal values being less than 5 ng/ml in males and less than 10 ng/ml in females. Growth hormone exerts its effects on peripheral tissues indirectly via **somatomedins** — polypeptides produced primarily by the liver and fibroblasts. Serum somatomedin C is a more accurate indicator of growth hormone bioactivity than the serum growth hormone levels. Provocative tests of growth hormone secretion are useful in confirming acromegaly. Most patients with acromegaly do not show the normal suppression of growth hormone following glucose load. Other provocative tests utilise thyrotrophin releasing hormone and growth hormone releasing hormone.

The investigation of Cushing's disease involves the measurement of ACTH by radioimmunoassay, either in the peripheral blood or, as more recently advocated, by sampling the petrosal sinus. A dexamethasone suppression test will help diagnose Cushing's syndrome and its cause. The urine- and plasma- free cortisol is measured and is normally suppressed following administration of low dose dexamethasone (0.5 mg 6 hourly). The levels will be suppressed following high dose dexamethasone (2 mg 6 hourly) in the pituitary dependent Cushing's disease. There will be a failure of depression of the levels with high dose dexamethasone if the Cushing's syndrome is due to other than pituitary causes.

Radiological investigations

High resolution CT scanning using thin slices and intravenous contrast is the appropriate investigation. Pituitary microadenomas are usually hypodense and may cause upward bulging and convexity of the upper border of the gland in adults, deviation of the pituitary stalk and thinning of the sellar floor on the side of the tumour (Fig. 8.7). High quality CT scanning is able to demonstrate tumours as small as 4 mm in diameter. Macroadenomas enhance after intravenous contrast and the exact nature of the extrasellar extension can be best appreciated with direct coronal scans (Fig. 8.8).

Magnetic resonance imaging has improved the identification of microadenomas, which appear as low density focal lesions on the T1 weighted scans and high intensity on the T2 weighted scans (Fig. 8.9). Macroadenomas usually appear as isointense on the T1 weighted images and moderately hyperintense on the T2 images. Haemorrhage into a tumour,

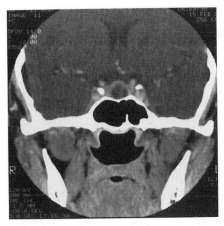

Fig. 8.7 Hypodense microadenoma in pituitary gland.

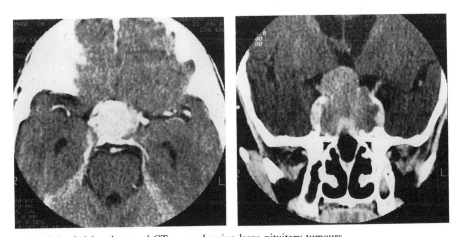

Fig 8.8 Axial and coronal CT scans showing large pituitary tumours.

such as occurs following pituitary apoplexy, shows as high intensity areas because of methaemoglobin on the T1 and T2 weighted scans intermingled with low density regions due to haemosiderin (see Figs. 8.5 and 8.9).

Plain skull X-rays may show enlargement of the sella with thinning erosion or bulging of its contours (Fig. 8.10).

Intra-arterial digital subtraction angiography is usually performed to exclude incidental aneurysms and to determine the position of the internal carotid arteries in the cavernous sinuses, although this information can usually be obtained from the MR scan.

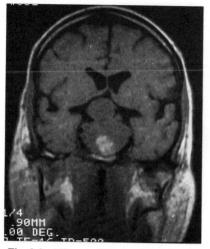
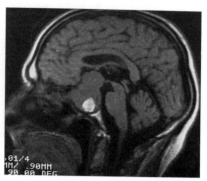

Fig. 8.9 MR scan (Tl) showing large pituitary tumour with area of recent haemorrhage.

Differential diagnosis

The major differential diagnoses are:

• Craniopharyngioma
• Suprasellar meningioma (arising from the tuberculum sella).

Uncommon masses around the suprasellar region also include optic nerve and hypothalamic glioma (Fig. 8.11), giant aneurysm from the carotid artery, suprasellar germinomas and chordomas.

Treatment

The objectives of treatment of patients with pituitary tumours depends on whether the patient has presented with features of endocrine disturbance or problems related to compression of adjacent neural structures. The methods of treatment used are:

1. Operative procedures
   a. transphenoidal excision
   b. transcranial excision
2. Radiotherapy
3. Medical treatment with antisecretory drugs.

Surgical excision. This will be used as the primary method of treatment for:

• Large tumours causing compression of adjacent neural structures, particularly the visual pathways

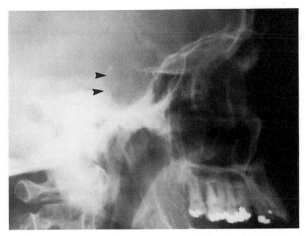

Fig. 8.10 Plain lateral skull X-ray showing thinning of the dorsum sellae and destruction of the pituitary fossa in a patient with a lárge pituitary tumour.

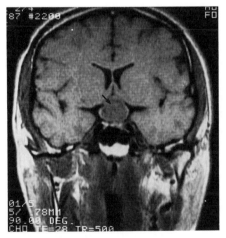

Fig. 8.11 Hypothalamic glioma.

- Growth hormone secreting tumours causing acromegaly
- ACTH secreting tumours causing Cushing's disease
- The occasional treatment of a prolactin secreting adenoma, either microadenoma or macroadenoma confined within the sella, when the medical treatment using bromocriptine is not tolerated.

Most tumours can be excised via the transphenoidal approach to the pituitary fossa (Fig. 8.12). The development of the surgical microscope and fluoroscopic radiography has made this a safe procedure. The sphenoid

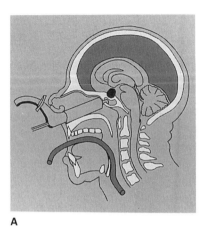
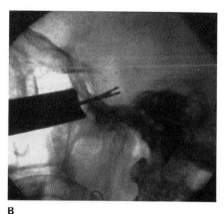

A   B

Fig. 8.12 (A) Diagram of operative exposure in transphenoidal resection of pituitary tumour. A self-retaining retractor is inserted and the anterior wall of the sphenoid sinus is removed. (B) Intra-operative X-ray showing the retractor in position and the forceps in the pituitary fossa.

sinus is usually entered using a trans-septal approach, with the incision either in the nasal mucosa or sublabially. The mucosa is reflected from the nasal septum and floor and the sphenoid is opened. The anterior wall of the sella is removed and the pituitary fossa entered. Microadenomas (tumours less than 10 mm diameter) may be evident on the surface of the gland or may become evident only once the gland is incised. These tumours can be completely excised, preserving pituitary function. The suprasellar extension of the tumour can be gently coaxed down into the pituitary fossa by slightly raising the intracranial pressure or by the anaesthetist injecting small increments of nitrous oxide and oxygen mixture into the lumbar theca until the intracranial pressure forces the suprasellar tumour into the operative field. This will also have the additional benefit that the intracranial gas will provide a pneumoencephalogram, outlining the remaining suprasellar extension of tumour.

Occasionally, a transcranial operation is necessary, particularly where there is a subfrontal or retroclival extension of the tumour.

Postoperative management requires careful attention to the fluid balance and hormonal status. Endocrine deficiency in the immediate postoperative period will require replacement with parenteral hydrocortisone and possibly the use of vasopressin for the treatment of transient diabetes insipidus, which commonly occurs after the excision of a large pituitary tumour. In the early postoperative period aqueous vasopressin (Pitressin®) should be given by intramuscular or subcutaneous injection and, if the diabetes insipidus persists, by the intranasal route. Other long-term hormonal replacements may include cortisone acetate (12.5–25 mg twice daily), thyroxine and testosterone.

Radiotherapy. Postoperative radiotherapy is used if there has been a sub-total excision of the tumour or if the postoperative endocrine studies demonstrate residual excessive hormone secretion.

Medical treatment. Treatment of patients with pituitary adenomas is undertaken:

— To restore the endocrine status of the patient by replacement of the pituitary hormone itself or by replacement of the hormone of the pituitary dependent glands. This will be a necessary pre-operative procedure in patients with evidence of hypopituitism and will frequently be necessary after the surgical excision of a macroadenoma.
— The treatment of prolactin secreting pituitary tumours by bromocriptine, a dopamine agonist. This is the preferred treatment for a symptomatic prolactin secreting microadenoma and may be used as either the definitive treatment of larger prolactin secreting tumours or in conjunction with surgery. Some patients show poor tolerance to bromocriptine, as it may cause intractable nausea, vomiting and postural hypotension, and these patients will require surgical treatment of the tumour.

CRANIOPHARYNGIOMA

This tumour may occur at any age, although nearly half occur in the first 20 years of life. They are thought to arise from the epithelial remnants of Rathke's pouch.

The tumours occur in the region of the pituitary fossa and extend through the suprasellar cisterns to the hypothalamus. The majority are cystic, and the fluid is often yellow and sparkling with cholesterol crystals. The cyst may be larger than the solid component, which is often pale and crumbly, consisting of epithelial debris.

Clinical presentation

Clinical features include:

• Raised intracranial pressure
• Visual impairment
• Endocrine dysfunction.

Raised intracranial pressure. This is common, particularly in children who present with headache, vomiting and papilloedema.

Visual impairment. This is due to papilloedema, chiasmal compression or a combination of both. Papilloedema is due to hydrocephalus as a result of 3rd ventricular obstruction by the tumour. The visual field defect is frequently similar to that produced by a pituitary tumour, a bitemporal hemianopia, but homonymous defects are more common than in pituitary adenoma.

Endocrine abnormalities. These are frequent in children and consist of:

- Hypogonadism
- Stunting of growth
- Diabetes insipidus.

Endocrine failure due to craniopharyngioma arising in adults is essentially similar to that caused by a pituitary tumour, except that diabetes insipidus occurs more commonly in patients presenting with craniopharyngioma.

Investigations

The CT scan usually shows a cystic tumour in the suprasellar region with calcification (Fig. 8.13). Tumours in adults may be solid and are less calcified than those seen in younger patients.

Changes in the sella turcica are seen in approximately 50% of patients. Suprasellar tumours and the associated hydrocephalus press downwards on the dorsum sellae and anterior clinoids and may enlarge the sella. Nearly 90% of tumours in children have radiographically identifiable calcification in the tumour, whereas only 40% of adults have radiologically demonstrable calcification. The calcification consists of aggregates of small flecks of calcium and may be curvilinear, outlining a portion of the cyst wall.

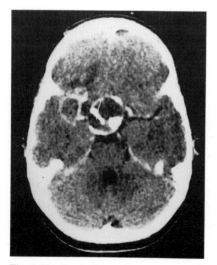
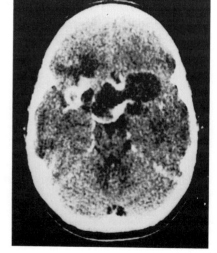

Fig. 8.13   Craniopharyngioma.

Treatment

Pre-operative visual and endocrine assessment is essential. The standard treatment for craniopharyngioma is operative, with an attempt at maximal resection of the tumour. However, complete resection may not be possible due to the extent of the tumour and the intimate attachment to hypothalamic vital structures.

The usual surgical approach is through a frontotemporal or pterional craniotomy but tumours extending into the 3rd ventricle may also need to be approached through the corpus callosum.

The role of postoperative radiotherapy in patients with a subtotal resection is controversial but radiotherapy may be beneficial in decreasing the production of cyst fluid and delaying recurrence of the tumour.

EMPTY SELLA SYNDROME

The empty sella refers to a communicating extension of the subarachnoid space into the pituitary fossa (Fig. 8.14). This may occur as a result of an incomplete anatomical formation of the diaphragma sellae which allows the arachnoid to herniate directly into the pituitary fossa or as a secondary phenomenon following either pituitary surgery or radiotherapy.

There is good reason to regard the empty sella as an anatomical variant rather than a syndrome. Bergland showed the presence of subarachnoid space within the sella in 20%, and anatomical defects of the diaphragma

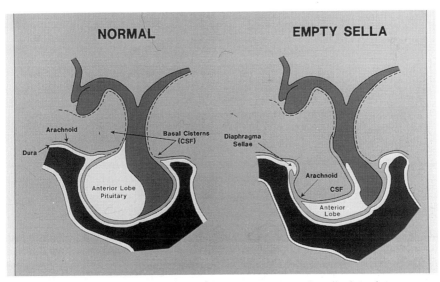

Fig. 8.14 Empty sella. The subarachnoid space is able to enter the sella through an incomplete diaphragma sella.

sellae of 5 mm or more in nearly 40%, of an autopsy series without pituitary disease. However, defects in the diaphragma are not the only requirement for formation of an empty sella. Increased intracranial pressure associated with benign intracranial hypertension or long-standing hydrocephalus will cause herniation of the subarachnoid space into the sella and will result in the remodelling of the pituitary fossa to produce the classic globular appearance on plain X-ray and CT scan (Fig. 8.15). It is possible that the normal variations in CSF pressure may be transmitted into the fossa through an incompetent diaphragma and so result in the bony changes.

Clinical presentation

Most patients with the radiological features of an empty sella are asymptomatic. The majority of patients presenting with symptoms are obese, middle-aged, hypertensive women. Headache is the most common symptom associated with the empty sella but the features are so varied that their relevance to the intrasellar subarachnoid space is dubious without an underlying cause for possible raised intracranial pressure.

Visual field defects and endocrine abnormalities are subtle and uncommon in patients with primary empty sella syndrome. In patients with a secondary empty sella, e.g. following surgery or radiotherapy, field defects may be more pronounced but are rarely severe.

The most serious consequence of an empty sella is spontaneous cerebrospinal fluid rhinorrhoea. This usually occurs only if there has been an underlying cause of raised intracranial pressure, such as benign intracranial hypertension. It is managed by repairing the leak in the floor of the sella with crushed muscle and fascia lata and performing a CSF shunt.

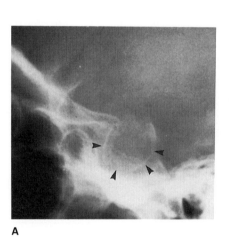
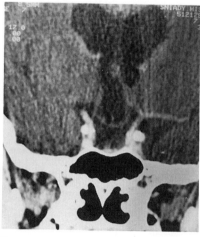

A   **B**

Fig. 8.15   Empty sella. (A) The classical globular enlarged sella. (B) CSF within the sella.

FURTHER READING

Abboud C F, Laws E R 1988 Diagnosis of pituitary tumours. In: Young W F, Klee G G
(eds) Endocrinology and metabolism clinics of North America. W B Saunders,
Philadelphia, vol 17: 241–277
Bergland R M, Ray B S, Torak R M 1968 Anatomical variations in the pituitary gland and
adjacent structures in 225 human autopsy cases. Journal of Neurosurgery 28: 93–99
Black P McL, Zervas N T, Candia G 1987 Incidence and management of complications of
transphenoidal operation for pituitary adenomas. Neurosurgery 20: 920–924
Cushing H 1912 The pituitary body and its disorders. Clinical states produced by disorders
of the hypophysis cerebri. J B Lippincott, Philadelphia.
Ebersold M J, Laws E R, Scheithauer B W, Randle R V 1983 Pituitary apoplexy treated
by transphenoidal surgery. An clinicopathological and immunocytochemical study.
Journal of Neurosurgery 58: 315–320
Hardy J 1968 Transphenoidal microsurgery of the normal and pathological pituitary.
Clinical Neurosurgery 16: 185–217
Kaufman B 1968 The 'empty' sella turcica: a manifestation of the intrasellar subarachnoid
space. Radiology 90: 931–941
Kaye A H, Galbraith J E K, King J 1981 Intracranial pressure in patients with empty sella
syndrome without benign intracranial hypertension. Journal of Neurosurgery 55: 453–456
Kovacs K, Horvath E 1985 Morphology of adenohypophyseal cells and pituitary adenomas.
In: Imura H (ed) The pituitary gland. Raven Press, New York
Laws E R, Randle R V, Abboud C F 1982 Surgical treatment of acromegaly: results in
140 patients. In: Givens J R (ed) Hormone secreting pituitary tumours. Year Book
Medical Publishers, Chicago
Ross D, Wilson C B 1988 Results of transphenoidal microsurgery for growth hormone
secreting pituitary adenoma in series of 214 patients. Journal of Neurosurgery 68: 854–867
Scheithauer B W 1984 Surgical pathology of the pituitary: The adenomas part I. In:
Sommers S C, Rosen P P (eds) Pathology annual part I. Appleton-Century-Crofts,
Connecticut, pp 317–374
Scheithauer B W 1984 Surgical pathology of the pituitary: The adenomas part II. In:
Sommers S C, Rosen P P (eds) Pathology annual part I. Appleton-Century-Crofts,
Connecticut, pp 269–329
Trumble H C 1951 Pituitary tumours: observations on tumours which have spread widely
beyond the confines of the sella. British Journal of Surgery 39: 7–24
Wilson C B 1984 A decade of pituitary microsurgery. Journal of Neurosurgery 61: 814–833
The intrasella subarachnoid space (Editorial article) 1982 Lancet July 31, pp 249–250

9. Subarachnoid haemorrhage

The sudden onset of a severe headache in a patient should be regarded as subarachnoid haemorrhage until proven otherwise.

Subarachnoid haemorrhage occurs when bleeding is primarily within the subarachnoid space rather than into the brain itself. It represents about 5–10% of all non-traumatic intracranial haemorrhage with an incidence of approximately 15/100 000 population. Apoplectic death has been mentioned in the earliest medical writings but its relationship to intracranial haemorrhage and cerebral aneurysm was not established until the latter part of the seventeenth century. The introduction of cerebral angiography by Moniz and de Lima in Lisbon in 1927 allowed the diagnosis of cerebral aneurysm to be made in living patients who had sustained subarachnoid haemorrhage. Pioneering surgery in the 1930s and 1940s, by Krayenbuhl in Switzerland and Dandy in North America, showed that aneurysms could be treated operatively, although at that time with considerable morbidity and mortality. Consequent improvements in microsurgical techniques and neuroanaesthesia have considerably improved the safety of surgery.

CAUSES OF SUBARACHNOID HAEMORRHAGE

The most common cause of subarachnoid haemorrhage in adults is rupture of a berry aneurysm. Subarachnoid haemorrhage in children is much less common than in the adult population and the most common paediatric cause is rupture of an arteriovenous malformation. Cerebral aneurysm as a cause of subarachnoid haemorrhage becomes more frequent than arteriovenous malformations over the age of 20 years. Rare causes of subarachnoid haemorrhage include bleeding from a tumour, bleeding disorders, blood dyscrasias and rupture of a spinal arteriovenous malformation (Table 9.1). The aetiology of subarachnoid haemorrhage remains undiscovered in approximately 15% of cases after thorough clinical and radiographic study. These patients often have associated intracranial vascular atherosclerosis and hypertension.

Table 9.1   Causes of subarachnoid haemorrhage (%)

Cerebral aneurysm	70
Arteriovenous malformation	10
Undiscovered	15

Other rare causes
  Spinal arteriovenous malformation
  Tumour
  Blood dyscrasia
	5

Table 9.2   Subarachnoid haemorrhage — presenting features

Headache
Diminished conscious state
Meningism   Neck stiffness, vomiting, photophobia, fever

Focal neurological signs
  Intracerebral haemorrhage
  Focal pressure by aneurysm
  Vasospasm

Fundal changes
  Subhyaloid haemorrhage
  Retinal haemorrhage
  Papilloedema

SUBARACHNOID HAEMORRHAGE — PRESENTING FEATURES (Table 9.2)

Headache

The sudden onset of a severe headache of a type not previously experienced by the patient is the hallmark of subarachnoid haemorrhage. A relatively small leak from an aneurysm may result in a minor headache, sometimes referred to as the 'sentinel headache', as this may be the warning episode of a subsequent major haemorrhage from the aneurysm. Naturally recognition of a possible minor 'warning' haemorrhage is essential to avert a possible later catastrophic bleed, although many are only recognised in retrospect.

Diminished conscious state

Most patients have some deterioration of their conscious state following sub-arachnoid haemorrhage. This varies from only a slight change when the haemorrhage has been minor to apoplectic death resulting from massive haemorrhage. It is a common cause of sudden death in young adults.

Meningism

Blood in the subarachnoid cerebrospinal fluid will cause the features of meningism – headache, neck stiffness, photophobia, fever and vomiting. Irritation of the nerve roots of the cauda equina, which occurs when the blood extends down to the lumbar theca, may result in sciatica type pain and low back discomfort.

Focal neurological signs

Focal neurological signs may occur in subarachnoid haemorrhage due to concomitant intracerebral haemorrhage, the local pressure effects of the aneurysm itself, or cerebral vasospasm.

A cerebral aneurysm usually lies within the subarachnoid cisterns but the aneurysm may become adherent to the adjacent brain parenchyma due to adhesions, frequently resulting from previous leakage of blood. A haemorrhage from an aneurysm in these circumstances may also extend into the brain and the position of the intracerebral haematoma will determine the type of neurological deficit. A middle cerebral artery aneurysm frequently ruptures into the temporal lobe, resulting in hemiparesis and aphasia if the dominant hemisphere is involved (Fig. 9.1). Anterior communicating artery aneurysms may haemorrhage into the frontal lobes with subsequent akinetic mutism (Fig. 9.2). Defective conjugate ocular movement may result from haemorrhage into a frontal lobe, persistent deviation usually being towards the side of the lesion and purposeful gaze defective away from that side.

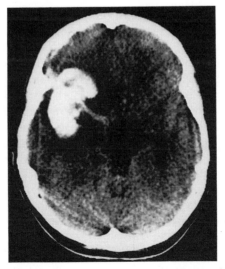

Fig. 9.1 Intracerebral haematoma in temporal lobe due to rupture of a middle cerebral artery aneurysm.

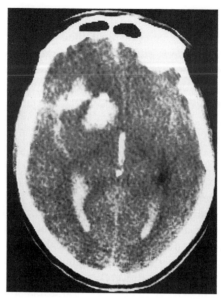

Fig. 9.2 Frontal intracerebral haematoma with blood in the sylvian fissure and ventricles from a ruptured anterior communicating artery aneurysm.

Occasionally, an aneurysm may also rupture into the subdural space, resulting in a subdural haematoma and brain compression causing lateralising neurological signs. An arteriovenous malformation usually lies at least partially within the brain parenchyma, so that when it ruptures intracerebral bleeding is frequently associated with the subarachnoid haemorrhage.

Focal neurological signs may result from the position of the aneurysm itself. An aneurysm arising from the internal carotid artery at the origin of the posterior communicating artery (known as a posterior communicating artery aneurysm) may cause pressure on the 3rd cranial nerve. Patients with an enlarging aneurysm in this position may present with features of a 3rd cranial nerve palsy (ptosis, pupil dilatation, extra ocular muscle palsy) prior to a subarachnoid haemorrhage. It is vital that the correct diagnosis of an enlarging cerebral aneurysm is made in this situation, so as to avoid the possible catastrophic effects of subarachnoid haemorrhage. The major differential diagnosis of the aetiology of an apparently isolated 3rd cranial nerve palsy is an ischaemic lesion such as those resulting from diabetes mellitus or atherosclerosis. Pupil size is a useful guide in differentiating between these causes. The pupil is usually dilated, with an expanding aneurysm which compresses the superior aspect of the nerve that contains the parasympathetic pupillary fibres arising from the nucleus of Edinger–Westphal in the mid-brain. An expanding aneurysm usually results in more pain than the ischaemia associated with diabetes mellitus, although this is an unre-

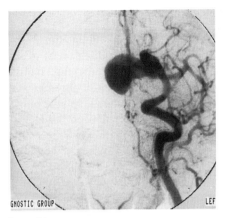

Fig. 9.3 Giant internal carotid artery aneurysm.

liable guide. If there is *any* doubt about the cause of the 3rd nerve palsy then angiography must be performed expeditiously. In a patient with impaired conscious state, or in one with other abnormal neurological signs suggesting a massive haemorrhage, 3rd cranial nerve palsy may be secondary to temporal lobe herniation.

A giant aneurysm (defined as larger than 2.5 cm diameter) may cause compression of adjacent neural structures resulting in focal signs (Fig. 9.3). A large aneurysm of the internal carotid artery or anterior communicating artery will cause compression of the optic nerve or chiasm, respectively, resulting in visual failure. Large vertebrobasilar aneurysms may cause brain stem compression.

Cerebral vasospasm following subarachnoid haemorrhage dose not usually result in clinical manifestations for 2 or 3 days after the initial bleed so that, although it may be the cause of subsequent focal signs resulting from brain ischaemia, it is not the cause of focal signs immediately after the haemorrhage.

Optic fundi

Mild papilloedema is common within the first few days of haemorrhage because of the sudden elevation of intracranial pressure resulting from hydrocephalus or cerebral oedema. A transient communicating hydrocephalus often occurs after subarachnoid haemorrhage due to blood blocking the arachnoid villi. In about 10% of cases the hydrocephalus persists and is severe enough to require a CSF shunt.

Ophthalmoscopy may reveal fundal haemorrhages, particularly in severe subarachnoid haemorrhage. Small, scattered retinal haemorrhages usually resolve satisfactorily, although the large subhyaloid haemorrhages may break into the vitreous, resulting in permanent visual defect.

CLINICAL ASSESSMENT

The diagnosis is usually obvious when the history is obtained from the patient, relative or friend. The classic sudden onset of severe headache with features of meningism and decreased conscious state is characteristic of a subarachnoid haemorrhage. However, difficulty may occur when the haemorrhage has been minor and, tragically, a subarachnoid haemorrhage may be misdiagnosed as either migraine or tension headache. A full neurological examination should be performed with particular attention given to the presence of neck stiffness, altered conscious state, pupillary and fundal changes and focal neurological signs in the limbs. A careful general examination should be undertaken, to assess in particular the blood pressure, respiratory state and the possible underlying cause for the haemorrhage.

A number of grading classifications have been proposed for patients with subarachnoid haemorrhage. These have been based on the severity of the headache and neck stiffness and on the level of conscious state. The two major systems are the Hunt and Hess classification and the Botterell system (Table 9.3).

Table 9.3 Subarachnoid haemorrhage grading systems

Hunt and Hess grading system*

Grade	Description
1	Asymptomatic, or minimal headache and slight nuchal rigidity
2	Moderate to severe headache, nuchal rigidity, no neurological deficit (except cranial nerve palsy)
3	Drowsiness, confusion or mild focal deficit
4	Stupor, moderate to severe hemiparesis, possible early decerebrate rigidity and vegetative disturbances
5	Deep coma, decerebrate rigidity, moribund

Botterell grading system

Grade	Description
1	Conscious patient with or without signs of blood in subarachnoid space
2	Drowsy patient without significant neurological deficit
3	Drowsy patient with neurological deficit and probable intracerebral clot
4	Patients with major neurological deficit, deteriorating because of large intracerebral clots, or older patients with less severe neurological deficit but pre-existing degenerative cerebrovascular disease
5	Moribund or nearly moribund patient with failing vital centres and extensor rigidity

* Serious systemic disease such as hypertension, diabetes, severe arteriosclerosis, chronic pulmonary disease, and vasospasm on angiography result in placement in next less favourable category

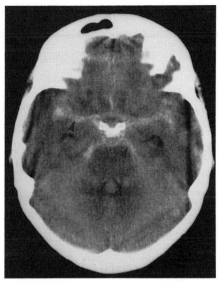

Fig. 9.4 Blood in the sylvian fissure and basal cisterns indicative of subarachnoid haemorrhage.

Investigations

The major differential diagnosis is meningitis, although a minor haemorrhage is often misdiagnosed as migraine. Confirmation of the clinical diagnosis of subarachnoid haemorrhage should be undertaken as soon as possible. Computerised tomography (CT) scanning (Fig. 9.4), if readily available, is the best initial investigation as it will confirm the diagnosis in over 80% of cases. It will also provide additional information on associated pathology such as intracerebral haemorrhage and hydrocephalus, and on the position of the haemorrhage, which is helpful if there is more than one aneurysm. Arteriovenous malformation causing subarachnoid haemorrhage can frequently be diagnosed on the CT scan. If there is any doubt that subarachnoid blood is present on the CT scan, as may occur following more minor haemorrhages, a lumbar puncture is essential. The presence of xanthochromia (yellow staining) in the cerebrospinal fluid will confirm subarachnoid haemorrhage. Xanthochromia resulting from breakdown of haemoglobin in the red blood cells occurs within 6–8 hours after the initial haemorrhage and it will confirm that the blood in the CSF is not due to trauma from the lumbar puncture needle. A further method frequently suggested to exclude trauma from the passage of the lumbar puncture needle as a cause of bloody CSF is to allow the CSF to drip into three consecutive tubes; if the blood fails to 'clear' in the last tube subarachnoid haemorrhage is confirmed. However, this method will result in many false positive diagnoses. The CSF should also be immediately examined for the presence of white blood cells and organisms.

Cerebral angiography will confirm the cause of the subarachnoid haemorrhage and will determine the subsequent treatment. Intra-arterial digital subtraction angiography has considerably reduced the risks of conventional angiography and should be undertaken in most cases as soon as the diagnosis has been confirmed and it is clear that the patient will survive the initial haemorrhage.

CEREBRAL ANEURYSM

Cerebral aneurysms are the most common cause of subarachnoid haemorrhage in the adult population, with a maximal incidence in the 4th and 5th decades of life, although they can occur at any age.

Surgical anatomy

The great majority of aneurysms arise at the branch points of two vessels, usually at an acute angle, and are situated mainly on the circle of Willis and the trunks of the large arteries which supply it. A few arise from its immediate branches but aneurysms on peripheral vessels are rare (Fig. 9.5). The majority of aneurysms occur in constant positions on the circle of Willis and about 85% occur on the anterior half of the circle. Aneurysms arise at approximately equal frequency from the internal carotid artery, anterior communicating artery and middle cerebral artery. Those associated with the internal carotid artery most frequently arise at the origin of the posterior communicating artery (the so-called posterior communicating artery aneurysm), less frequently at the terminal bifurcation and occasionally at the origin of the ophthalmic artery, anterior choroidal artery or in the cavernous sinus. Middle cerebral artery aneurysms arise from the middle cerebral artery at its bifurcation or trifurcation in the sylvian fissure (Fig. 9.6). Less commonly an aneurysm may arise from the pericallosal artery at the genu of the corpus callosum.

Approximately 15% of aneurysms arise from the posterior half of the circle of Willis, the most common position being the basilar artery, most frequently at the terminal bifurcation into the posterior cerebral arteries. However, an aneurysm may arise from any of the main branches of the vertebral or basilar arteries, in particular the posterior inferior cerebellar artery, anterior inferior cerebellar artery, or superior cerebellar artery (Fig. 9.7).

Multiple aneurysms

Aneurysms occur in more than one position in approximately 15% of cases.

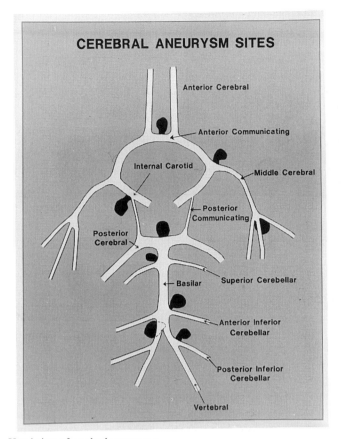

Fig. 9.5   Usual sites of cerebral aneurysms.

Table 9.4   Position of cerebral aneurysm

Anterior circle of Willis
   Anterior communicating artery
   Middle cerebral artery — bifurcation or trifurcation
   Internal carotid artery
      posterior commuicating artery
      terminal bifurcation
      anterior choroidal artery
      ophthalmic artery
      intracavernous
   Pericallosal artery

Posterior circulation (15%)
   Terminal basilar artery — most common
   Vertebrobasilar junction
   Posterior inferior cerebellar artery
   Anterior inferior cerebellar artery
   Superior inferior cerebellar artery
   Posterior cerebral artery

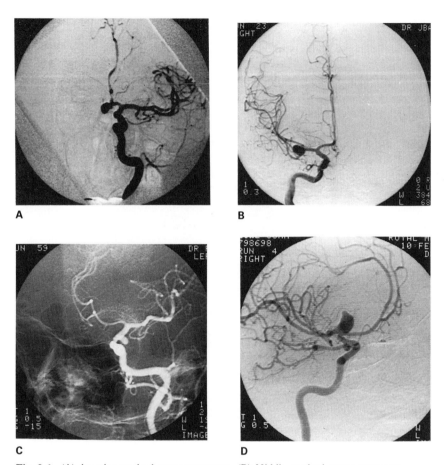

A   B

C   D

Fig. 9.6 (A) Anterior cerebral artery aneurysm. (B) Middle cerebral artery aneurysm. (C) Posterior communicating artery aneurysm. (D) Terminal internal carotid artery aneurysm.

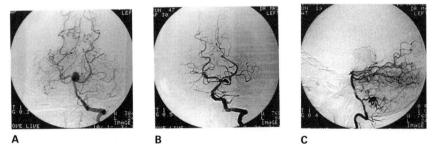

A   B   C

Fig. 9.7 (A) Terminal basilar artery aneurysm. (B) Aneurysm arising from junction of basilar artery and superior cerebellar artery. (C) Posterior inferior cerebellar artery aneurysm.

Pathogenesis of cerebral aneurysms

The common type of cerebral aneurysm resulting in a subarachnoid haemorrhage is a **saccular** aneurysm, which is also known as a **berry** or **congenital** aneurysm. **Fusiform** aneurysms occur on the intracranial circulation, particularly on the vertebrobasilar arteries or internal carotid arteries and are due to diffuse atheromatous degeneration of the arterial wall, frequently associated with hypertension. Mycotic aneurysms result from septic emboli. They may be situated on peripheral vessels, are frequently multiple and have a high risk of haemorrhage.

The saccular or berry aneurysm arises at the junction of vessels where there is a congenital deficiency in the muscle coat. The elastic layer in cerebral arteries, in contrast with arteries elsewhere, is limited to the internal lamina, making these vessels more susceptible to weakening effects of degeneration. Fragmentation and dissolution of the internal elastic membrane occurs at the site of aneurysm development. The combination of the muscle defect and the discontinuity of the underlying internal elastic membrane is probably necessary for the formation of a saccular aneurysm. Other factors that increase the risk of aneurysm formation include atheroma and hypertension. There is an increased incidence of atheroma in the vessels of the circle of Willis and hypertension in patients with ruptured aneurysms. It is probable that these factors play a role in the growth of the aneurysm and its subsequent rupture in some patients.

Related diseases

There is no hereditary basis to the development of intracranial aneurysms, although aneurysms do occur in association with hereditary syndromes such as Ehlers–Danlos syndrome, coarctation of the aorta and polycystic kidney disease.

Management of ruptured cerebral aneurysm

The management of patients following rupture of a cerebral aneurysm is determined by three major factors:

1. Severity of the initial haemorrhage
2. Rebleeding of the aneurysm
3. Cerebral vasospasm.

Severity of the initial haemorrhage. About 30% of all patients suffering a subarachnoid haemorrhage from a ruptured aneurysm either have an apoplectic death or are deeply comatose as a result of the initial haemorrhage.

Rebleeding. This occurs in about 50% of patients within 6 weeks and 25% of patients within 2 weeks of the initial haemorrhage. About half the patients that have a subsequent haemorrhage will die as a result of the

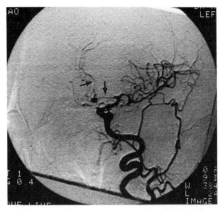

Fig. 9.8   Spasm of the anterior cerebral arteries following subarachnoid haemorrhage from an anterior communicating artery aneurysm.

rebleed. After the first year the risk of a further haemorrhage from the aneurysm is about 2–3% per year.

The only certain way to prevent an aneurysm rebleeding is to surgically occlude it from the circulation. Antifibrinolytic agents (such as epsilon amino capoic acid or tranexamic acid) decrease the risks of rebleeding but, as they are associated with increased incidence of thrombosis (such as deep vein thrombosis and pulmonary embolus) and an increased risk of cerebral thrombosis associated with vasospasm, these agents are now rarely used.

Cerebral vasospasm. Angiographic vasospasm (Fig. 9.8) occurs in about 50% of patients following subarachnoid haemorrhage and in 25% it results in serious neurological complications. There is a direct correlation between the amount of blood noted in the basal cisterns on the CT scan, the risk of developing vasospasm and its severity. Although the spasm may principally affect the vessels most adjacent to the ruptured aneurysm, generalised vasospasm occurs frequently. The clinical manifestations resulting from vasospasm will be determined by the vessels which are most severely affected. Spasm of the internal carotid artery and middle cerebral arteries produce hemiparesis and aphasia in the dominant hemisphere. Vasospasm of the anterior cerebral vessels causes paralysis of the lower limbs and akinetic mutism. Severe vasospasm may cause widespread cerebral ischaemia so that the patient may become obtunded; if the vasospasm is sufficiently severe it will result in death. Vasospasm does not usually occur until 2 or 3 days after the initial haemorrhage and its onset is rarely delayed beyond 1 to 14 days. The cause of delayed cerebral vasospasm remains obscure but it is certainly related to vasoconstrictor substances in the CSF as a result of the haemorrhage. Vasoactive substances isolated from both the blood clot surrounding the spastic vessels and from the adjacent CSF include serotonin, prostaglandins (F2-alpha and E2) angiotensin and histamine. In addition, unidentified vasoconstrictor substances have been isolated from incubates of fibrinogen, platelets, erythrocytes and blood/CSF mixtures.

Until recently there has been no satisfactory treatment for cerebral vasospasm. If the aneurysm has been surgically occluded from the circulation then hypertensive therapy combined with hypervolaemia may overcome the hypoperfusion due to narrowing of the cerebral blood vessels and reverse the ischaemic effects. Calcium channel blocking agents such as nimodopine and nifedipine are at present being evaluated for their use in subarachnoid haemorrhage to prevent and treat vasospasm. Nimodopine, a substituted 1,4-dihydropyridine, is a calcium 'antagonist' that blocks the influx of extracellular calcium, the primary source of calcium for contraction of large cerebral arteries. Trials in North America and Scandinavia have shown promising results when the calcium channel blocking agents are used prophylactically.

Surgery for ruptured aneurysm

The **timing** of the operation is critical for obtaining optimal results following subarachnoid haemorrhage. Although better operative results may be achieved when the surgery is delayed, the longer the operation is deferred the greater the risk that the aneurysm will rebleed. However, surgery should be avoided when the patient has clinical or angiographically severe vasospasm. Surgery is not performed on patients who are very drowsy, comatose or have features of a decerebrate posturing response unless the CT scan shows a large intracerebral haematoma resulting from the ruptured aneurysm which needs to be evacuated. Otherwise the operation is performed:

- Within the first 72 hours of the haemorrhage, prior to the onset of vasospasm
- If the patient presents after the first 72 hours in a satisfactory neurological condition, the operation may be performed at that time provided there is no clinical or radiological evidence of vasospasm
- The operation may be delayed until about 10 days after the haemorrhage if the patient presents after the first 72 hours and there are radiological features of cerebral vasospasm.

Preoperative management. In those patients where it has been elected to delay surgery either due to the patient's condition or because of the presence of clinical or angiographic vasospasm, the management should include careful attention to the following:

— **Posture**—the patient should lie flat in a quiet room with subdued lighting. Every attempt should be made to avoid environmental situations which could cause sudden elevation of the patient's blood pressure and thus increase the risk of rupture of the aneurysm. Sedation using barbiturates or diazepam may be necessary if the patient is agitated.

— **Blood pressure control** — the blood pressure is frequently elevated immediately after the haemorrhage and should be carefully controlled. Initially this should be done using intravenous medication and utilising vasodilating agents (such as hydralazine or glyceryl trinitrate) and beta blockers. Although it is essential to control high blood pressure, as this may lead to rupture of the aneurysm, excessive hypotension may result in cerebral ischaemia, particularly when vasospasm is present. The appropriate desirable blood pressure will depend upon the premorbid level.

— **Fluids and electrolytes** — correct hydration is essential to avoid electrolyte disturbance; in addition, over hydration may precipitate cerebral oedema and insufficient fluids may increase the risk of cerebral thrombosis associated with vasospasm. Electrolyte disturbances may also occur following subarachnoid haemorrhage due to inappropriate antidiuretic hormone (ADH) secretion, which results in hyponatremia.

— **Pain relief** — simple analgesic medication or codeine phosphate is best used for controlling the headaches resulting from subarachnoid haemorrhage.

Surgical procedures

The surgical procedures available are:

- Occlusion of the neck of the aneurysm
- Reinforcement of the sac of the aneurysm
- Proximal ligation of a feeding vessel.

Haemorrhage from an aneurysm is due to rupture of the fundus of the aneurysmal sac. Therefore, the best surgical procedure is to occlude the neck of the aneurysm, thereby isolating the aneurysm from the circulation. In brief, the operation involves a craniotomy which is usually based on the pterion (pterional craniotomy) for aneurysms of the anterior circulation. This type of craniotomy may also be used for aneurysms arising from the terminal basilar artery, although many surgeons prefer an approach under the temporal lobe via a temporal craniotomy. Microsurgical techniques, utilising the operating microscope and microneurosurgical instruments, are employed. Access to the basal cisterns may be aided by withdrawing CSF either from the lumbar theca or using a ventricular drain. The arachnoid around the basal cisterns is opened, the neck of the aneurysm identified and dissected and a clip placed across the neck to exclude the aneurysm from the circulation. During the dissection of the aneurysm it is essential that vital adjacent vessels, including the perforating arteries, are not injured, as damage to these vessels may result in severe neurological disability.

Occasionally it is not possible to place a clip across the neck of the aneurysm safely, usually as a result of branches of the parent vessel either arising from the aneurysm or being inseparable from the fundus. In this case the wall of the aneurysm may be reinforced by a number of techniques, including wrapping the wall with crushed muscle, gauze or cotton wool or a combination of these. Rapidly solidifying polymer (aneurysm cement) may be poured around the aneurysm to provide it with a solid covering.

Although ligation of the common or internal carotid artery in the neck was commonly used for treatment of aneurysms of the internal carotid artery, improved microneurosurgical techniques have made this operation almost obsolete. The procedure has also been used for intracavernous aneurysms but these are now best treated by balloon occlusion, usually performed by a radiologist. Ligation of the internal carotid artery may be performed for a giant internal carotid artery aneurysm which is not amenable to direct surgery, but an extracranial–intracranial bypass procedure may need to be performed prior to the occlusion to prevent cerebral ischaemia.

Postoperative management. The usual postcraniotomy operative management applies, with special attention to be given to the neurological state, hydration, posture, oxygenation and blood pressure. Anticonvulsant medication is recommended for 6 months to 1 year. Steroid medication is frequently used in the initial postoperative course to control cerebral oedema, although its effectiveness is not proven.

The major specific postoperative problem results from delayed cerebral vasospasm. As indicated previously, prophylactic calcium channel blocking agents may be of use in preventing this complication. The transcranial doppler, utilising non-invasive ultrasound, may give useful information on the degree of intracranial vasospasm. Symptomatic vasospasm can be treated using hypervolaemic hypertensive therapy, but this treatment entails careful monitoring and requires the transfer of the patient to an intensive care unit.

Following the initial postoperative course the patient may require transfer to a rehabilitation unit for further rehabilitation and, if necessary, retraining for appropriate employment.

Management of an unruptured aneurysm

Multiple aneurysms occur in 15% of patients who present following subarachnoid haemorrhage. In general, an unruptured aneurysm will be clipped at the same time as the surgery for the ruptured aneurysm, provided it can be performed through the same craniotomy. The indications for surgery are controversial for an unruptured aneurysm occurring either in a patient who has suffered a subarachnoid haemorrhage from another aneurysm or an unruptured aneurysm found incidentally. The risk of haemorrhage from an unruptured aneurysm is approximately 2–3% per year. Consequently, surgery is advisable in a younger patient, with an accessible aneurysm, but could be reasonably avoided in the elderly patient.

ARTERIOVENOUS MALFORMATION

Arteriovenous malformations are the most common cause of subarachnoid haemorrhage in children. Other types of vascular malformations of the brain include:

- Capillary telangiectasia—bleed infrequently but may result in fatal haemorrhage, particularly in the pons
- Cavernous angioma—often cause minor local extravasations of blood but major haemorrhage is uncommon. Frequently presents following an epileptic seizure.
- Venous malformations.

The arteriovenous malformation is the most common vascular malformation. Although it accounts for approximately 60% of all subarachnoid haemorrhage in children by the 3rd decade it is responsible for 20% and by the 5th decade, for less than 5%.

Clinical presentation

Haemorrhage. This is the most frequent first symptom of an arteriovenous malformation and, although the bleeding may be subarachnoid, there is commonly an intracerebral component. The arteriovenous fistulous communication results in the development of aneurysms within the lesion, enlargement of the arteries which feed the malformation and, consequently, the possible secondary development of saccular aneurysms on the major feeding vessels. The haemorrhage associated with an arteriovenous malformation may quite often be due to rupture of a saccular aneurysm on the feeding vessel.

Epilepsy. This is the second most common presenting manifestation of an arteriovenous malformation.

Headache. Migraine characteristics are particularly associated with headache due to arteriovenous malformation.

Progressive neurological deficit. For example, a slowly progressive hemiparesis, may occur in a large malformation due either to local ischaemia induced by the shunt or to increasing size of the lesion.

Surgical anatomy

Most arteriovenous malformations are situated in the cerebral hemispheres, although they may occur in the posterior fossa involving either the cerebellum or brain stem; they show considerable variation in size. The malformations involving the cerebral hemispheres frequently form a pyramidal mass, the base of which may reach the cortical surface with the apex pointing towards the lateral ventricle. There are frequently multiple, enlarged arteries feeding the malformation and arterialised draining veins

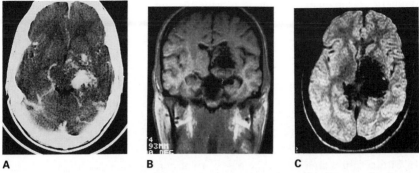

Fig. 9.9   (A) The arteriovenous malformation enhances vividly on the CT scan after i.v. contrast and the major dilated feeding vessels can be seen. (B) The MRI shows the position of the malformation in coronal and axial planes and further information about the feeding vessels and draining veins (C).

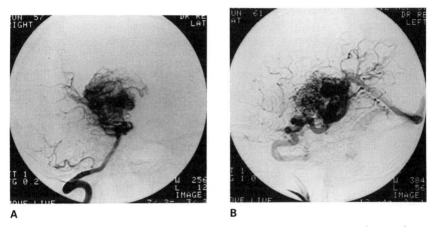

Fig. 9.10   Cerebral angiography (digital subtraction angiogram) demonstrates the vascular anatomy of the arteriovenous malformation. (A) The major feeding vessels are shown on the arterial phase. (B) The drain veins are demonstrated on the venous phase.

extend superficially to the superior saggittal sinus or transverse sinus or deeply into the internal cerebral vein system.

Radiological investigations for arteriovenous malformations (Figs. 9.9 and 9.10)

An arteriovenous malformation is often apparent on the CT scan because of the vivid enhancement of the enlarged feeding vessel and arterialised draining veins after intravenous contrast. Cerebral angiography is best performed using digital subtraction angiographic techniques and is essential for adequate evaluation of the malformation. Precise determination of the position of the major feeding and draining vessels is vital prior to surgery.

Magnetic resonance imaging is a valuable aid in determining the exact position of the arteriovenous malformation and the vessels.

Pre-operative occlusion of accessible major feeding vessels close to the malformation by an interventional radiologist may be useful if the procedure is technically feasible. A flow directed catheter is positioned in the artery, which is occluded using cyanoacrylate glue or a polymerising collagen mixture.

Management

As with cerebral aneurysms the aim of treatment is to avoid either an initial haemorrhage or rebleed from the malformation. There has been controversy over the risk of haemorrhage and the morbidity and mortality associated with rupture of an arteriovenous malformation. Recent studies have shown that the chance of haemorrhage for both ruptured and unruptured arterio-venous malformations is about 3% each year and that the combined morbidity and mortality of each haemorrhage is at least 40%. However, unlike cerebral aneurysms, haemorrhage from an arteriovenous malformation rarely causes symptomatic vasospasm.

Surgical excision, provided it is technically feasible and would not result in disabling neurological deficit, should be performed if the malformation has haemorrhaged.

Unruptured arteriovenous malformations should be considered for excision if surgery is unlikely to produce significant neurological deficit.

Surgery for arteriovenous malformations

The principles of the operation involve isolation and occlusion of the principal feeding arteries followed by meticulous dissection of the malformation, with occlusion and division of the numerous small feeding vessels. The draining veins should be ligated only after all the feeding vessels have been occluded, since premature obstruction to the arterialised venous outflow will result in a precipitous swelling and rupture of the vascular mass.

The surgical management of giant arteriovenous malformations is fraught with considerable risk. The lesions may be surrounded by chronically ischaemic brain due to a 'steal' by the malformation and abrupt occlusion of the shunt has led in some cases to oedema and haemorrhage in the adjacent brain, a phenomenon first described by Spetzler and which was called the 'normal perfusion pressure breakthrough' theory. Methods that have been employed to avoid this complication include pre-operative and intra-operative embolisation and staged excision of the malformation.

The use of radiosurgical techniques involving either the gamma knife (a highly focussed cobalt source of irradiation) or stereotactic radiosurgery using a linear accelerator has recently been investigated for the treatment of small, unruptured and surgically inaccessible arteriovenous malformations. The early results are encouraging but, as the radiotherapy effect is slow, the patient remains at risk from haemorrhage for some time.

Vein of Galen malformation

This unusual malformation results when arteries feed directly into the vein of Galen and produces distinct clinical syndromes depending on the age at which the disease presents:

- Neonates present shortly after birth with cyanosis and heart failure due to the shunt through the malformation
- Infants and young children present with seizures and hydrocephalus due to obstruction of the cerebral aqueduct
- Adults may present with multiple subarachnoid haemorrhage.

SUBARACHNOID HAEMORRHAGE OF UNKNOWN AETIOLOGY

In about 15% of patients the cause of subarachnoid haemorrhage remains unclear, despite clinical and radiological investigation. Many of these patients are hypertensive and have evidence of intracranial arterial atherosclerosis, although this is not inevitable. Most patients make a good recovery following the subarachnoid haemorrhage and rebleeding is uncommon.

Management

It is essential to exclude a cause for the subarachnoid haemorrhage and this may entail repeating the cerebral angiography, particularly if the initial angiography has been in some way imperfect and especially if not all the major vessel branches have been shown adequately. Systemic causes for the subarachnoid haemorrhage must be excluded, as well as rare causes such as pituitary apoplexy.

The patient is managed symptomatically with bed rest until the headache has settled.

FURTHER READING

Chyatte D, Fode N, Sundt T 1988 Early versus late intracranial aneurysm surgery in subarachnoid haemorrhage. Journal of Neurosurgery 69: 326–331
Drake C J 1984 Early times in aneurysm surgery. Clinical Neurosurgery 32: 41–50
Heros R C, Tu Y K 1987 Is surgical therapy needed for unruptured arteriovenous malformations? Neurology 37: 279–286
Heros R C, Zervas N T, Varsos V 1983 Cerebral vasospasm after subarachnoid haemorrhage: an update. Annals of Neurology 14: 599–603
Jane J A, Kassell N F, Torner J C, Winn H R 1985 The natural history of aneurysms and arteriovenous malformations. Journal of Neurosurgery 62: 321–323
Ljunggren B, Brandt L 1985 Timing of aneurysm surgery. Clinical Neurosurgery 33: 147–176

10. Stroke

Stephen Davis

Stroke is the third most common cause of death in Western countries and is the most important cause of chronic neurological morbidity. There has been a progressive decline in the incidence of stroke over the past 25 years. This has been attributed chiefly to the effective recognition and treatment of hypertension and other risk factors. Stroke is generally regarded as a disease of ageing, but young adults are also affected, with a different pathological spectrum.

The terminology used in descriptions of cerebrovascular disease is confusing and punctuated by misleading or outdated terms such as 'CVA' (cerebrovascular accident) and 'RIND' (reversible ischaemic neurological deficit). The term **'stroke'** is used to describe a sudden neurological deficit of vascular aetiology lasting more than 24 hours. A **transient ischaemic attack** (TIA) indicates a transient neurological deficit of vascular origin lasting less than 24 hours, although many patients with TIAs have suffered minor strokes.

Stroke is categorised as **cerebral infarction**, signifying ischaemic brain damage or **cerebral haemorrhage**, where the primary pathology involves vascular rupture and extravasation of blood into the surrounding tissues or compartments. The term **'haemorrhagic infarction'** is used to describe an infarct into which there has been a secondary extravasation of blood.

RISK FACTORS AND ASSOCIATED DISEASES (Table 10.1)

The major risk factors for stroke and associated disease are:

- Age and sex
- Hypertension
- Heart disease
- Diabetes
- Smoking
- Polycythaemia
- Alcohol

Age and sex

In general, the incidence of stroke increases with advancing age, although there are important differences between subtypes of stroke. For example, patients with subarachnoid haemorrhage are usually aged 30–60 years; this condition typically affects young and middle-aged adults in their productive years. Conversely, cerebral infarcts due to extracranial vascular disease affect older individuals. Among middle-aged and older patients there is a slightly higher rate of stroke in males.

Hypertension

Hypertension is the most important risk factor for both cerebral infarction and haemorrhage. Numerous population studies have demonstrated an increased frequency of stroke in patients with both systolic and diastolic hypertension, and the presence of hypertension can be correlated with common pathogenetic stroke mechanisms. These include cardiac disease with the risk of cerebral embolism, intracerebral small vessel disease (producing lacunar infarction), extracranial atherosclerosis (producing thromboembolism) and rupture of deep perforating vessels (producing intracerebral haemorrhage). A large number of randomised controlled trials have shown that the effective treatment of hypertension is associated with a reduction in the incidence of stroke.

Heart disease

Cardiogenic cerebral embolism is the second most common type of cerebral infarction, after thromboembolism from extracranial vascular disease. Valvular heart disease, from a congenital or rheumatic cause, has long been recognised as a cause of cerebral embolism and the decline in the incidence of rheumatic heart disease has probably contributed to the reduction in the rate of stroke. Attention has recently been focused on other forms of cardiac disease, particularly non-valvular atrial fibrillation, which is the most common cause of cardiogenic cerebral infarction and is associated with a five-fold increase in risk of stroke. Recent clinical trials have demonstrated a significant reduction in the rate of stroke in patients with non-valvular atrial fibrillation treated with warfarin. One of these also showed a therapeutic benefit with aspirin.

Diabetes

Diabetes mellitus is associated with an approximately three-fold increase in the rate of stroke. This is principally due to accelerated atherogenesis in the extracranial arteries and also to the development of small vessel, lacunar infarcts. Diabetes is also associated with intravascular factors that potentiate stroke, such as increased blood viscosity. The prognosis of stroke in diabetic and other hyperglycaemic patients is probably worse than in those with normal blood sugar levels, probably as a result of the production of excessive lactate and increased tissue damage.

Smoking

Smoking is recognised as an important specific risk factor for stroke and for coronary and peripheral atherosclerosis. Like diabetes, smoking accelerates atherogenesis; it also has intravascular effects on platelet adhesion and viscosity. Chronic smoking lowers cerebral blood flow and is associated with coronary artery disease and hence with risk of cardiogenic embolism due to either acute myocardial infarction or atrial fibrillation.

Other risk factors

Hyperlipidaemia, and in particular, hypercholesterolaemia, appears to be a relatively weak risk factor for stroke, but is an important risk factor for associated diseases, including ischaemic heart disease.

Heavy alcohol use is associated with an increased risk of both ischaemic and haemorrhagic stroke, particularly subarachnoid haemorrhage.

Polycythaemia is an important and treatable risk factor for cerebral infarction. It would appear that an elevated haematocrit, even in the upper 'physiological' range, is associated with increased stroke risk and severity.

Obesity, physical inactivity and psychological stress have not been specifically associated with increased stroke risk.

TRANSIENT ISCHAEMIC ATTACKS

Definition and clinical significance

Transient ischaemic attacks (TIAs) are brief and clinically reversible episodes of cerebral or retinal vascular dysfunction, lasting less than 24 hours by accepted definition. The majority of TIAs are very brief, with 75% lasting less than 1 hour. Using various brain imaging techniques, including computerised tomographic (CT) scanning and positron emission tomography (PET) it is now recognised that many TIAs in fact produce tissue damage and, that TIAs and strokes are part of a pathological spectrum.

For more than 40 years it has been recognised that TIAs are a prodrome of ischaemic stroke. The risk of stroke after a TIA is approximately 5–10% per year, compared with about 1% in a control population. The risk is greatest in the first few weeks after the initial event — transient ischaemic attacks are also a strong predictor of myocardial infarction.

Aetiology

The aetiology of transient ischaemic attacks is heterogeneous. Transient ischaemic attacks are most commonly related to extracranial vascular disease via microembolism from atheromatous plaques or via haemodynamic mechanisms with distal reduction in perfusion due to proximal arterial stenosis. Rarer causes include cardiogenic embolism and small vessel lacunar disease.

Multiple short-lived TIAs with a similar clinical pattern are often due to haemodynamic mechanisms. Single TIAs of prolonged duration are often due to an underlying cardiac source. A flurry of transient episodes of pure motor hemiplegia, due to small vessel disease, can precede the development of a lacunar infarct in the posterior limb of the internal capsule.

Clinical features

Transient ischaemic attacks are subdivided into those affecting the carotid and those affecting the vertebrobasilar territory. This distinction has important implications for both investigation and management.

Carotid territory TIAs. These are due to transient ischaemia in the retina or cerebral hemisphere. Transient monocular blindness ('amaurosis fugax') is due to a transient reduction in retinal perfusion produced by embolism or haemodynamic factors. The patient typically describes a 'shade' pulled down over one eye. In clinical practice it is vital to determine whether a visual disturbance is truly monocular, indicating retinal ischaemia, or binocular, implicating the vertebrobasilar circulation. Hemispheric symptoms most commonly consist of transient dysphasia and varying degrees of hemiparesis or hemisensory disturbance, either singly or in combination.

Vertebrobasilar TIAs. These are often more complex than carotid territory events and usually include two or more of the following symptoms:

- Binocular visual disturbance
- Vertigo
- Diplopia
- Ataxia
- Bilateral weakness or paraesthesiae
- Deafness
- Tinnitus
- Amnesia
- Occasional loss of consciousness.

These symptoms are produced by transient ischaemia of the brain stem, occipital and medial temporal lobes and upper spinal cord.

Differential diagnosis

The differential diagnosis of TIAs is of great clinical importance and includes:

- Focal epilepsy
- Migraine
- Vestibular disorders
- Syncope
- Hypoglycaemia

- Drop attacks
- Transient global amnesia.

Isolated **syncopal attacks** without other vertebrobasilar symptoms should not be regarded as vertebrobasilar TIAs. The term '**drop attacks**' describes a syndrome in which sudden falls to the ground occur without warning or actual loss of consciousness, typically affecting middle-aged or elderly women. These spells have a benign natural history and are of unknown cause. Similarly, the condition '**transient global amnesia**', where there is loss of memory and associated confusion, usually lasting a few hours and without other vertebrobasilar symptoms, is also a benign condition of unknown aetiology and should not be regarded as a brain stem ischaemic event.

Investigation of transient ischaemic attacks

History and examination

The investigation and management of patients with TIAs is based on a careful history and examination which is directed at:

- Delineating the arterial territory
- Determining the number and frequency of episodes
- Looking for evidence of atherosclerosis or cardiac disease
- Identification and treatment of risk factors.

For example, a prolonged TIA in a patient with chronic atrial fibrillation suggests a cardiac embolic source and the need for cardiac assessment, which may include echocardiography. The finding of a cholesterol embolus or carotid bruit on fundoscopic examination of a patient with attacks of amaurosis fugax suggests the presence of a carotid arterial source and the need for carotid investigation. Vertebrobasilar TIAs are usually due to localised atherosclerosis in the large vessels or branch arteries and are less often due to cardiogenic embolism.

CT scanning

CT scanning is usually performed in patients with TIAs to detect any evidence of infarction or other structural lesions, such as cerebral tumour or subdural haematoma, which may occasionally produce transient neurological deficits.

Digital subtraction angiography

The investigation of patients with TIAs due to suspected carotid atherosclerosis has undergone a revolution in the last decade. The introduction of the safer digital subtraction angiography (DSA) technique has virtually replaced conventional catheter angiography. Digital subtraction angiography can be performed by the intravenous or arterial route. The arterial route is favoured as it appears to be virtually as safe as intravenous DSA and produces far better spatial resolution, particularly of intracranial vessels. The technique utilizes a fine catheter and a small volume of contrast medium, and is often performed as an outpatient procedure.

Doppler ultrasonography

The development of various non-invasive carotid evaluation techniques includes the imaging of the vessel wall by B-mode Doppler ultrasound and the evaluation of arterial flow and any turbulence at the common carotid bifurcation by Doppler frequency analysis. Initial DSA is to be generally recommended in a patient with a carotid territory TIA or minor infarct, who is likely to have carotid disease and who is being considered for carotid endarterectomy. Duplex scanning (the combination of B-mode ultrasound imaging and Doppler frequency analysis) can be performed as a screening technique for patients with atypical histories, completed strokes and in patients where the distinction between a cardiac and carotid source is difficult.

Vertebrobasilar TIA

Vertebrobasilar TIAs are most commonly due to localised atherosclerosis in the distal vertebral and basilar arteries. This disease is surgically inaccessible. Vertebrobasilar angiography is sometimes performed in patients with vertebrobasilar TIAs to detect the presence of stenotic lesions in the distal vertebral and basilar arteries; these carry a poor prognosis. Anticoagulation with warfarin is sometimes used for these cases, when antiplatelet therapy has failed to stop the episodes.

Therapeutic options

Medical

Several large, multicentre, randomised controlled trials have shown that aspirin reduces the incidence of stroke in patients with transient ischaemic attacks. Aspirin exerts its antiplatelet effect by inhibition of cyclooxygenase, but the effective clinical dosage remains controversial. The earlier clinical trials used 'large dose' aspirin (1200–1300 mg/day) which is associated with a significant incidence of side-effects, chiefly gastrointestinal haemorrhage. Smaller doses of aspirin (50–300 mg/day) exert a more selective effect on the thromboxane A_2 (platelet aggregant) pathway than on the prostacyclin (platelet anti-aggregant) pathway and are of theoretical benefit, as well as being associated with a lower incidence of side-effects. Similar efficacy for high dose and low dose regimens has been demonstrated and it is now usual, therefore, to use the lower dose range of aspirin in stroke prevention.

Oral anticoagulation with warfarin is used for patients with a cardioembolic source, in some patients with vertebrobasilar TIAs and underlying atherosclerotic occlusive disease and in selected patients with inaccessible carotid or middle cerebral lesions.

Surgical

Carotid endarterectomy. While carotid endarterectomy has been used for 35 years as a stroke prevention technique, its benefit for stroke prevention has not been proved. Concern has been expressed about the selection criteria used to determine which patients receive carotid endarterectomy. The inclusion of asymptomatic patients or those with non-carotid territory symptoms, has caused particular concern, as have the unacceptably high morbidity and mortality rates being reported from some centres. This has led to the organisation of several large, multicentre, randomised trials designed to evaluate the precise place of carotid endarterectomy in stroke prevention. While the results of these studies are awaited we will continue to consider patients for carotid endarterectomy when they have major stenosis and/or ulceration in an internal carotid artery and ipsilateral ischaemic symptoms.

Transcranial bypass anastomosis. Extracranial–intracranial (EC–IC) arterial anastomosis for patients with TIAs or small strokes and inaccessible carotid or middle cerebral disease has now largely been abandoned after the negative results of a randomised, controlled North American study. Nonetheless, there are those who believe that this operation may still have a place in a very small subset of patients with inaccessible haemodynamic lesions, where conservative methods have failed.

Surgery for vertebrobasilar TIAs. Vertebral endarterectomy and posterior circulation (EC–IC) anastomoses have both fallen out of favour, but an occasional patient with vertebrobasilar TIAs and severe, bilateral, haemodynamic carotid disease may be considered for carotid endarterectomy to improve overall cerebral perfusion.

Asymptomatic carotid bruit and stenosis

Prevalence and significance

Carotid bruits occur in at least 4% of asymptomatic adults over the age of 40 years. They are associated with a mild increase in stroke risk, and are a stronger predictor of myocardial infarction. Investigation and management of patients with asymptomatic carotid bruits and stenoses remains controversial, with a number of unresolved issues. These include the natural history of varying degress of internal carotid artery disease, the role of prophylactic endarterectomy for those with severe stenosis, the efficacy of any medical therapy and the management of patients with asymptomatic carotid disease contralateral to carotid endarterectomy or in patients undergoing major surgery.

Natural history

A number of follow-up studies of patients with carotid bruits and internal carotid stenosis using Doppler ultrasound techniques have found a relatively small rate of unheralded ipsilateral infarcts, in the order of 2% per year without preceding TIAs. While severe stenosis appears to be associated with a higher risk of stroke than non-stenotic plaque, it is highly questionable whether carotid endarterectomy is beneficial, once the morbidity and mortality of the procedure is considered, even in experienced hands.

Management

Most neurologists would advocate a conservative approach until the results of a large, randomised, North American study evaluating endarterectomy for asymptomatic carotid stenosis become available. There is little evidence to suggest that an asymptomatic carotid bruit or stenosis increases the perioperative stroke risk in patients undergoing major surgery, including coronary artery bypass grafting where most strokes are due to cardiogenic embolism.

CLASSIFICATION AND PATHOGENESIS OF STROKE

Cerebral infarction

Cerebral infarction accounts for approximately 80% of stroke patients and may be classified according to anatomical location or pathogenesis. It is useful to incorporate both classifications when considering stroke in a particular patient.

Anatomical classification (Table 10.1)

The anatomical location refers to the specific arterial territory (e.g internal carotid versus vertebrobasilar, anterior cerebral versus middle cerebral) or specific location within the brain (e.g lateral medullary syndrome, ventral pontine infarction or internal capsular infarction). Infarction most commonly occurs in the middle cerebral arterial territory and can be classified as cortical or deep (subcortical). The cortical middle cerebral syndromes depend on whether a small branch has been occluded, or involve one or

Table 10.1   Typical clinical stroke syndromes

Arterial territory	Stroke syndrome
Internal carotid artery occlusion	May be asymptomatic. Mixture of middle and anterior cerebral artery syndromes
Middle cerebral artery occlusion	Contralateral hemiplegia, hemianaesthesia, homonymous hemianopia, aphasia, inattention, cortical sensory loss
Anterior cerebral artery occlusion	Hemiparesis, chiefly in the leg
Posterior cerebral occlusion	Homonymous hemianopia, disconnection syndromes, hemianaesthesia, amnesia, midbrain and thalamic syndromes
Vertebrobasilar thrombosis (basilar occlusion)	Quadriparesis, bulbar paralysis, impaired gaze, coma
Ventral pontine infarction	Quadriparesis. Absent horizontal but retained vertical gaze. Normal conscious state ("Locked In" syndrome)
Lateral medullary syndrome	Ipsilateral ataxia, Horner's syndrome, 9th and 10th nerve palsies, nystagmus, facial numbness. Contralateral spinothalamic loss

both of the main two divisions of the middle cerebral artery, the superior or inferior division (Fig. 10.1).

Subcortical infarcts occur in the territory of the deep perforating vessels supplying the internal capsule, thalamus, basal ganglia and brain stem (Fig. 10.2). The occlusion of a single perforating vessel produces a small infarct, less than 1.5 cm in diameter, called a **lacunar infarct**. The obstruction of the origins of several of the deep perforating branches can produce a larger subcortical infarct, sometimes called a **striatocapsular infarct**.

Pathogenetic classification

In the past, stroke classification was largely based on elegant clinical–pathological correlations, with the delineation of neuroanatomical syndromes. From a therapeutic viewpoint, greater emphasis is now placed on the pathogenesis of cerebral infarction. The three chief pathogeneses include, in order of frequency:

1. Extracranial atherosclerosis
2. Cardiogenic embolism
3. Lacunar infarction.

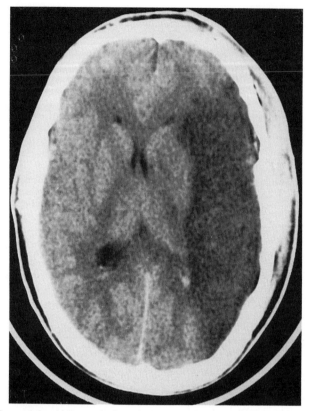

Fig. 10.1 Severe left middle cerebral cortical infarction. Note sparing of anterior and posterior cerebral arterial territories.

Extracranial atherosclerosis/thromboembolism. The development of extracranial atherosclerotic plaque, which most commonly occurs at the common carotid bifurcation, produces a progressive stenosis of the proximal internal carotid artery. (Fig. 10.3). Subsequent plaque complications include the development of ulceration, intraplaque and subintimal haemorrhages and superimposed platelet–fibrin thrombus formation. Various mechanisms can then lead to the syndromes of either transient cerebral ischaemia or completed infarction. These include the development of thrombus followed by propagation and distal thrombo-embolism into the intracranial vessels, embolism composed of atheromatous debris, and haemodynamic dysfunction due to the reduction of cerebral perfusion in the distal cerebral vessels. Primary intracranial atherothrombosis is rare and suggestive of a hypercoagulable state, such as seen with thrombotic thrombocytopenic purpura, sickle cell anaemia or polycythaemia.

Cardiogenic embolism. A variety of cardiac diseases affecting the cardiac walls, valves or chambers can lead to cerebral embolism (Fig. 10.4):

- Non-valvular atrial fibrillation
- Valvular heart disease
- Myocardial infarction with ventricular thrombus formation
- Postcardiac surgery (either valvular surgery or coronary artery bypass grafts)
- Prosthetic cardiac valves
- Infective endocarditis
- Atrial myxoma
- Cardiomyopathy
- Septal defect with paradoxical embolism.

The first five items listed above are the most common causes of cerebral embolism. It is now recognised that occlusion of cerebral vessels from these

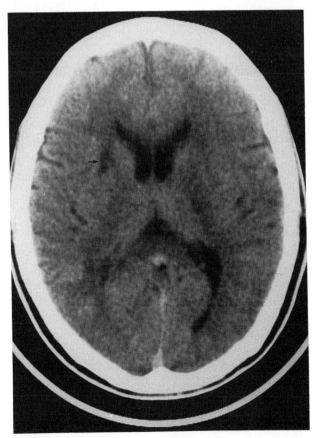

Fig. 10.2   Infarct in anterior limb of internal capsule.

embolic sources is often clinically 'silent'. Cerebral infarction due to cardiogenic embolism is more likely to be haemorrhagic than infarction due to extracranial atherosclerosis.

Lacunar infarction. The occlusion of single deep perforating arteries supplying the internal capsule, basal ganglia or brain stem can lead to the development of small lacunar infarcts (Fig. 10.3). These are most commonly the result of hypertensive disease, which produces localised arterial wall pathology, termed lipohyalinosis, in these small penetrating arteries. Other mechanisms, including localised micro-atheroma, are sometimes relevant. It is generally accepted that lacunar infarcts are rarely due to embolism from a proximal source such as extracranial atherosclerosis or intracardiac thrombus.

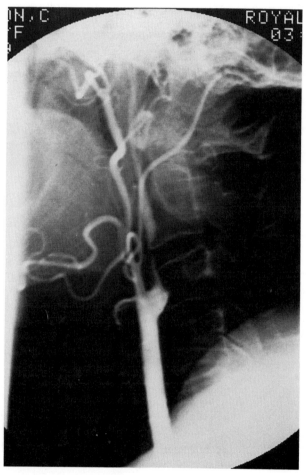

Fig. 10.3 Severe internal carotid stenosis. The external carotid is of normal calibre.

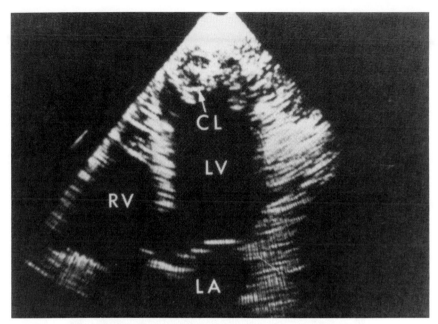

Fig. 10.4 Echocardiogram demonstrating clot (CL) in left ventricle (LV).

Cerebral haemorrhage

Cerebral haemorrhage can also be classified into anatomical and pathological subtypes.

Intracerebral haemorrhage

Non-traumatic (primary) intracerebral haemorrhage is most commonly due to hypertension, which leads to rupture of deep perforating arteries in the putamen, thalamus, central white matter, brain stem and cerebellum. The precise mechanism of this vascular rupture is uncertain, but it has been related to the development of small Charcot–Bouchard micro-aneurysms on the vessel walls of these penetrating arteries (Fig. 10.5).

'Lobar haemorrhage' refers to superficial vascular rupture within the cerebral lobes, outside these deep arterial territories. It is sometimes due to an underlying structural lesion, such as an arteriovenous malformation, cerebral aneurysm, tumour or vasculopathies, particularly **amyloid angiopathy**, which is an increasingly recognised cause of lobar cerebral haemorrhage in elderly patients and is due to amyloid deposition in the walls of the cerebral arteries. These haemorrhages may be multiple and typically occur in patients who are normotensive and who may show features of an Alzheimer's-type dementia (Fig. 10.6).

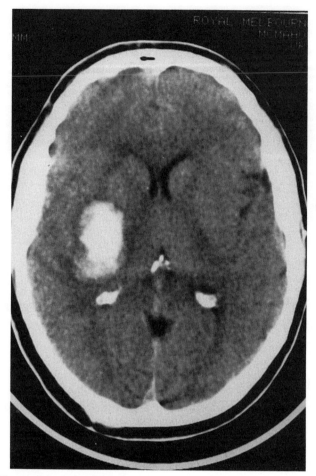

Fig. 10.5   Haemorrhage in basal ganglia

Subarachnoid haemorrhage

Subarachnoid haemorrhage is classified according to pathological cause and site (Ch. 9). The two most important identifiable causes include rupture of a berry aneurysm and arteriovenous malformation but, in up to 15% of cases, no bleeding site can be identified at angiography.

DIAGNOSIS AND MANAGEMENT OF COMPLETED STROKE

The following questions should be considered in the management of any patient with a presumed stroke:

- Is it a stroke?
- Is it an infarct or haemorrhage?

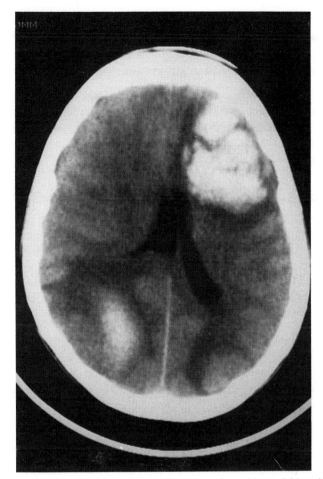

Fig. 10.6 Frontal and occipital lobar haemorrhages in patient with amyloid angiopathy.

- What is the arterial or anatomical localisation and pathogenesis?
- Is the stroke process static or progressing?
- How to prevent recurrent stroke?

Stroke and pseudostroke

While the diagnosis of stroke is generally regarded as easy, other pathologies ('pseudostroke') such as cerebral tumour, subdural haematoma, abscess, migraine, metabolic disturbances and epilepsy can mimic the stroke process. All patients with suspected stroke should therefore have a CT scan to exclude non-cerebrovascular disorders, which often require urgent therapy. Lumbar puncture is reserved for those cases where meningitis is considered (usually after a CT scan) or where the diagnosis of subarachnoid haemorrhage is still contemplated after a normal CT scan.

The distinction between infarct and haemorrhage

The distinction between cerebral haemorrhage and infarction is vital, as some haemorrhages are considered for surgical evacuation and some patients with cardiogenic or progressive infarcts are candidates for anticoagulation. The differentiation between haemorrhage and infarction is based on clinical, CT scan and, occasionally cerebrospinal fluid, criteria.

Clinical features

Cerebral haemorrhages are more commonly associated with an immediate rise in intracranial pressure, so that early depression of conscious state and, to a lesser extent, the presence of headache, vomiting and sometimes meningismus, point to a haemorrhagic process. In contrast, a patient with a history of TIAs who develops the gradual onset of a neurological deficit is very likely to have a cerebral infarct due to extracranial atherosclerosis with thrombosis.

Cerebral imaging

Clinical pointers, however, are often unreliable and an early CT scan will demonstrate all clinically significant haemorrhages, except for small brain stem bleeds. The CT scan is often normal in the first 12–24 hours after cerebral infarction, but is still regarded as superior to MRI in the diagnosis of acute stroke, as MRI may not detect acute haemorrhage. However, MR scanning is more sensitive for the early changes associated with cerebral infarction and has a particular role in diagnosis of small infarcts in the brain stem, where the CT scan is relatively insensitive and is hampered by bone-induced artefacts.

Lumbar puncture

Lumbar puncture should not be used to distinguish infarct from haemorrhage, as the technique is both unreliable in this differentiation and can lead to transtentorial herniation ('coning') and death due to the elevated intracranial pressure associated with acute stroke.

Location and pathogenesis

Infarction

Cortical infarcts. Based on the clinical examination, a distinction should be made between an infarction in the carotid or in the vertebrobasilar territory. With regard to carotid territory infarction, the presence or absence of cortical signs are of foremost importance. The presence of one of the following cortical deficits — dysphasia, apraxia, anosognosia (unawareness or denial of the stroke), sensory, motor or visual agnosia (inattention), acalculia, right/left confusion, dysgraphia or cortical sensory loss (loss of two point discrimination, astereognosis, dysgraphaesthesia) — suggests an embolic source from either the extracranial vessels or the heart. Thrombo-embolism from the extracranial vessels is suggested by the presence of a carotid bruit, the slow or 'stuttering' onset of the neurological deficit and the prodromal occurrence of TIAs in the same arterial territory. The clinical finding of a cardiac source, such as atrial fibrillation or valvular heart disease, suggests the likelihood of cardiogenic embolism, which is typically of sudden onset. Embolism may have occurred previously in other cerebral or peripheral arterial territories.

Subcortical infarcts. Subcortical infarcts in the carotid territory are sometimes large and due to embolism from a proximal source (striatocapsular infarcts) but they are more commonly due to small vessel lacunar infarcts, particularly if one of the classic lacunar syndromes is present. The most common pattern is termed 'pure motor stroke', indicating an isolated hemiparesis that affects the face, arm and leg in a symmetrical manner, usually due to a lacunar infarct in the posterior limb of the internal capsule. The other major lacunar syndromes reflect small vessel occlusions in the internal capsule, thalamus and brain stem and include pure sensory stroke, sensorimotor stroke, ataxic hemiparesis and dysarthria — clumsy hand syndrome.

Investigations. In addition to CT scan, an early electrocardiogram should be performed on all stroke patients. This may confirm the presence of atrial fibrillation, or recent myocardial infarction. Duplex Doppler scanning is of value in the diagnosis of large vessel atherosclerosis, while echocardiography may be of use in the diagnosis of intracardiac thrombi and valvular or cardiac wall kinetic abnormalities. Routine blood tests should include urea and electrolytes, a random blood glucose, a full blood count and erythrocyte sedimentation rate.

Haemorrhage

Intracerebral haemorrhage. The rapid onset of a stroke with early depression of conscious state favours the diagnosis of a primary intracerebral haemorrhage. Primary intracerebral haemorrhage and aneurysmal subarachnoid haemorrhage overlap in their clinical presentations. For example, a berry aneurysm can rupture primarily into the brain parenchyma, presenting as an intracerebral haemorrhage, whereas a primary brain haemorrhage can rupture directly into the ventricular system and present with marked meningeal features due to subarachnoid blood.

Subarachnoid haemorrhage. (Ch. 9)

Investigations

The diagnosis of both primary intracerebral haemorrhage and subarachnoid haemorrhage should be confirmed by CT scanning. Lumbar puncture is reserved for those patients with suspected subarachnoid haemorrhage, but where the CT scan shows no evidence of blood in the basal cisterns or cerebral sulci. Patients with subarachnoid haemorrhage require early angiography to determine whether they have a cerebral aneurysm or arteriovenous malformation. Angiography is performed in patients with cerebral haemorrhage when there is the suggestion that there may be an underlying abnormality, typically suspected in a normotensive patient with a lobar haemorrhage.

Management of the stable stroke patient

General measures

If the patient has a stable deficit, whether partial or complete, initial management consists of skilled nursing care rather than any specific medical or surgical intervention. The head of the bed should be elevated if there are features of raised intracranial pressure. The patient should be hydrated normally, since hypovolaemia can result in impaired cerebral perfusion. If the patient's bulbar function is compromised, fluid maintenance, via either an intravenous line or nasogastric tube, will be required.

While it is commonplace to administer oxygen via an intranasal catheter or oxygen mask, there is little scientific evidence to support this practice. In general, further management of the stable stroke patient is directed towards the prevention of recurrent stroke and treatment of non-neurological complications such as pneumonia, deep venous thrombosis and electrolyte disorders.

Management of hypertension

The treatment of hypertension in acute stroke is controversial, but it is generally agreed that aggressive reduction of blood pressure is rarely warranted. As cerebral autoregulation is impaired in acute stroke, sudden reduction of blood pressure will result in a fall in cerebral blood flow and potentially increased tissue damage. Stroke is often associated with a sudden increase in arterial blood pressure. This tends to subside spontaneously in the 24–48 hours after onset with bed rest and continuation of routine or additional oral antihypertensive therapy, given via a nasogastric tube if necessary. In patients with hypertensive encephalopathy or in aneurysmal subarachnoid haemorrhage, more rapid blood pressure reduction is required with the use of parenteral agents and close monitoring, often via an arterial line.

Rehabilitation

Once a stroke patient has stabilised, and if no other intervention is being considered, a coordinated rehabilitation programme should be commenced. Physiotherapy should be started at an early stage, to prevent complications such as chest infection or muscular contractures and to initiate mobilisation and motor relearning as early as practicable. Speech therapist involvement helps in the assessment and management of bulbar dysfunction and also helps the patient, nursing staff and family to understand the implications and problems of dysphasia. In practice, many hospitals have developed specialised areas dedicated to the care of stroke patients or have stroke teams or services, whereby a coordinated group of doctors, nurses and therapists are involved in the management of each patient.

Management of the progressing stroke patient

Infarction

Cerebral oedema and the role of steroids. Up to 30% of patients with cerebral infarction deteriorate after hospital admission, with extension of their neurological deficit and/or depression of conscious state. Excluding recurrent thromboembolism from either the heart or extracranial vessels, the chief cause is the development of cerebral oedema. The most common cause of mortality in both infarct and haemorrhage patients is this progressive rise in intracranial pressure leading to transtentorial herniation. While steroid therapy is very effective for the vasogenic oedema associated with cerebral tumours, the cytotoxic oedema due to cerebral infarction is not responsive to steroids, and although other agents, particularly mannitol, are sometimes used to reduce intracranial pressure, they also are of little value.

Anticoagulation. In some patients with a progressing stroke due to extracranial atherosclerosis and thromboembolism, the deterioration is thought to be due to recurrent embolism or propagation of intraluminal thrombus. This is the rationale for the use of heparin in some patients with progressing infarction. Although the efficacy of this therapy is unproven, it is widely used in selected patients with progressing infarction which is assumed to be due to either carotid or vertebrobasilar atherosclerosis and thrombo-embolism.

Urgent carotid surgery. Urgent carotid thrombo-endarterectomy in patients with acute stroke is associated with an unacceptably high morbidity and mortality and is rarely indicated. Because the causes of deterioration in stroke patients are heterogeneous, other factors should be considered. These include electrolyte disturbances, particularly hyponatraemia and systemic complications including pneumonia and pulmonary embolism.

New strategies for treatment of cerebral infarction

While there is currently no firmly established 'salvage therapy' for acute ischaemic stroke, there have been recent advances based on experimental brain stroke models and studies in acute stroke patients with physiological brain imaging using positron emission tomography, which allows measurement of regional cerebral blood flow and metabolism. A large number of randomised, controlled clinical trials have been reported, or are currently in progress, aimed at the evaluation of acute therapy.

Pathophysiological changes in acute infarction. There is a rim of tissue, of borderline viability, surrounding the core of infarcted tissue in patients with ischaemic stroke; this is termed the '*ischaemic penumbra*'. It has been postulated that many of the cells in this border zone area are in a critical state of cerebral perfusion during the infarct process and hence might be benefited by measures to increase regional cerebral blood flow. This concept has been supported by evaluation of the pathophysiological stages of cerebral infarction using PET scanning.

During the early stage of the infarct process, many patients have a state of relative hypoperfusion, out of proportion to the metabolic requirements of the cerebral tissues. In this state, cerebral metabolism is initially maintained by increasing the cellular oxygen extraction fraction from the failing regional cerebral blood flow. Eventually, oxygen metabolism cannot be sustained, because of the severity of ischaemia, and irreversible infarction occurs. Thrombolytic therapy, haemodilutional therapy and the use of calcium channel blockers have all been postulated as methods to increase cerebral perfusion at this critical stage of the infarct process.

Thrombolytic therapy. The earlier studies with thrombolytic agents, particularly streptokinase, were performed via the intravenous route, before the advent of CT scanning, and were associated with unacceptable rates of intracranial haemorrhage. There has been renewed interest in the early use of thrombolytic therapy. A number of small studies have reported benefit from intra-arterial thrombolytic therapy. Large, randomised multicentre studies are now underway to evaluate the safety (the risk of intracranial haemorrhage) and efficacy (evidence of arterial recanalisation at repeat angiography) of thrombolytic therapy with tissue plasminogen activator.

Haemodilution therapy. The use of haemodilution therapy, with agents such as low molecular weight dextran, combined with venesection can reduce blood haematocrit and increase cerebral perfusion, particularly if the hypervolaemic technique is used. While there have been conflicting results from various clinical trials using differing protocols, this type of therapy holds promise in selected patients and is being subjected to further study.

Calcium channel blockers. Calcium channel blockers, particularly nimodipine, act as arteriolar vasodilators and also counter the effects of free radicals — cytotoxic by-products of the tissue damage produced by the infarct process. Nimodipine is of proven value in the therapy of cerebral vasospasm due to aneurysmal subarachnoid haemorrhage. Its efficacy in cerebral infarction has been recently reported and is being subject to further trial at present.

Cerebral haemorrhage

Medical therapy. Deterioration in patients with cerebral haemorrhage is usually due to a progressive rise in intracranial pressure and impairment of vital centres. As for infarcts, medical therapies to reduce intracranial pressure are largely ineffective.

Surgery for supratentorial haemorrhage. The role of surgical evacuation in the treatment of supratentorial cerebral haematoma is controversial, but is considered under certain conditions. It is generally agreed that patients with large haemorrhages and who are comatose with severe neurological deficits are not benefited by evacuation of haemorrhage. Similarly, there is no evidence that patients who are either neurologically stable or are improving, are benefited by surgery. Surgical evacuation of supratentorial haematoma should be considered when the patient is in 'reasonable' neurological condition on admission and then undergoes subsequent deterioration, presumed to be due to the mass effect of the haemorrhage. While the precise indications for surgery remain uncertain, patients with lobar or superficial lobar haemorrhages are preferred candidates.

Cerebellar haemorrhage. The importance of surgical evacuation of cerebellar haematoma has been recognised for over 30 years. These patients often present with the sudden onset of:

- Vomiting
- Vertigo
- Profound ataxia.

Patients rarely have hemiparesis in the early stages. Excepting those with small haematomas, these patients are at high risk of deterioration and death from brain stem compression. Urgent surgical treatment should be considered in all cases (Fig. 10.7).

Prevention of recurrent stroke

Infarction

Extracranial atherosclerosis. Patients who have had a cerebral infarct due to extracranial vascular disease are at risk of recurrent infarction and are thought to follow the same natural history as those who have had a TIA. Carotid endarterectomy should be considered in selected patients who make a reasonably good neurological recovery and who have major ipsilateral

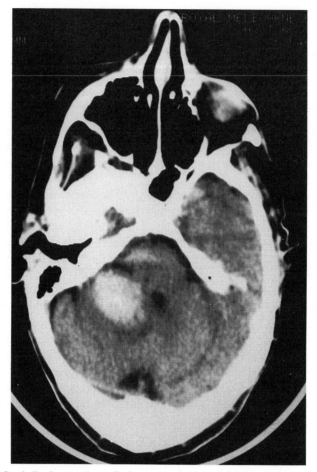

Fig. 10.7   Cerebellar haemorrhage. Brain stem and 4th ventricle are compressed.

carotid disease. It is useful to delineate this subset of patients with the use of Duplex Doppler techniques and subsequent DSA.

Where carotid endarterectomy is planned it is usual to defer surgery for 4–6 weeks in those patients with a significant deficit, as early surgery when the infarct is unstable is associated with increased risk due to secondary haemorrhage. Patients with a very small deficit are often treated earlier and managed along the lines of TIA patients. As a prelude to surgery, or where surgery is not appropriate, aspirin should be used as prophylactic treatment. Some patients with severe stenosis may be anticoagulated while awaiting surgery.

Cardiogenic embolism. Recurrent stroke in this group is a significant problem, estimated to occur in up to 20% of patients with cerebral infarction due to atrial fibrillation within the first 3 weeks after the initial event. Early anticoagulation should always be considered for this group, although there is controversy over the timing and duration of therapy. These patients have a propensity to develop haemorrhagic 'transformation' of the initially bland infarct, particularly in those with large regions of infarction.

Our policy is to use heparin acutely in patients with small or medium-sized cardio-embolic infarcts, based on clinical and CT criteria, where the CT scan shows no suggestion of haemorrhagic transformation. In patients with large neurological deficits we delay anticoagulation for at least a few days. Warfarin is usually used for longer term prophylaxis, although there is controversy about the duration of therapy, given the significant risks of anticoagulant induced intracranial or gastrointestinal haemorrhage.

Lacunar infarction. The diagnosis of lacunar infarction has several implications. There is a very low mortality rate because of the absence of significant oedema and patients rehabilitate extremely well because of the lack of cortical deficits. These infarcts are considered to be due to local small vessel disease, so that a search for a proximal embolic source with angiography is not warranted unless there is diagnostic uncertainty. Preventive treatment is directed at the hypertension — the chief cause of the small vessel arteriopathy.

Cerebral haemorrhage

Intracerebral haemorrhage. Prevention of recurrent haemorrhage depends on the cause of the presenting bleed. In most cases this is due to hypertension and rupture of deep perforating vessels and prophylactic therapy therefore consists of effective, long-term antihypertensive management. Patients with an underlying, identifiable structural lesion, such as an arteriovenous malformation or aneurysm, are then considered for specific treatment, including surgery, embolisation or stereotactic radiotherapy.

Subarachnoid haemorrhage. (Ch. 9).

YOUNG ADULT AND RARE TYPES OF CEREBRAL INFARCTION

Cerebral infarction in young adults is due to a wide spectrum of causes, including:

- Migraine
- Oral contraceptive pill
- Mitral valve prolapse
- Cerebral vasculitis
- Extracranial arterial dissection

- Fibromuscular dysplasia
- Moya-moya disease
- Hypercoagulability states.

Consequently, these patients require more intensive investigation than many older patients with stroke, with cerebral angiography and echocardiography virtually mandatory in all cases. Many patients will also require a lumbar puncture, to look for evidence of an underlying inflammatory condition, and detailed haematological investigations directed at the elucidation of a hypercoagulability state.

Migraine

Migraine is a common cause of stroke in young adults but the precise mechanism of infarction is unclear. Although vasospasm is usually postulated it has only rarely been demonstrated on cerebral angiography in patients with migraine and stroke. The diagnosis of migraine as the cause of infarction should only be made in a migraineur who has a persisting neurological deficit, in the wake of a classic attack and where other causes have been excluded by detailed investigations, including angiography and echocardiography.

Oral contraceptive pill

Oral contraceptive agents, particularly the higher dosage oestrogen containing forms which can increase blood coagulability, have been linked to stroke.

However, the relative risk of the oral contraceptive pill is probably small, and should not be assumed to be the cause of a young adult stroke without exclusion of other causes.

Cardiac causes

Mitral valve prolapse is a common echocardiographic finding in young women, but also figures prominently in clinical series of young adult stroke patients. While the risk of cerebral infarction is extremely remote in an individual patient with this condition, it would appear that some patients have strokes due to cardiogenic embolism related to the valvular abnormality or consequent arrhythmias.

Another putative cardiac embolic source in young adults is *patent foramen ovale* with paradoxical embolism from the venous circulation. The investigation of young adult stroke patients with contrast echocardiography not infrequently shows these septal defects at a higher rate than those seen in a control population, but the precise significance and therapeutic implications of this finding remain uncertain.

Cerebral vasculitis

Cerebral vasculitis used to be commonly seen in patients with an underlying basal meningitis due to tuberculosis or syphilis but it is now seen mainly with aseptic, inflammatory conditions. These include multisystem disorders such as systemic lupus erythematosus or polyarteritis nodosa.

Isolated central nervous system angiitis (granulomatous angiitis) is an aseptic vasculitis associated with multifocal cerebral infarcts and a high mortality. The cause is unknown. As with the other types of intracranial arteritis, some patients have 'beading' of arteries on angiography, an excess of CSF lymphocytes and an elevated erythrocyte sedimentation rate. Definitive diagnosis depends on brain biopsy. High dose steroids are used for these conditions, sometimes in combination with other immunosuppressive agents, such as cyclophosphamide.

Arteritis has been identified in illicit drug use with heroin, oral or intravenous amphetamines, cocaine and other agents. Giant cell arteritis (temporal arteritis) is seen in older patients with extracranial artery inflammation, headache, systemic symptoms and an elevated erythrocyte sedimentation rate. The chief complication is ischaemic optic neuropathy due to infarction of the optic nerve but cerebral infarction occasionally occurs due to involvement of the vertebral arteries.

Ophthalmic herpes zoster can be followed by middle cerebral arteritis and infarction.

Dissection of the extracranial arteries

Dissections are usually due to trauma, although the preceding injury may be extremely mild. Recognised causes include motor car accidents with torsional neck or seat belt injuries, and cervical manipulation. Spontaneous dissections also occur, some of these cases having an underlying arteriopathy such as fibromuscular dysplasia.

Carotid artery dissection is associated with ocular pain and Horner's syndrome. Neurological deficits may occur due to intimal thrombus superimposed on the ruptured lining of the artery and distal thrombo-embolism. The lateral medullary syndrome is a common clinical presentation of vertebral artery dissection. Diagnosis is made by angiography which shows a narrowed or tapered artery, the 'string sign', sometimes with the formation of an arterial aneurysm. Therapy is controversial but anticoagulation is frequently advocated to prevent subsequent thrombo-embolic events.

Fibromuscular dysplasia

This arteriopathy chiefly affects females and most commonly involves the distal portions of the extracranial carotid artery. It may be associated with renal fibromuscular dysplasia. It is usually asymptomatic, but is associated with an increased risk of both TIAs and cerebral infarcts, as well as cerebral haemorrhages due to associated berry aneurysms. The ischaemic events are probably due to thrombo-embolism and occasionally arterial dissection. Angiography demonstrates a classic 'saw-tooth' appearance. Treatment is usually conservative with aspirin.

Moya-moya disease

Moya-moya disease is a rare obliterative arterial condition where the terminal internal carotid arteries are occluded and there is a fine, telangiectatic web of anastomotic, intracranial vessels which produces the classic angiographic 'puff of smoke' appearance (Fig. 10.8). The posterior circulation is usually spared. It is associated with an increased risk of either cerebral infarction due to brain ischaemia or haemorrhage due to rupture of the abnormal telangiectatic vessels. The cause of the condition is unknown and medical therapy is ineffective. Surgical treatment, including transcranial bypass anastomosis, is used in selected patients.

Hypercoagulability states

Disorders of blood haemostasis and coagulation are sometimes recognised as the cause of stroke in young adults. Various rare abnormalities of the coagulation process have been identified in some patients. The lupus anticoagulant, an antiphospholipid antibody, has been implicated as an important cause of young adult stroke. This has been associated with a wide range of disorders, including systemic lupus erythematosus. It is more common in

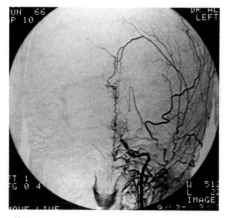

Fig. 10.8 Moya-moya disease.

females and is associated with recurrent spontaneous abortions, false positive syphilitic serology and other manifestations of hypercoagulability, such as deep venous thrombosis.

Cerebral venous thrombosis

Cerebral venous thrombosis is a rare type of stroke with variable clinical manifestations. Septic and aseptic syndromes are recognised. Septic thrombosis most commonly involves the cavernous sinus but can also affect the superior sagittal and lateral sinuses, with sources of infection including the face, paranasal sinuses, middle ear infection and bacterial meningitis. Aseptic cerebral venous thrombosis is most commonly seen in conditions associated with hypercoagulability states such as pregnancy, presence of the lupus anticoagulant or the oral contraceptive pill.

Clinical features include the insidious development of headache and papilloedema, focal syndromes in the cavernous sinus region, hemiplegia, depressed conscious state, fever, sinus tachycardia and co-existent venous thrombosis in the limbs and meningismus. Computerised tomography scanning and, more recently, MRI have led to earlier diagnosis of this entity. Therapy in septic cases is directed against the causative infection. Treatment in aseptic cases involves the use of early anticoagulation and high dose steroids.

FURTHER READING

Ackerman R H, Alpert N M, Correia J A et al 1984 Positron imaging in ischemic stroke disease. Annals of Neurology 15(Suppl): 126–130
Adams R D, Victor M 1985 Cerebrovascular diseases. In: Principles of Neurology, 3rd edn. McGraw-Hill, New York
Barnett H J M, Mohr J P, Stein B M, Yatsu F M 1986 Stroke: pathophysiology, diagnosis and management. Churchill Livingstone, New York
Caplan L R, Stein R W 1986 Stroke: a clinical approach. Butterworths, Boston
Grotta J C 1987 Current medical and surgical therapy for cerebrovascular disease. New England Journal of Medicine 317: 1505–1516
Hachinski V, Norris J W 1985 The acute stroke, Contemporary Neurology Series. F A Davis, Philadelphia

11. Developmental abnormalities

There are a number of neurosurgical conditions that are developmental in origin and that involve the cranium, intracranial contents and spinal column. The more important of these will be described in this chapter.

ARACHNOID CYST

Arachnoid cysts are benign developmental cysts that occur along the craniospinal axis.

Bright (after whom Bright's disease was named) was the first to accurately describe the condition in 1831. In 1964, Robinson described a large series of middle cranial fossa arachnoid cysts and erroneously postulated that the primary defect was agenesis of the temporal lobe; he later revised his opinion and recognised that the cysts were arachnoid malformations. In 1958, Starkman recognised that the cysts were developmental, 'intra-arachnoid' in location and that they resulted from splitting and duplication of the arachnoid membrane.

The cysts contain clear, colourless fluid which resembles normal CSF; they occur in characteristic locations:

- Sylvian fissure   50%
- Cerebellopontine angle   10%
- Quadrigeminal   10%
- Suprasellar   10%
- Vermian   8%
- Cerebral convexity   5%
- Other   7%

Clinical features

The presenting features depend on the position of the arachnoid cyst.

Sylvian fissure

The sylvian fissure is the most common site for arachnoid cysts and symptoms may become manifest at any age. There is a marked male predominence. The most common presenting features are:

1. Raised intracranial pressure
   a. headaches
   b. nausea
   c. vomiting
2. Seizures.

However, as with arachnoid cysts in any other location, the cyst may remain asymptomatic throughout life.

Cerebellopontine angle

The clinical features are similar to those of an acoustic neuroma, with sensorineural hearing loss as the most common initial symptom. A large cyst may cause minor impairment of 5th nerve function, with depression of the corneal reflex and, rarely, ataxia due to cerebellar compression.

Suprasellar arachnoid cysts

The majority of cysts in this position present in children and adolescents and the clinical manifestations are due to:

- Hydrocephalus
- Visual impairment
- Endocrine dysfunction.

The hydrocephalus results from protrusion of the cyst into the 3rd ventricle and occlusion of the foramen of Munro. Visual failure results from compression of the optic pathways, as well as long-standing raised intracranial pressure causing optic atrophy. Endocrine dysfunction may be due to intrasellar extension of the cyst and compression of the pituitary gland, or long-standing pressure on the hypothalamus, and is manifest as hypopituitarism, growth retardation or isosexual precocious puberty.

Cerebral convexity

In adults, arachnoid cysts over the convexity present with seizures, headaches or a progressive hemiparesis. The presenting feature in infants may be asymmetric enlargement of the head.

Convexity and sylvian fissure cysts slightly predispose the patient to subdural haematoma formation.

Quadrigeminal cistern

The cysts arising in the supracollicular region mimic pineal masses and the most common presenting symptom is obstructive hydrocephalus with raised intracranial pressure.

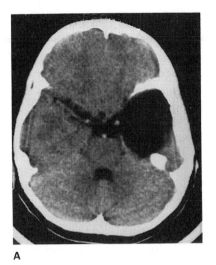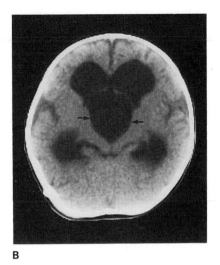

A　　　　　　　　　　　　**B**

Fig. 11.1 (A) Arachnoid cyst arising in the sylvian fissure. (B) Suprasellar arachnoid cyst causing obstructive hydrocephalus.

Radiological investigations

The CT scan will show the cyst in the characteristic position and the fluid will have the same density as CSF (Fig. 11.1). The bone windows on the CT scan or the plain skull X-rays may show remodelling and erosion of adjacent bone. The sylvian fissure arachnoid cyst is characteristically associated with expansion of the middle cranial fossa, elevation of the lesser wing of the sphenoid and outward expansion and thinning of the squamous portion of the temporal bone.

The suprasellar arachnoid cyst extending into the 3rd ventricle and causing hydrocephalus may be difficult to differentiate from a dilated 3rd ventricle due to aqueduct stenosis. Magnetic resonance imaging, particularly sagittal views, will help to differentiate the conditions.

Treatment

Arachnoid cysts are frequently diagnosed as an incidental finding on CT scan. Surgery is not necessary if they are completely asymptomatic, with no distortion or enlargement of the ventricular system; the patient should be carefully reviewed at regular intervals.

The two major surgical procedures for arachnoid cysts are:

1. Craniotomy, excision of the cyst wall and opening of the membranes to allow drainage into the basal cisterns
2. Shunting of the cyst into the peritoneal cavity.

The type of surgical procedure will depend on the position of the cyst, the presenting features and the surgeon's preference.

CHIARI MALFORMATIONS AND SYRINGOMYELIA

Chiari malformations and syringomyelia are complex developmental malformations with a wide spectrum of severity; they may present at any stage of life. The conditions are linked closely both through their underlying pathophysiology and their clinical presentation.

The Chiari malformation results from abnormalities at the craniocervical junction involving the caudal cerebellum, medulla and upper cervical region. In 1881 and 1885, Chiari reported the anomaly of the cerebellum and medulla oblongata and described three type of malformation. The **type I malformation** consists of caudal displacement of the cerebellar tonsils below the foramen magnum into the upper cervical canal. The **type II malformation** comprises caudal displacement of the cerebellar vermis, 4th ventricle and medulla oblongata below the foramen magnum. This is similar to the case reported by Arnold in 1894 and consequently is also known as the 'Arnold–Chiari malformation' (Fig. 11.2). The **type III malformation** involves caudal displacement of the cerebellum and brain stem into a high cervical meningocele. Chiari also described a type IV abnormality, comprising two cases of hypoplastic cerebellum.

It is usual for the Chiari type I malformations to present clinically in adults and many of the presenting features are related to the common association of syringomyelia. The Chiari type II malformation has an even

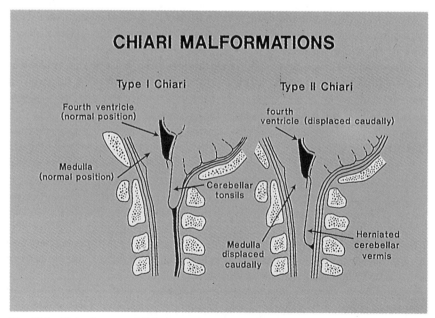

Fig. 11.2 Major features of Chiari types I and II malformation.

higher incidence of association with syringomyelia and it is almost invariably present in patients with myelomeningocele. Other frequent associations are hydrocephalus due to aqueduct stenosis, atresia or forking of the aqueduct, fusion of the superior and inferior colliculi on both sides into a single 'beaked' structure and a small and 'crowded' posterior fossa. Supratentorial anomalies include enlargement of the massa intermedia, microgyria and heterotopias, which may involve both the cerebral hemispheres and cerebellum. Cranial lacunae or mesodermal defects of the skull (Luckenschadel) are common and the radiographic appearance is of multiple 'punched out' areas which usually resolve in the first 6 months of life. The Chiari type II malformation may also be associated with anomalies of the cardiovascular system, gastrointestinal system (imperforate anus) and genitourinary system.

Syringomyelia is cavitation within the spinal cord. However, the cavitation occurring in association with the Chiari malformation is now usually called hydromyelia, as it is a dilatation of the central canal which is lined by ependyma. The term syringomyelia is reserved for the cavitation lying outside the central canal area and lined by glial tissue.

Aetiology

Gardner popularised the hydrodynamic theory of the origin of syringomyelia (hydromyelia) associated with Chiari malformation. In brief, the theory proposes that the CSF is unable to pass freely out of the 4th ventricle as the normal pathways have either failed to open or are obliterated due to the 'crowding' in the posterior fossa. The normal pulsations of CSF are consequently transmitted down the central canal of the spinal cord. The close association of the Chiari type II malformation and meningomyelocele led to a theory that spinal cord tethering resulted in the caudal displacement of the cranial structures as a result of growth. Alternatively, the malformation may result from hind brain maldevelopment during early fetal life.

Williams has proposed a differential pressure between the intracranial and intraspinal fluid compartments as another mechanism for the development of the malformation. With a Valsalva manoeuvre, the engorgement of the spinal epidural veins causes a rise in the intraspinal pressure. The spinal subarachnoid space is compressed and a pressure wave moves into the intracranial cavity. When the spinal pressure returns to normal the reverse should occur, with flow from the intracranial cavity into the spinal cavity. If this equalisation of pressures is impaired and delayed by adhesions and tissue in the foramen magnum, a pressure differential is created between the intracranial and intraspinal fluid compartments and alternative pathways develop, such as through a patent obex into the spinal central canal. In addition, the pressure differential promotes progressive caudal displacement of cerebellar tissue through the foramen magnum.

Clinical presentation

The clinical features of the Chiari type II malformation present in infancy, childhood or adolescence. A Chiari type I malformation causes symptoms presenting in adolescence and adulthood.

In infancy the abnormality will be apparent with its association with myelomeningocele. Progressive hydrocephalus may develop. Severe brain stem dysfunction may result in episodic apnoea, depressed gag reflex, nystagmus and spastic paresis of the upper limbs.

In childhood the type II malformation may be manifest by nystagmus, spastic paralysis and bulbar dysfunction.

In adolescence the symptoms may be due to either a type I or type II Chiari malformation. The features will involve a progressive spastic paralysis of the upper and/or lower limbs and may also include the features of syringomyelia, including suspended thermo-anaesthesia sensory loss, atrophic changes in the hands and upper extremities and bulbar problems either due to extension of the syrinx into the lower brain stem or to the direct pressure from the Chiari type II malformation itself.

Adult symptoms are primarily due to a combination of the Chiari type I malformation and syringomyelia. The characteristic symptoms include occipital headache, exacerbated by coughing, and neck and arm pain. Nystagmus is common and may be either horizontal or vertical. Downbeat nystagmus, exacerbated by the patient looking down and out, is characteristic of a craniocervical junction abnormality.

The characteristic clinical features resulting from syringomyelia include:

- Dissociated sensory loss (loss of pain and temperature sensation with preservation of joint position sense) occurring in a 'cape-like' distribution (Fig. 11.3). The sensory loss will often result in painless injury of the fingers or hands and Charcot joints may develop
- Weakness and wasting of the small muscles of the hand
- Progressive long tract signs resulting in spastic paresis of the lower limbs and paralysis of the upper limbs
- Bulbar features, if the syrinx extends into the lower brain stem.

Radiological investigations

Magnetic resonance imaging has revolutionised the radiological investigations of craniocervical junction abnormalities. The sagittal and coronal scans will show displacement of the cerebellum into the upper cervical canal, with caudal displacement of the 4th ventricle and brain stem in the type II malformation. It will also show the other associated intracranial abnormalities (Fig. 11.4). However, MRI may not adequately demonstrate the underlying anatomy of the bone structures.

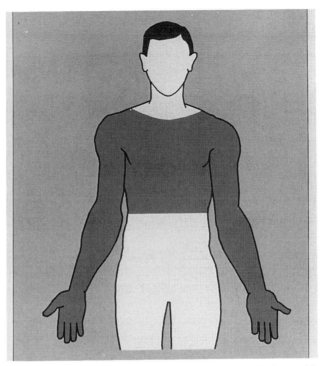

Fig. 11.3 'Cape-like' distribution of pain and temperature loss typically resulting from syrinx or other intramedullary lesion in the cervical and upper thoracic regions.

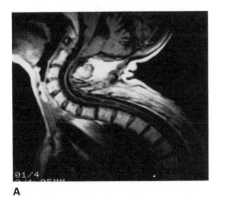

A

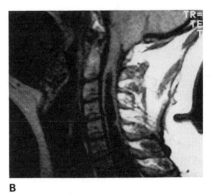

B

Fig. 11.4 (A) Chiari type II malformation with dysplastic cerebellum extending through foramen magnum to C2 level and caudal displacement of 4th ventricle and medulla. There is a syrinx (hydromyelia) in the cervical and upper thoracic spinal cord. (B) Chiari type I malformation with cervical syrinx (hydromyelia).

Magnetic resonance imaging has virtually replaced CT scanning with intrathecal contrast, and myelography is no longer necessary.

Syringomyelia (hydromyelia)

As discussed earlier, intraspinal cavitation can be either **hydromyelia**, where the syrinx is a dilatation of the central canal and there is usually communication with the CSF pathways, or the non-communicating **syringomyelia**, where the syrinx is separate from the central canal.

Hydromyelia (communicating syringomyelia) results from Chiari type I and type II malformations and occasionally from basilar arachnoiditis. The non-communicating syringomyelia may be due to previous trauma, neoplasms or associated with spinal arachnoiditis. Occasionally, no underlying abnormality can be found as a cause of the syrinx.

The most valuable radiological investigation is MRI, which will show the extent of the syrinx and associated abnormalities. This investigation has almost completely replaced the use of CT scan with water based contrast injected into the subarachnoid space. Delayed CT scanning shows intramedullary opacification as well as the enlarged cord.

Treatment

The two major surgical procedures are:

1. Posterior fossa decompression
2. Shunting of the intramedullary cavity.

The posterior fossa operation involves decompression by removing the posterior rim of the foramen magnum, posterior arch of the atlas and laminae of the upper cervical spine, extending down to below the level of the descent of the cerebellar tissue. The dura is opened widely, as it often acts as a constricting band, particularly at the level of the foramen magnum. A variety of other procedures may be performed at that time, including dissection of the subarachnoid adhesions, opening of the foramen of Majendie into the 4th ventricle, plugging the enlarged opening of the central canal at the obex with tissue and placing a stent through the foramen of Majendie. These procedures must be done with meticulous microsurgery techniques to avoid further damage to this extremely sensitive area. The dura is closed using a graft of nuchal ligament.

The syringomyelia (hydromyelia) may be shunted into either the subarachnoid space or the peritoneal or pleural cavity. Some surgeons prefer to carry out this procedure at the same time as the posterior fossa decompression but others prefer to perform the operation only if there is continuing progression of neurological disability.

CRANIOVERTEBRAL JUNCTION ABNORMALITIES

The craniovertebral junction region involves the foramen magnum, the adjacent occipital bone and the atlas and axis vertebrae. Numerous congenital or acquired abnormalities occur in this region, these may result in compression of the underlying neural structures. Some abnormalities, including spina bifida of the anterior or posterior arch of the atlas, remain asymptomatic.

Basilar invagination (impression)

Basilar invagination is a deformation of the basi-occiput in which there is an upward indentation or invagination of the base of the skull, including the rim of the foramen magnum, occipital condyles and neighbouring bone, into the posterior fossa. The clivus is often shortened and the invagination reduces the diameter of the foramen magnum. The odontoid process frequently projects into the anterior part of the foramen magnum, so that its diameter is reduced still further. There is a frequent association with congenital fusion of the cervical vertebrae to each other or to the occiput.

Acquired basilar impression may be due to softening of the bone by disease. The most common cause is Paget's disease but it may also occur in osteomalacia, hyperparathyroidism and osteogenesis imperfecta.

The clinical features resulting from basilar impression are due to compression of the neural structures at the cervicomedullary junction — the medulla oblongata, the cranial nerves, the cervical roots and the spinal cord.

The clinical features may include a progressive quadriparesis, dysphagia, respiratory difficulties, nystagmus (sometimes downbeat) and suboccipital headache due to irritation of the 2nd cervical nerve.

The useful radiological investigations include CT scan (with sagittal reconstruction and intrathecal contrast) (Fig. 11.5), MRI and plain X-rays. Various measurements at the base of the skull can be used to diagnose the anomaly. Chamberlain's line joins the tip of the dorsal lip of the foramen magnum to the dorsal margin of the hard palate and, on a lateral skull X-ray or the sagittal MRI, should normally lie above the tip of the odontoid pro-

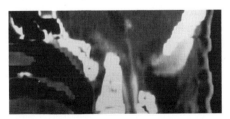

Fig. 11.5   Sagittal reconstruction of CT scan (with intrathecal contrast) demonstrating the odontoid process extending through the foramen magnum.

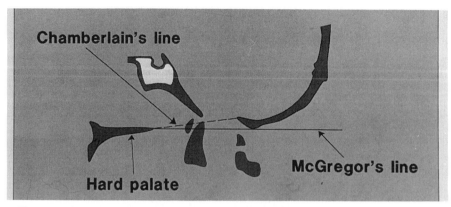

Fig. 11.6   Plain X-ray measurement for basilar invagination.

cess of the axis and pass through the ventral lip of the foramen magnum. McGregor's line joins the hard palate to the most caudal portion of the occipital curve. In basilar invagination the tip of the odontoid lies more than 4.5 mm above this line (Fig. 11.6).

Platybasia

Platybasia is sometimes erroneously used synomously with basilar impression. Platybasia refers to an obtuse basal angle joining the plane of the clivus with the plane of the anterior fossa of the skull; it is said to be present if the angle exceeds 145°.

Although platybasia is often present with basilar impression it causes no symptoms by itself.

Atlantoaxial dislocation

Dislocations at the atlanto-axial joint can result from congenital malformations, involving in particular the congenital fusion of the occiput to the atlas and fusions of C2 and C3. Multiple congenital cervical fusions occur in the Klippel–Feil syndrome. These types of fusions will increase the strain on the ligaments of adjacent vertebrae, resulting in instability. Atlanto-axial dislocation may also result from inflammatory conditions such as rheumatoid arthritis or following trauma (Fig. 11.7).

DANDY–WALKER CYST

The Dandy–Walker cyst is a cystic enlargement of the 4th ventricle, usually associated with hypoplasia or partial agenesis of the cerebellum and hydrocephalus of the 3rd and lateral ventricles.

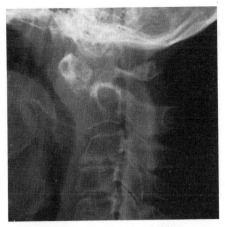

Fig. 11.7   Atlanto-axial subluxation in rheumatoid arthritis.

It is probable that the primary cause is an embryological failure of the foramen outlets of the 4th ventricle to open, resulting in cystic enlargement of the 4th ventricle and hydrocephalus. However, the Dandy–Walker cyst is sometimes associated with other congenital abnormalities, such as agenesis of the corpus callosum and aqueduct stenosis, and it has been suggested that it may represent a cerebellar dysraphism.

The clinical features are usually apparent in infancy and result primarily from hydrocephalus.

The cyst may be diagnosed in childhood, particularly if it does not produce significant hydrocephalus and the major presenting features are ataxia and delayed motor development.

The diagnosis is made by CT scan (Fig.11.8) or MRI. The standard treatment is now shunting of the cyst but, if aqueduct stenosis is present, a ventricular shunt may also need to be inserted.

SPINAL DYSRAPHISM

Spinal dysraphism results from incomplete or faulty closure of the dorsal midline embryological structures. The major forms of spinal dysraphism are:

1. Myelomeningocele
2. Meningocele
3. Lipomyelomeningocele
4. Occult spinal dysraphism
   a. dermoid tumours
   b. diastematomyelia
   c. intraspinal lipoma
   d. hypertrophic filum terminalae.

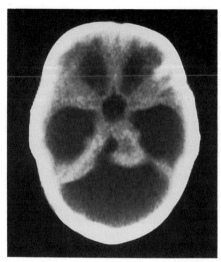

Fig. 11.8 Dandy–Walker cyst in posterior fossa with hydrocephalus of lateral and third ventricles.

Spina bifida occulta is a bony deficit usually found in the laminae of the lumbosacral spine and due to a midline fusion defect. It is an incidental radiological finding and is present in up to 20% of adults. In the vast majority there is no neurological involvement and the lesion is asymptomatic throughout life.

Myelomeningocele

Myelomeningocele is the most common and important form of spinal dysraphism presenting during the neonatal period (Fig.11.9). It is characterised by the neural elements protruding through a vertebral defect into a meningeal lined sac. Typically, the cord at this level is not fused and is in its flattened embryological state, with the nerve roots arising from the ventral surface and the open central cord lying dorsally. The major disability from this condition results from the irreversible neurological deficit caused by this spinal cord abnormality. Depending on the level of the defect the spinal cord or conus and cauda equina may be involved. Although myelomeningocele may occur at any level, it is most common in the lumbar and lumbosacral segments.

This disorder occurs in approximately 2/1000 live births. There is a greater frequency among whites than blacks, and a slight female predominance. There is a familial incidence, if one member of a family is affected the risk of the disorder occurring in subsequent offspring is about 5%. Seasonal outbreaks of myelomeningocele have been reported and there are ethnic differences, with a higher incidence of the condition in the United Kingdom, Northern India and Egypt.

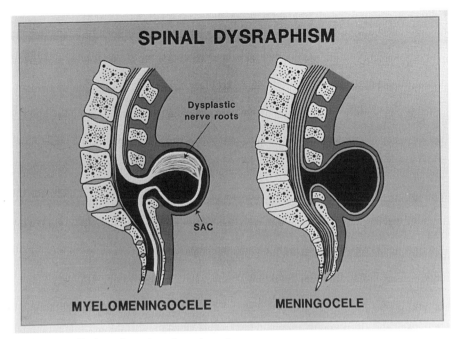

Fig. 11.9   Myelomeningocele and meningocele.

Prenatal diagnosis of myelomeningocele and other open neural tube disorders is possible by measuring α-1-fetoprotein in the amniotic fluid at 14–16 weeks and by prenatal ultrasound examination.

Myelomeningocele is frequently associated with other congenital abnormalities, most commonly the Chiari type II malformation, aqueduct stenosis (forking) and hydromyelia (syringomyelia).

The management of myelomeningocele involves:

1. Assessment of the sac and its coverings
2. Neurological evaluation
3. Examination for other associated conditions
   a. within the central nervous system, e.g. hydrocephalus
   b. associated extracranial anomalies, e.g. gastrointestinal, urinary
4. Counselling and careful discussions with the parents
5. Surgical procedures.

The decisions concerning which patient should have a surgical procedure with closure of the sac are among the most difficult in neurosurgical practice. On the one hand, the child has a right to life but there is also a right that the life should be of sufficient quality that it is worth living. The immediate decision is whether to close the myelomeningocele sac. In 1959 physicians in Sheffield undertook a programme of immediate closure in all neonates, with aggressive treatment of the hydrocephalus and other malformations. However, when the series was examined, only 7% 'had less than grossly crippling disability and may be considered to have a quality of life not inconsistent with self respect, earning capacity, happiness and even marriage'. Consequently, selective criteria were developed and the children excluded from treatment were those with:

- Paralysis at L2 to L3 or above
- Marked hydrocephalus
- Kyphosis
- Other major congenital abnormalities or birth injuries.

However, although when these criteria are used, a large number of untreated infants do not live long, a significant minority do, and there is great concern about their quality of life.

The initial operation aims to:

- Preserve all the neural tissue and reduce it into the intervertebral canal; untether the spinal cord
- Obtain a watertight closure of dura lining the sac
- Cover the defect with muscle, fascia and skin.

It will subsequently be necessary to make decisions concerning the treatment of hydrocephalus and other associated malformations.

The continued care of these children requires a multidisciplinary approach including urologists, orthopaedic surgeons, physicians, physiotherapists and social workers. The children frequently have severe urological problems, which may result in renal failure as adolescents. The musculoskeletal disorders, including talipes and hip dislocation, require careful orthopaedic management to maximise any residual lower limb function.

Lipomyelomeningocele

This is a much less common disorder than myelomeningocele. The mass is covered by skin and the lipomatous tissue extends intradurally and is intimately interwoven with the rootlets of the cauda equina and the conus medullaris, which is not usually fused. The neurological examination is usually normal at birth and progressive neurological deficits occur, resulting from growth and tethering of the spinal cord. The most common symptoms include bladder and bowel disturbance, back pain and progressive paralysis in the legs with foot deformities and loss of sensation.

Surgery is delayed until about 4 months. The lipoma is removed as completely as possible without endangering the neural tissue, the primary surgical aim is to untether the spinal cord.

Meningocele

This is much less common than myelomeningocele and is characterised by a cystic lesion containing only meninges and CSF; it does not contain any neural tissue.

Occult spinal dysraphism

Occult spinal dysraphism includes a number of spinal disorders, the vast majority of which are situated in the lumbar region and produce progressive neurological dysfunction, often as a result of tethering of the spinal cord. The more common lesions include:

- Intraspinal lipomas (and lipomyelomeningocele)
- Dermoid tumours
- Diastematomyelia.

The underlying intraspinal lesion can often be suspected from an overlying skin lesion such as a dimple, sinus tract, fatty mass, haemangioma, or abnormal tuft of hair. The neurological symptoms are usually first noted in childhood or adolescence. There is usually a slowly progressive neurological dysfunction involving:

- Bowel and bladder disturbance
- Progressive weakness of the legs and foot deformities
- Back pain
- Sensory disability in the lower limbs
- Progressive scoliosis.

Depending on the level of the abnormality, the neurological examination will show evidence of either a lower and/or upper motor neuron damage.

Lipomas are the most frequent form of occult spinal dysraphism. The lumbosacral lipoma presents at birth as a soft subcutaneous mass, usually in the midline and covered by skin. In its most severe form — lipomyelomeningocele — the lipoma will involve neural tissue and will extend through a spina bifida. Less severe abnormalities will be associated with a low lying conus and with tethering of the cord by an enlarged filum terminale or fatty tissue.

Diastematomyelia is a condition in which the spinal cord is bifid and the two hemicords are separated by a bony spur or dural band. Progressive neurological dysfunction will occur due to traction on the cord that is transfixed during growth periods.

The cord is occasionally tethered by a shortened, thickened filum terminale — hypertrophic filum terminale — and the only associated abnormalities are spina bifida occulta and an occasional hairy patch over the lower spine.

Radiological assessment will utilise plain X-rays, CT scan (with intrathecal contrast) and MRI. Plain X-rays will show a range of vertebral abnormalities including spina bifida, hemivertebrae, abnormal spinal curves, diastematomyelic spurs and widened interpedicular distances.

The surgical treatment is aimed at:

- Removing the underlying pathological cause while preserving neural tissue
- Untethering the cord.

CRANIOSYNOSTOSIS

Craniosynostosis is premature closure of cranial sutures. It may occur as a condition involving a single cranial suture or as part of a complex syndrome involving multiple fusion abnormalities.

The posterior fontanelle has usually closed by 2–3 months of age and the anterior fontanelle by about 16–18 months. The brain ceases to grow at 10–12 years of age, at which time the cranial sutures are obliterated by firm fibrous tissue. Complete ossification of the sutures does not occur until after the 3rd decade of life.

The clinical features of craniosynostosis are related to:

- The cranial deformity
- Underlying brain compression
- Presence of associated congenital abnormalities.

Sagittal synostosis

This is by far the most common type of primary craniosynostosis, the incidence is greater than that of all other types of craniosynostosis combined. Males are most commonly affected and the condition is usually not associated with other congenital abnormalities.

Premature fusion of the sagittal suture results in the head expanding in the occipitofrontal diameter and produces a long narrow head (scaphocephaly). Compensatory growth along the metopic and coronal sutures causes the forehead to expand laterally (frontal bossing).

Coronal synostosis

Coronal synostosis occurs more commonly in females. The head expands superiorly and laterally (brachiocephaly). This produces a short anterior cranial fossa, shallow orbits, hypertelorism and elevation of the forehead. Choanal atresia is common.

Bilateral coronal synostosis commonly occurs as one of several congenital defects in Crouzon's and Apert's syndromes.

If only one coronal suture fuses prematurely there will be an asymmetric cranial deformity.

Metopic synostosis

Metopic synostosis produces a narrow, triangular forehead (trigonocephaly) associated with hypotelorism.

Lambdoid synostosis

Lamboid synostosis is uncommon. There is symmetrical flattening of the posterior cranium.

Operative treatment

Surgery is performed to:

- Correct the cranial deformity
- Relieve the effects of cranial compression.

If only one suture is fused, compensatory growth along the open suture lines will reduce the risk of raised intracranial pressure. However, if two or more cranial sutures fuse prematurely there is a risk of increased intracranial pressure as growth proceeds. This may lead to mental and motor retardation and to optic atrophy.

Surgery is usually best delayed until the child is 4–6 weeks old, but if two or more cranial sutures are fused then it may be undertaken earlier to minimise the effects of brain compression.

The operation involves resection of the affected sutures. It should be carefully planned and meticulously performed to minimise blood loss.

FURTHER READING

Barbaro N M, Wilson C B, Gutin P H, Edwards M S B 1984 Surgical treatment of syringomyelia: favourable results with syringoperitoneal shunting. Journal of Neurosurgery 61: 531–538

Delashaw J B, Pershing J A, Broaddus W C, Jane J A 1989 Cranial vault growth in craniosynostosis. Journal of Neurosurgery 70: 159–166

Dyste G N, Menezes A H, Vanglider J C 1989 Symptomatic Chiari malformations. An analysis of presentation, management and long term outcome. Journal of Neurosurgery 71: 159–168

Gardner W J 1965 Hydrodynamic mechanism of syringomyelia: its relationship to myelocoele. Journal of Neurology, Neurosurgery and Psychiatry 28: 247–259

Hockley A D, Wake M J, Goldin H 1988 Surgical management of craniosynostosis. British Journal of Neurosurgery 2: 307–314

Hoffman H J, Hendrick E B, Humphreys R P 1976 The tethered spinal cord: its protean manifestations, diagnosis and surfical correction. Child's Brain 2: 145–151

Hoffman H J, Hendrick E B, Humphreys R P, Armstrong E A 1982 Investigation, management of suprasellar arachnoid cysts. Journal of Neurosurgery 57: 597–602

Hoffman H J, Hendrick E B, Humphreys R P 1975 Manifestations and management of Arnold Chiari malformation in patients with myelomeningocoele. Child's Brain 1: 255–259

Humphreys R P 1985 Spinal dysraphism. In: Wilkins R H, Rengochary S S (eds) Neurosurgery. McGraw Hill, New York, ch 258, pp 2041–2052

Levy W J, Mason L, Hahn J F 1983 Chiari malformation presenting in adults: A surgical experience in 127 cases. Neurosurgery 12: 377–390

Little J R, Gomez M R, McCarty C S 1973 Infratentorial arachnoid cysts. Journal of Neurosurgery 39: 380–386

Lorber J 1971 Results of treatment of myleomeningocoele: An analysis of 524 unselected cases, with special reference to possible selection for treatment. Developmental Medicine and Child Neurology 18: 279–303

Matson D D 1969 Neurosurgery in infancy and childhood. Charles C Thomas, Springfield

Milhorat T H 1978 Paediatric neurosurgery. Contemporary Neurology Series. F A Davis, Philadelphia

Robinson R G 1964 The temporal lobe agenesis syndrome. Brain 87: 87–106

Robinson R G 1971 Congenital cysts of the brain: arachnoid malformations. Progress in Neurological Surgery 4: 133–174

Shillito J, Matson D D 1968 Craniosynostosis: a review of 519 surgical patients. Paediatrics 41: 829–853

Starkman S P, Brown T C, Linell E A 1958 Cerebral arachnoid cysts. Journal of Neuropathology and Experimental Neurology 17: 480–500

Williams B 1980 On the pathogenesis of syringomyelia: a review. Journal of the Royal Society of Medicine 73: 298–806

12. Infections of the central nervous system

Infections involving the nervous system present in a variety of ways, many of which result in death or severe morbidity if not diagnosed and treated promptly. The infections usually occur as the result of haematogenous spread or direct extension from adjacent bone, soft tissue or sinuses. A large variety of pathogens are involved, including viruses, fungal agents and bacteria. The most common infections involving the neurosurgeon are:

- Acute bacterial meningitis
- Cerebral abscess.

Neurosurgeons are involved in the management of nervous system infections because patients frequently present with manifestations of a rapidly progressive neurological illness, as well as the systemic manifestations of sepsis.

Infection may involve any part of the nervous system or its coverings and can be classified in the following way:

1. Cranial vault
2. Extradural
3. Subdural
4. Meningitis
5. Brain
   a. brain abscess
   b. encephalitis.

MENINGITIS

Bacterial meningitis is a serious life-threatening infection of the meninges. Viral meningitis is the more common infection but is usually self-limiting, and the neurosurgeon is rarely involved.

Most of the common organisms which cause bacterial meningitis are related to the patient's age and to the presence and nature of any underlying predisposing disease. Although a few types of bacterial organisms account for most cases of acute pyogenic meningitis there is a wide range of organ-

Table 12.1 Common organisms causing primary bacterial meningitis related to age

Age	Organism
Neonate (0–4 weeks)	Group B Streptococcus, *Escherichia coli*
4–12 weeks	Group B streptococcus, *Streptococcus pneumoniae, Salmonella, Haemophilus influenzae, Listeria monocytogenes*
3 months–5 years	*Haemophilus influenzae, Streptococcus pneumoniae, Neisseria meningitidis*
Over 5 years and adults	*Streptococcus pneumoniae, Neisseria meningitidis*

isms that may be responsible. Table 12.1 shows the most common causes of bacterial meningitis related to age.

The bacteria reach the meninges and CSF by three main routes:

1. Haematogenous spread from extracranial foci of infection
2. Retrograde spread via infected thrombi within emissary veins from infections adjacent to the central nervous system, such as sinusitis, otitis or mastoiditis
3. Direct spread into the subarachnoid space, such as from osteomyelitis of the skull, infections of the paranasal sinuses

The CSF is a good culture medium which will support the growth of many microorganisms. Normal CSF contains very low concentrations of immunoglobulins and complement components and is devoid of polymorphonuclear phagocytes. Furthermore, phagocytosis is impaired by the low opsonic activity of CSF and organisms such as *Streptococcus pneumoniae, Haemophilus influenzae* type B, Group B streptococci, *Escherichia coli* and *Klebsiella pneumoniae* have a polysaccharide capsule that hinders phagocytosis.

Clinical presentation

Bacterial meningitis is usually an acute illness with rapid progression of clinical signs. Many cases are preceded by symptoms of an upper respiratory tract infection. The major presenting features are:

- High fever
- Meningismus, including headaches, neck stiffness, photophobia and vomiting.

Although patients are usually alert at the commencement of the illness they will frequently become drowsy and confused and, if treatment is not commenced promptly, there may be further deterioration of the conscious state as a result of a direct septic effect on the underlying brain, septic thrombosis of the cerebral arteries and veins or the development of hydro-cephalus. Focal neurological signs may develop as a result of cortical infarction secondary to thrombosis.

In infants and neonates the presentation of bacterial meningitis may be different. Neck stiffness and fever are often absent and the presentation includes listlessness and irritability.

A careful search should be made for a skin rash. Meningococcal infection frequently has a co-existing petechial rash, which occurs less frequently in other bacterial (e.g. staphylococcal bacteraemia, *H. influenzae* infection) or viral infections. The original source of infection, e.g. sinusitis, bacterial en-docarditis, otitis media or mastoiditis, may be evident and many patients have evidence of a pharyngitis — bacterial meningitis sometimes follows an upper respiratory tract infection.

Diagnosis

The diagnosis is made by CSF examination obtained by lumbar puncture which should be performed immediately the diagnosis is suspected. If the patient is drowsy, has other signs of raised intracranial pressure or if there are focal neurological signs, an urgent CT scan must be performed prior to the lumbar puncture to exclude an intracranial space occupying lesion.

The CSF features on lumbar puncture are:

- Raised cell count. This is usually in excess of 500 cells/mm^{3}and is predominantly a polymorphonuclear leucocytosis
- The protein level is greater than 0.8 g/l; it is often substantially higher
- The glucose level is less than 2 mmol/l, frequently much lower. A useful index is the CSF : serum ratio which is less than 0.4 in bacterial infection
- The Gram stain will be positive in over 70% if common pathogens are involved, and in approximately 50% for Gram-negative bacilli.

Other tests which should be performed on the CSF include:

- Examination for *Cryptococcus neoformans* using an India ink preparation and an agglutination test for cryptococcal antigen
- Investigation for *Mycobacterium tuberculosis* (Ziehl–Nielsen stain for acid-fast bacilli) and amoebae.

Difficulties arise in diagnosis of partially treated bacterial meningitis be-cause the CSF culture is often negative.

Other investigations include:

- Blood cultures
- Radiological investigations to detect the source of infection — chest X-ray, CT scan or skull X-ray for sinusitis.

The differential diagnosis includes:

1. Other types of meningitis
   a. viral
   b. fungal (*Cryptococcus neoformans*)
   c. amoebic
   d. tuberculosis
   e. carcinomatosis (Ch. 6)
2. Subdural empyema
3. Subarachnoid haemorrhage (Ch. 9)
4. Viral encephalitis (especially herpes simplex encephalitis)

Treatment

High dose intravenous antibiotic therapy should be commenced immediately and the selection of the antibiotic depends on:

- The initial expectation of the most likely organism involved, taking into account the age of the patient and the source of infection
- CSF microbiology studies
- The antibiotic that has the best penetration into the CSF.

There are many antibiotic regimes but if there is no obvious site of infection initial therapy should commence immediately as follows:

- Neonates (under 4 months) — amoxycillin plus gentamicin
- Four months–5 years — amoxycillin plus chloramphenicol
- Children over 5 years and adults — penicillin G plus chloramphenicol.

When the organism has been identified the most appropriate antibiotic should be used, depending on sensitivities and the ability of the antibiotic to penetrate into the CSF. Table 12.2 shows the CSF penetration of antibiotics.

Table 12.2 Antibiotic penetration into cerebrospinal fluid

Good penetration with or without meningeal inflammation	Good penetration only with meningeal inflammation	Fair to poor penetration
Chloramphenicol	Penicillins	Cephalosporins
Metronidazole	Penicillin Amoxycillin	Aminoglycosides
'Third generation' cephalosporins Moxalacatam Cefotaxime	Flucloxacillin Rifampicin	Gentamicin Tobramycin
	Trimethoprim/sulphamethoxazole	

The usual specific antimicrobial therapy following identification of the organism is:

— *Pneumococcus* or *meningococcus* — penicillin (70 000 units/kg i.v. 8 hourly for neonates and 50 000 units/kg i.v. 4 hourly for adults). Chloramphenicol is used if there is penicillin allergy (25 mg/kg i.v. 6 hourly in adults). About half the patients with meningococcal meningitis have petechiae or purpura. Subclinical or clinical disseminated intravascular coagulation often accompanies meningococcaemia and may progress to haemorrhagic infarction of the adrenal glands, renal cortical necrosis, pulmonary vascular thrombosis, shock and death. The antibiotic therapy must be accompanied by intensive medical supportive therapy
— *H. influenzae* — amoxycillin plus chloramphenicol. A test for penicillinase production is performed and therapy can be modified by stopping either the amoxycillin or chloramphenicol according to the result
— Listeria — penicillin.

Complications of bacterial meningitis

Complications are more likely to occur if treatment is not commenced immediately. The major complications are:

- Cerebral oedema
- Seizures
- Hydrocephalus — communicating hydrocephalus. This may occur early in the disease or as a late manifestation
- Subdural effusion — particularly in children. Most resolve spontaneously but some may require drainage
- Subdural empyema. A rare complication that usually requires drainage
- Brain abscess — occurs as a rare complication of meningitis.

Bacterial meningitis following neurosurgical procedures

Bacterial meningitis may complicate any intradural neurosurgical procedure, often with devastating consequences. It is a much feared complication following insertion of a CSF shunt (Ch. 3).

The majority of shunt infections are caused by *Staphylococcus epidermidis* and diphtheroids, species that are present in the normal skin flora. However, other pathogens such as *Staph. aureus*, *Pneumococcus* and *Haemophilus* species may also be involved. Unlike primary bacterial meningitis, the clinical presentation is frequently subacute or chronic and the patients present with a low grade fever before developing the more overt signs of meningitis. There is frequently a co-existing ventriculitis.

The diagnosis is confirmed by examination of the CSF obtained either by withdrawal through the shunt and/or lumbar puncture. The treatment consists of administration of antibiotics and removal of the shunt.

The most frequently isolated organisms in meningitis following neurosurgical operations are *Staph. aureus*, *Staph. epidermidis* and Gram-negative aerobic bacilli. The clinical features of bacterial meningitis may be masked, or confused with the underlying neurosurgical illness and operation. Although the meningitis may present as a rapidly fulminating infection, it is also possible for the clinical features to evolve slowly. The diagnosis must be suspected if there is unexplained fever, impaired conscious state, seizures or neck stiffness following surgery.

Cerebrospinal fluid must be obtained and treatment with the appropriate antibiotics commenced. However, it may be difficult to identify the causative organism, as perioperative prophylactic antibiotics may make isolation of the organism difficult.

BRAIN ABSCESS

Cerebral abscess may occur at any age, be single or multiple and, although most are supratentorial, can also occur in the cerebellum or brain stem.

Pathogenesis

Pyogenic inflammation of the brain leading to cerebral abscess may result from:

- Haematogenous spread from a known septic site or occult focus
- Direct spread from an adjacent infected paranasal or mastoid sinus
- Trauma causing a penetrating wound.

The metastatic brain abscesses arising by haematogenous dissemination of infection are frequently multiple and develop at the junction of white and grey matter. The incidence in each part of the brain is proportional to its regional blood flow, so that most abscesses occur in the distribution of the middle cerebral artery, principally the parietal lobe, although they can also be found in the cerebellum and brain stem.

The most common sites of infection include skin pustules, chronic pulmonary infection (e.g. bronchiectasis), diverticulitis, osteomyelitis and bacterial endocarditis. Patients with congenital heart disease and who have a right to left shunt are particularly prone to brain abscesses because their blood does not filter through the capillary beds within the lungs. The site of origin of the haematogenous spread is unknown in approximately 25% of patients.

Direct spread from paranasal sinuses, mastoid infection of the middle ear is the most common pathogenic mechanism in most series. Infection from the paranasal sinuses spreads, by retrograde thrombophlebitis, through the diploic veins into either the frontal or temporal lobe. The abscesses are usually single and are located superficially. Frontal sinusitis may cause a brain abscess in the frontal lobe, sphenoid sinusitis an abscess in either the frontal or temporal lobe, maxillary sinusitis an abscess in the temporal lobe and ethmoid sinusitis an abscess in the frontal lobe. Middle ear infection may spread into the temporal lobe and, uncommonly, a cerebellar abscess may result from infection spreading from the mastoid air cells. The mechanism of abscess formation is either by erosion of the adjacent bone and spread through the dura or due to retrograde septic thrombophlebitis in an emissary vein.

A cerebral abscess may result from craniocerebral trauma which has caused a penetrating brain injury, particularly if foreign bodies such as bone or hair have been implanted in the brain. A less common, but well documented cause of brain abscess results from infection spreading from skull tongs used for skeletal traction for cervical dislocation.

Histopathology

The abscess begins as a small area of focal inflammation — **cerebritis** — consisting of polymorphonuclear leucocytes, lymphocytes and plasma cells, which migrate from the peripheral blood circulation and which surround the area of developing infective necrosis. The necrotic centre enlarges and pus is formed by the release of enzymes from the inflammatory cells. At the periphery of this necrotic centre fibroblasts lay down a reticulin network and, as the abscess enlarges, a collagen capsule develops. The wall of the abscess develops more slowly on the ventricular side because of the poorer vascularity of the deep white matter compared with the cortical grey matter. Consequently, the abscess tends to enlarge into the deep white matter, and it may rupture into the lateral ventricle.

Bacteriology

In the pre-antibiotic era brain abscess was caused predominantly by *Staph. aureus* and streptococci. After the introduction of antibiotics the incidence of staphylococcal abscesses declined and most abscesses were thought to be due to streptococci, although up to 50% of culture results in some series were 'sterile'. When improved anaerobic culture techniques became available the incidence of positive cultures increased, and many of the abscesses previously thought to be sterile were found to have been caused by anaerobic organisms, particularly streptococci and *Bacteroides* species. Meticulous culture techniques have resulted in considerable improvement in the definition of the bacterial spectrum in brain abscesses and confirmed that streptococci are the most common organisms isolated in brain abscesses of all origins, but the exact bacterial flora depends on the cause of the abscess (Table 12.3).

Streptococci are isolated from approximately 80% of brain abscesses. The

Table 12.3   Cerebral abscess — pathogenesis and principal organisms

History	Site of abscess	Predominant organism
Sinusitis — frontal	Frontal lobe	Aerobic streptococci *Streptococcus milleri* *Haemophilus* species
Mastoiditis, otitis	Temporal lobe	Mixed flora Aerobic and anaerobic streptococci Enterobacteria *Bacteroides fragilis* *Haemophilus* species
Haematogenous, cryptogenic	Brain	Aerobic streptococci Anaerobic streptococci Enterobacteria
Trauma	Brain	*Staphylococcus aureus*

most common single species is the α-haemolytic carboxyphilic *Streptococcus milleri*, a micro-aerophilic streptococcus which grows in anaerobic culture and also 10% carbon dioxide. The major habitat of *Strep. milleri* is the alimentary tract, including the mouth and dental plaque. The association between frontal lobe abscesses, *Strep. milleri* and sinusitis indicates that the source of infection in many brain abscesses is the upper respiratory tract, the organism passing into the brain from the paranasal sinuses.

Otogenic abscesses usually yield a mixed flora, including bacteroides (*Bacteroides fragilis*), various streptococci and members of the Enterobacteriaceae (*Esch. coli, Proteus* and *Pseudomonas* species).

Metastatic haematogenous infection may be due to various aerobic and anaerobic streptococci, enterobacteria and other Gram-negative bacilli.

Staph. aureus is often the pathogen in abscesses resulting from trauma.

Presenting features

Patients present with features of:
1. An intracranial mass
   a. raised intracranial pressure
   b. focal neurological signs, e.g. hemiparesis, dysphasia
   c. epileptic seizures
2. Systemic toxicity — fever and malaise
3. Clinical features of the underlying source of the infection — sinusitis, bacterial endocarditis, diverticulitis

The clinical features develop over 2–4 weeks, although a slower progression is not unusual. If the abscess involves an eloquent intracerebral location it may present when quite small. Alternatively, an abscess in the frontal lobe may reach a large size before producing any major neurological deficit.

About half the patients with brain abscess have systemic symptoms, including fever at the time of the diagnosis. Marked toxic symptoms may be attributable to the abscess rupturing into the ventricle or associated meningitis.

Diagnosis

Computerised tomography scanning has been responsible for a dramatic reduction in the mortality of cerebral abscess because of its ability to diagnose single and multiple abscesses and to localise the lesion accurately.

The CT scan appearance is typically a ring enhancing mass often surrounded by considerable oedema (Figs. 12.1, 12.2 and 12.3). The enhancing capsule is usually thinner adjacent to the ventricle compared with the more superficial capsule. The lesions may be multiple (Fig. 12.2B) or multiloculated (Fig. 12.3). In the early stages of development of the abscess, when the infection is localised as 'cerebritis', the CT scan appearance will be an area of low density which enhances after intravenous contrast but without the typical 'ring' appearance and usually with marked adjacent oedema. If the abscess is due to haematogenous spread it is usually located at the grey/white matter junction (Fig. 12.1).

Peripheral blood examination may show a leucocytosis. Raised erythrocyte sedimentation rate and positive blood cultures may be obtained if there is a co-existing septicaemia.

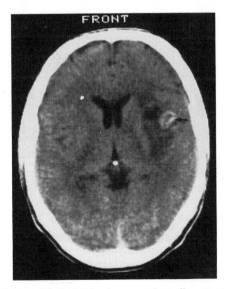

Fig. 12.1 Cerebral abscess early in its development. A small contrast-enhancing lesion surrounded by low density cerebral oedema.

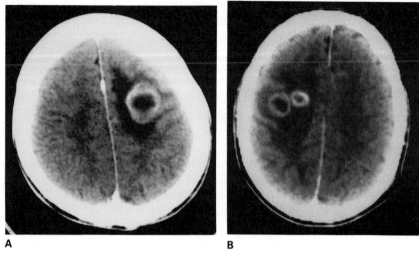

Fig. 12.2 (A) Typical ring-enhancing cerebral abscess in the frontal lobe with surrounding cerebral oedema. (B) Multiple cerebral abscesses.

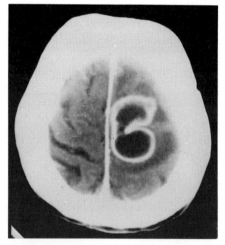

Fig 12.3 Multiloculated cerebral abscess.

Management

The principles of treatment are to:

- Identify the bacterial organisms
- Institute antibiotic therapy
- Drain or excise the abscess.

A specimen of the pus is essential for accurate identification of the organism so that the appropriate antibiotic therapy can be commenced. Occasionally, the organism can be identified from a positive blood culture or other obvious source of infection.

Surgical treatment. Surgical treatment of the abscess involves either:

1. Aspiration of the abscess through a burr hole, with repeated aspirations as required
2. Excision of the abscess.

Drainage of the abscess through a burr hole, if necessary using CT guided stereotaxis, is a safe, effective way of obtaining the pus and emptying the abscess. It is frequently necessary to repeat the aspirations and this is best evaluated by follow-up CT scans.

The surgical excision of the abscess should be considered if:

- There is persistent re-accumulation of pus despite repeated aspirations
- The abscess is in an accessible site
- There is a well formed fibrous capsule which fails to collapse despite repeated aspirations
- There is a cerebellar abscess.

Antibiotic therapy. As soon as pus has been obtained, antibiotic therapy should commence. The initial choice of antibiotic, before culture results are available, will depend on the probable cause of the brain abscess and the Gram stain. The usual initial treatment is high dose penicillin and chloramphenicol. *Strep. milleri* is the organism most frequently found in abscesses of sinusitic origin involving the frontal lobe; it is highly sensitive to penicillin. Chloramphenicol and metronidazole are active against the occasionally reported obligate anaerobes. Abscesses of otitic origin, usually occuring in the temporal lobe, are caused by a wide range of aerobic and anaerobic bacteria. A combination of penicillin with chloramphenicol or metronidazole should be used. Abscesses of metastatic or cryptogenic origin may be caused by streptococci or by a mixture of bacteria and broad spectrum therapy, including penicillin, should be used until bacteriological results are available. As many of the organisms are resistant to penicillin, it has been suggested that a penicillinase stable penicillin (e.g. flucloxacillin) should be substituted.

As soon as the culture results are available the appropriate antibiotic should be used intravenously in high doses and selection should be made bearing in mind the antibiotic's penetration into the brain and CSF.

Corticosteroid therapy (dexamethasone) may be necessary to reduce cerebral oedema and should be considered in patients who are drowsy or have a deteriorating neurological state despite surgery and antibiotic treatment.

Anticonvulsant medication should be commenced as there is an incidence of seizures in between 30–50% of cases.

Prognosis

The improvement in antibiotic therapy and CT scanning has dramatically reduced the mortality of bacterial abscesses from 50% to less than 10%.

EPIDURAL ABSCESS

Cranial epidural abscess results following:

- Trauma
- Surgery — craniotomy or insertion of skull traction tongs
- Paranasal sinusitis or mastoiditis.

The condition is frequently associated with osteomyelitis of the cranial vault.

Clinical features

The clinical features of an epidural abscess are primarily those of osteomyelitis, with acute localised pain and tenderness and localised pitting oedema of the scalp over the affected area, described by Percival Pott and known as 'Pott's puffy tumour'. There are usually systemic symptoms of infection.

The most common organisms are aerobic and anaerobic streptococci and *Staph. aureus*.

Treatment

Treatment involves evacuation of the pus, excision of any infected bone and surgical eradication of the underlying cause (e.g. sinus infection). High dose antibiotic therapy should be administered.

The diagnosis is made on CT scan, which will show the extradural collection of pus as well as osteomyelitis and the infected sinuses.

SUBDURAL ABSCESS

A subdural abscess is an uncommon but potentially life-threatening infection with possible serious neurological sequelae in the patients who survive. The abscess follows infection in the paranasal sinuses, particularly frontal sinusitis and, less commonly, infection in the mastoid air cells. The infection in the subdural space is an extension of the sinusitis through emissary veins and retrograde thrombophlebitis.

Subdural empyema may also result from penetrating wounds, or may follow surgery. In infants, subdural empyema may occur as an infection of the subdural space following meningitis.

Microbiology

The most common organism responsible for subdural empyema following frontal sinusitis is *Strep. milleri*. However, other aerobic and anaerobic streptococci, other anaerobes and *Staph. aureus* may also be responsible, with a pattern similar to that indicated for intracerebral abscesses.

Clinical presentation

In contrast to patients with extradural abscesses, patients presenting with subdural empyemas are usually seriously ill, being toxic and febrile, with features of meningeal irritation. They frequently have rapidly progressive neurological signs, including depressed conscious state, hemiparesis and dysphasia. Epileptic seizures occur in most patients.

The classic presentation is a patient with a history of acute frontal sinusitis who develops severe headaches, high fever and has a rapid neurological deterioration with seizures.

Diagnosis

The differential diagnosis includes:

- Viral encephalitis
- Bacterial meningitis
- Brain abscess
- Septic cavernous sinus thrombosis.

Investigations

Evidence of underlying sinusitis will be present on plain skull X-ray and CT scan. The CT scan findings may be subtle, as the abscess is usually iso- or hypodense. There may be contrast enhancement of the underlying inflamed membranes and evidence of underlying cerebral oedema, although these features are not universal.

Lumbar puncture should not be performed if the diagnosis is suspected clinically, as it is hazardous and frequently not diagnostic. There is usually a pleocytosis in the CSF with elevated protein, but the sugar may be normal and organisms usually cannot be cultured.

Treatment

Subdural empyema is a surgical emergency. The principles of treatment, as for any abscess are:

- Drain the abscess
- Identify the organism
- Treat with appropriate high dose antibiotics.

The surgical techniques used to drain the abscess are either multiple burr holes, craniotomy or craniectomy. The advantage of the multiple burr hole technique is that the pus may be widespread and bilateral and the patient is frequently seriously ill. However, it may be difficult to drain the pus adequately through burr holes, as the underlying oedematous brain may swell up to occlude the hole. In addition, it is difficult to provide adequate drainage for the parafalcine pus, which frequently lies between the falx and the medial aspect of the hemispheres, through burr holes.

The subdural space should be irrigated with antibiotic solution at the time of surgery and subdural catheters should be left in place for further drainage of pus and postoperative antibiotic irrigation. It is arguable whether the antibiotic irrigation is useful but it is probably worthwhile, in view of the seriousness of the situation.

High dose systemic antibiotic therapy should be commenced as soon as pus is obtained for culture. The initial therapy will depend on the underlying cause, as for cerebral abscess, bearing in mind that the most common infecting organism is penicillin sensitive *Strep. milleri* from frontal sinusitis. Further antibiotic therapy will depend on the results of the culture.

Anticonvulsant therapy is important as the patients have a high incidence of seizures.

TUBERCULOSIS

Tuberculosis involving the brain is unusual in Western countries but is not uncommon in India, Asia, the Middle East, South America and Eastern Europe.

The infection may occur as:

- Tuberculous meningitis
- Intracranial tuberculomas.

Tuberculous meningitis

Tuberculous meningitis is usually a subacute illness; patients present with headaches, confusion and features of meningitis. It occurs more frequently in children and will result in secondary pathological changes and neurological deficit, including:

- Basal arachnoiditis causing hydrocephalus
- Visual failure due to arachnoiditis around the optic pathways
- Multiple cranial nerve palsies due to the basal arachnoiditis
- Arteritis causing cerebral infarction.

CSF examination will show:

- Lymphocytic pleocytosis (100–500 cells/mm^3)
- Elevated protein (greater than 0.8 g/l)

- Low glucose (less than 2 mmol/l)
- Low chloride (less than 110 mmol/l)
- Acid fast bacilli in 20% of patients using a Ziehl–Nielsen stain.

The definitive diagnosis is often only made on culture of the mycobacterium tuberculosis, which may take up to 6 weeks.

Antituberculous therapy should be commenced if tuberculous meningitis is suspected, as it is invariably fatal within 6 weeks and is often more rapidly fatal. The antituberculous medication includes isoniazid and rifampicin.

Hydrocephalus should be treated with a ventriculoperitoneal shunt. Steroid therapy has been used to diminish the risk of arachnoid adhesions and arteritis but is probably of little benefit. A brief course may be indicated in patients with raised intracranial pressure. The serum sodium in older patients may drop, probably due to inappropriate antidiuretic hormone secretion, and should be treated by fluid restriction.

Intracranial tuberculoma

An intracranial tuberculoma originates by haematogenous spread from tuberculous lesions in other parts of the body, especially the lung. Tuberculomas are frequently multiple and are predominantly located in the posterior fossa in children and young adults, but may occur throughout the cerebral hemispheres.

The clinical presentation is similar to an intracranial tumour, with features of raised intracranial pressure, focal neurological signs and epileptic seizures. Systemic symptoms of tuberculosis, such as fever, excessive perspiration and lethargy, occur in less than 50% of cases.

The CT scan appearance of a tuberculous granuloma is an area of low attenuation with a contrast-enhancing capsule. There is usually surrounding oedema and the lesions may be multiple. The tuberculoma is occasionally calcified.

The pre-operative diagnosis is usually appreciated only after recognition of tuberculous foci elsewhere in the body.

The optimal treatment is surgical excision of the tuberculoma, if it is in a surgically accessible region, and antituberculous chemotherapy.

CEREBRAL CRYPTOCOCCOSIS

Cryptococcosis (torula) is a fungal infection which may involve the central nervous system.

C. neoformans is commonly found in avian habitats, and particularly among pigeons. The usual portal of entry is by inhalation of the airborne cryptococcus.

Up to half the patients with central nervous system involvement have an underlying predisposing condition such as sarcoidosis, lymphoma or prolonged steroid therapy, and some patients also have cryptococcal lesions in the lungs.

Cerebral cryptococcosis presents as:

- Meningitis
- Meningo-encephalitis
- Cerebral granuloma.

Meningitis. The most common presentation is meningitis, which is usually subacute, and the patients present with increasing headaches followed by vomiting, seizures and impaired conscious state. Papilloedema occurs in up to half the patients and cranial nerve palsies may develop.

Meningo-encephalitis. This will develop if the meningeal infection extends along the Virchow–Robin spaces into the brain.

Intracerebral granulomas. These are uncommon in cryptococcal infection but may develop in conjunction with meningitis or in isolation (Fig. 12.4).

The CSF studies will show:

- Elevated pressure
- Pleocytosis — usually lymphocytes
- Elevated protein
- Decreased glucose (in 50%)

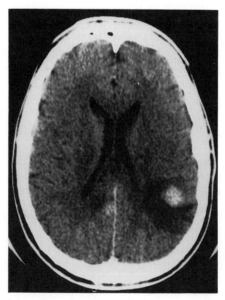

Fig. 12.4 Cryptococcal granuloma. A contrast-enhancing mass with surrounding oedema.

- *C. neoformans* on wet preparation stained with India ink
- Latex cryptococcal agglutination test which detects cryptococcal capsular antigen in CSF.

Treatment

Treatment consists of anticryptococcal therapy using amphotericin B, 5-fluorocytosine or fluconazole. Intracerebral granulomas may need to be excised and a thoracotomy may be necessary for a lung lesion.

Hydrocephalus is a common complication of cryptococcal infection of the central nervous system and should be treated with a shunt.

HYDATID

Hydatid disease is endemic in rural areas, particularly those involved with sheep and cattle raising such as the western region of Victoria in Australia, South America and South Africa. The *echinococcus granulosus* is a small tapeworm, about 6 mm long and with approximately four segments, which lives in the small bowel of canines. The ova are shed in the faeces of dogs and the intermediate hosts are cattle and sheep, although man may also serve in this capacity. Following ingestion the egg capsule is digested and the hexocanth oncosphere penetrates the intestinal mucosa and passes into the portal circulation. Most are trapped in the liver (65%) or lungs (20%) and less than 5% pass to the bone or central nervous system. The embryos lodge within the capillaries and will develop into cysts, which progressively increase in size. The cyst is filled with the clear hydatid fluid, around which is an inner nucleated germinative layer and an outer opaque non-nucleated layer with delicate laminations. Daughter cysts develop from the germinative layer (Fig. 12.5). The inflammatory reaction occurring in the tissue which surrounds the laminated layer does not usually occur in the brain.

The neurosurgeon is involved when the hydatid cyst lodges in the brain, vertebral or orbit.

Intracerebral hydatid cyst

Intracerebral hydatid cyst presents as a mass lesion with slowly developing neurological involvement. The CT scan (Fig. 12.6) shows a hypodense cyst with minimal or low enhancement around the margins.

The surgical treatment is excision and great care should be taken to remove the cyst intact. If the contents are spilled the hydatid disease may be disseminated through the central nervous system and anaphylactic shock has occasionally been reported.

Orbital involvement is usually manifest by unilateral proptosis. If the vertebral column is involved there will be destruction of cancellous bone with vertebral collapse and possible cord compression.

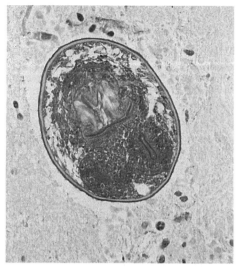

Fig 12.5   Hydatid daughter cyst or 'brood capsule'.

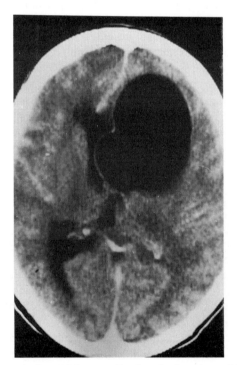

Fig. 12.6   Hydatid cyst in frontal lobe extending into the lateral ventricle.

If cerebral hydatid disease is suspected, clinical examination and radiological investigation may show involvement of the liver and lung. Serological investigations help in the diagnosis.

AIDS

Acquired immune deficiency syndrome (AIDS) is due to the T-cell lymphotrophic virus type III, also known as the human immunodeficiency virus (HIV) type I.

The virus attacks the patient's immune system, rendering the patient prone to opportunistic infection or malignancy. The virus is also neurotropic and can involve the central nervous system directly. Approximately 10% of patients are diagnosed due to central nervous system symptoms at presentation and up to 70% of patients have central nervous symptoms at death.

The central nervous system manifestations are due to:

— Secondary infection. The most common infection is *Toxoplasma gondii*, which is a mass lesion and may present with features indistinguishable from a tumour. The lesions may be solitary or multiple and are usually ring-enhancing on CT scan and MRI (Fig. 12.7). *C. neoformans* is the second most common cause of CNS infection and other infections include tuberculosis, *Candida albicans*, herpes simplex encephalitis (Fig. 12.8) and progressive multifocal leuco-encephalopathy.

— Malignant disease of the brain may be either primary CNS lymphoma, secondary lymphoma from systemic disease and secondary Kaposi's sarcoma.

— The AIDS virus may infect the nervous system directly, causing the AIDS dementia complex in over 90% of patients. This may present

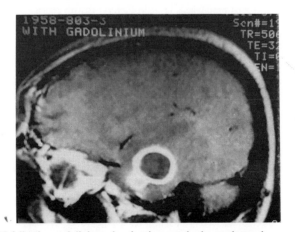

Fig 12.7 MRI following gadolinium showing intracerebral toxoplasmosis.

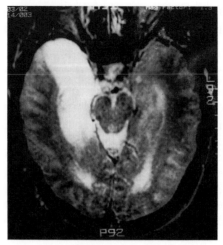

Fig 12.8 MRI of herpes simplex encephalitis with major involvement of the right temporal lobe and less severe changes in the left temporal lobe.

as a behavioural change similar to presenile dementia. Transverse myelitis and peripheral neuropathy may also occur.

The advisability of biopsy of intracerebral lesions in AIDS patients and the possible benefits are not clear at this stage, as there is no satisfactory treatment for the underlying disease process.

FURTHER READING

Becker G L, Knep S, Lance K P, Kaufman L 1980 Amoebic abscesses of the brain. Neurosurgery 6: 192–194
Bell W E 1981 Treatment of bacterial infections of the central nervous system. Annals of Neurology 9: 313–327
Brown E 1987 Antimicrobial prophylaxis in neurosurgery. British Journal of Neurosurgery 1: 159–162
Chan K H, Mann K S, Yue D P 1989 Neurosurgical aspects of cerebral Cryptococcosis. Neurosurgery 25: 44–48
Everett E D, Stausbaugh L J 1980 Antimicrobial agents and the central nervous system. Neurosurgery 6: 691–714
Garvey G 1983 Current concepts of bacterial infections of the central nervous system. Journal of Neurosurgery 59: 735–744
Gotvai P, De Louvis J, Hurley R 1987 The bacteriology and chemotherapy of acute pyogenic brain abscess. British Journal of Neurosurgery 1: 189–204
Haines S J 1989 Efficacy of antibiotic prophylaxis in clean neurosurgical operations. Neurosurgery 24: 401–405
Mampalam T J, Rosenblum M L 1988 Trends in the management of bacterial brain abscesses: a review of 102 cases over 17 years. Neurosurgery 23: 451–458
Mandel G L, Douglas R G, Bennett J E 1985 Principles and practice of infectious diseases, 2nd edn. John Wiley, New York
Richards P 1987 AIDS and the neurosurgeon. British Journal of Neurosurgery 1: 163–172
Rosenblum M L, Levy R M, Bredesen D E 1986 Neurological implications of the acquired immunodeficiency syndrome (AIDS). Clinical Neurosurgery 34: 419–445
Stephanov S 1988 Surgical treatment of brain abscesses. Neurosurgery 22: 724–730

13. Low back pain and leg pain

About 80% of the population suffer from low back pain at some time and 30% of these will develop leg pain due to lumbar spine pathology.

The critical factor in assessing patients with low back pain is whether there are also features of lumbosacral nerve root compression, such as leg pain or focal signs of neural compression in the lower limbs. In general, neurosurgeons are principally concerned with lumbar spine pathology that causes nerve root compression.

Sciatica is the clinical description of pain in the leg due to lumbosacral nerve root compression which is usually in the distribution of the sciatic nerve. Sciatica was first mentioned in an Egyptian manuscript dated 2500–3000 years BC. In 1934, Mixter and Barr established that a prolapsed lumbar intervertebral disc was commonly the cause of sciatica.

Lumbar canal stenosis, a narrowing of the lumbar spinal canal, is the other major spinal cause of leg pain. In 1949, Verbiest specifically defined the clinical significance of the narrow spinal canal and the syndrome of intermittent neurogenic claudication of the legs.

A lumbar disc prolapse can occur at any age in adults but is uncommon in teenagers. The symptoms of lumbar canal stenosis usually commence after the 5th decade. Although lumbar canal stenosis and lumbar disc prolapse may be present in the same patient, they each produce a distinct clinical entity which will be described separately.

SCIATICA

Aetiology (Table 13.1)

The most common cause of sciatica is a lumbar disc prolapse causing nerve root compression. Sciatica-type pain may also occur as a result of bony compression of the nerve root, usually by an osteophyte, and is often associated with lumbar canal stenosis or spondylolisthesis. Narrowing of the 'lateral recess' of the spinal canal may also occur in conjunction with lumbar canal stenosis, and may cause compression of a nerve root. Sciatica may occasionally be caused by tumours of the cauda equina or by pelvic tumours, such as spread from carcinoma of the rectum.

Table 13.1   Causes of sciatica

Prolapsed lumbar disc

Lumbar spondylosis (osteophyte)

Lumbar canal stenosis (lateral recess)

Lumbar spondylolisthesis

Cauda equina tumours (e.g. ependymoma)

Pelvic tumours (e.g. carcinoma rectum)

Spinal arteriovenous malformation (rare)

Anatomy and pathology

Nearly 75% of the lumbar flexion–extension and of total spinal movement occurs at the lumbosacral junction, 20% of lumbar flexion–extension occurs at the L4/5 level and the remaining 5% is at the upper lumbar levels. Consequently, it is not surprising that 90% of lumbar disc prolapses occur at the lower two lumbar levels; the most frequently affected disc is at the L5/S1 level.

The lumbar disc consists of an internal nucleus pulposus surrounded by an external laminar fibrous container — the annulus fibrosus. A disc prolapse may consist of the nucleus pulposus bulging with the annulus being stretched but intact. Alternatively, the nucleus may rupture through the annulus and sequestrate as a free fragment under the posterior longitudinal ligament or lie in the extradural space. Prolapse of the disc is usually in a posterolateral direction, as the posterior longitudinal ligament prevents direct posterior herniation. Infrequently, the disc may herniate laterally to trap the nerve in the neural foramen.

A prolapsed intervertebral disc causes compression of that nerve which runs along the posterior aspect of the disc and down under the pedicle of the vertebra below (Fig. 13.1). Consequently, an L4/5 posterolateral intervertebral disc prolapse will usually compress the L5 nerve root, which runs caudally across the disc to enter the interneural foramen below the L5 pedicle. Similarly, a lumbosacral (L5/S1) disc prolapse will usually affect the S1 nerve root. The infrequent lateral disc prolapse will cause compression of the nerve root at one level higher than expected (e.g. L4 nerve root compression due to L4/5 lateral disc prolapse). In the case of a large disc prolapse, there may be evidence of more than one nerve root compression.

Cauda equina compression may result if the disc herniation is sufficient to rupture the posterior longitudinal ligament and produce a posterior central disc prolapse.

Patient assessment

The patient suffering from sciatica will be in obvious discomfort, which will be reflected by movements and posture when lying supine. The patient lies

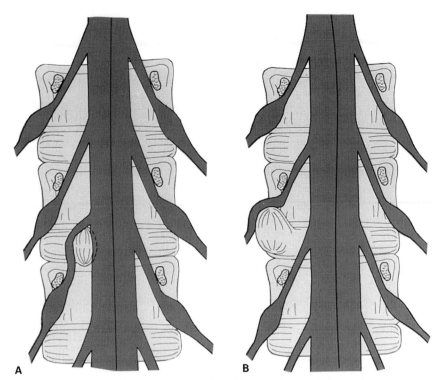

A   B

Fig. 13.1 The diagram shows (A) a posterolateral lumbar disc proplapse causing compression of lumbar nerve root passing across the disc to enter the neural canal below the pedicle and (B) a lateral disc prolapse causing compression of the nerve root passing beneath the pedicle above the disc proplapse.

tilted, usually to the side opposite to the sciatica, with the affected hip and knee slightly flexed taking pressure off the stretched nerve. The pain is worse on movement, coughing, sneezing or straining. Although back pain may be present, the important feature is the pain which radiates down the leg in the distribution of the affected nerve. The pain usually radiates into the buttock, along the posterolateral aspect of the thigh and calf into the foot (S1 nerve root), it may extend into the dorsum of the foot and great toe (L5 nerve root). An L3/4 disc herniation may produce pain in the posterior thigh but, as with an L2/3 disc prolapse, the pain is frequently along the anterior aspect of the thigh. L4 root pain frequently radiates into the anterior aspect of the lower leg. Depending on the degree of nerve root compression, the patient may complain of sensory disturbance such as numbness or tingling in the leg or foot, and weakness may be present. The history must include an assessment of sphincter function, as a large disc prolapse may cause cauda equina compression.

Examination features

Lumbar back movements may be restricted and a scoliosis may be seen, usually concave to the side of the affected leg. Straight leg raising (Lasègue's test) will be restricted on the affected side and, in severe cases, pain in the affected leg will be reproduced when the opposite leg is raised.

Examination of the neurological disability should proceed in an ordered fashion. Initially a search is made for 'wasting' in specific muscle groups — particularly the quadriceps, calf muscles, extensor digitorum brevis muscle and the small muscles of the foot. The patient is then examined for weakness in each of the muscle groups (Tables 13.2 and 13.3). Weakness of dorsiflexion of the foot and extension of the great toe (extensor hallucis longus) is most commonly caused by a prolapsed L4/5 intervertebral disc with involvement of the L5 nerve root; severe cases may result in complete foot drop.

Plantar flexion weakness is caused by compression of the S1 nerve root, usually due to a prolapsed lumbosacral disc. However, plantar flexion is a very strong movement and any weakness may be difficult to elicit unless tested by asking the patient to stand on the toes on the affected side. A

Table 13.2   Segmental innervation of lower limb musculature

L1	Psoas major; psoas minor
L2	Psoas major; iliacus; sartorius; gracilis; pectineus; adductor longus; adductor brevis
L3	Quadriceps; adductors (magnus, longus, brevis)
L4	Quadriceps; tensor fasciae latae; adductor magnus; obturator externus; tibialis anterior; tibialis posterior
L5	Gluteus medius; gluteus minimus; obturator internus; semimembranosus; semitendinosus; extensor hallucis longus; extensor digitorum longus and peroneus tertius; popliteus
S1	Gluteus maximus; obturator internus; piriformis; biceps femoris; semitendinosus; popliteus; gastrocnemius; soleus; peronei (longus and brevis); extensor digitorum brevis
S2	Piriformis; biceps femoris; gastrocnemius; soleus; flexor digitorum longus; flexor hallucis longus; some intrinsic foot muscles
S3	Some intrinsic foot muscles (except abductor hallucis; flexor hallucis; brevis; flexor digitorum brevis; extensor digitorum brevis)

Table 13.3   Segmental innervation of lower limb joint movements

Hip	Flexors, adductors, medial rotators	L1, 2, 3
	Extensors, abductors, lateral rotators	L5, S1
Knee	Extensors	L3, 4
	Flexors	L5, S1
Ankle	Dorsiflexors	L4, 5
	Plantar flexors	S1, 2
Foot	Invertors	L4, 5
	Evertors	L5, S1
	Intrinsic muscles	S2, 3

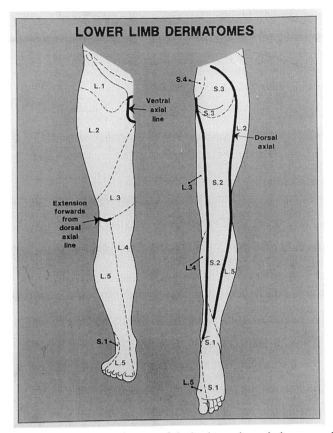

Fig. 13.2 Segmental distribution of nerves of the lumbar and sacral plexuses to the skin of the anterior and posterior aspect of the lower limb.

large prolapsed disc at the L4/5 level may result in some plantar flexion weakness because of compression of the S1 nerve root, and similarly a large lumbosacral disc prolapse may be associated with dorsiflexion weakness due to L5 nerve root compression.

The deep tendon reflexes should be carefully tested as they provide an objective sign of evidence of nerve root compression. The ankle jerk is depressed or absent when the S1 nerve root is compressed, usually by the lumbosacral disc prolapse. Sensation should be tested in the foot and leg (Figure 13.2).

At the end of the examination the patient should be turned prone so that the buttocks can be inspected for atrophy of the gluteal muscles, sensation can be tested along the back of the legs and in the perianal region, and anal tone can be assessed. A rectal examination should be performed if there are clinical features suggestive of a pelvic tumour.

Summary of clinical features

Clinical localisation of the disc prolapse should be possible in the majority of patients with sciatica. The following features are typical (but not invariable) for disc herniation:

L5/S1 prolapsed intervertebral disc

- Pain along the posterior thigh with radiation to the heel
- Weakness of plantar flexion (on occasion)
- Sensory loss in the lateral foot
- Absent ankle jerk.

L4/5 prolapsed intervertebral disc

- Pain along the posterior or posterolateral thigh with radiation to the dorsum of the foot and great toe
- Weakness of dorsiflexion of the toe or foot
- Paraesthesia and numbness of the dorsum of the foot and great toe
- Reflex changes unlikely.

L3/4 prolapsed intervertebral disc

- Pain in the anterior thigh
- Wasting of the quadriceps muscle
- Weakness of the quadriceps function and dorsiflexion of foot
- Diminished sensation over anterior thigh and medial aspect of lower leg
- Reduced knee jerk.

Management

Most patients with sciatica achieve good pain relief with simple conservative treatment and less than 20% will require surgery. The likelihood of symptomatic relief without surgery is related to the pathology of the disc prolapse. A 'bulging' disc is likely to settle with simple conservative measures, but sciatica due to a nucleus pulposus that has herniated out of the disc space and 'sequestrated' outside the annulus will probably need surgery for satisfactory relief of symptoms.

Conservative treatment

Most patients achieve good pain relief following strict bed rest, usually for a period of about 10 days, and the use of simple analgesic agents and non-steroidal anti-inflammatory medication. Although traction is sometimes recommended it probably has only limited benefit and may result in lower leg complications. Resolution of the pain is probably due to a combination of some resorption of the prolapsed disc material, the oedema of the nerve decreasing and possible adaptation of the pain fibres to pressure. Spinal manipulation is not recommended and the concept that a disc prolapse can be 'reduced' by manipulation is a myth. Initially, the only necessary investigations are a plain lumbar spine X-ray and an erythrocyte sedimentation rate (ESR). The lumbar spine X-ray will diagnose an associated spondylolisthesis which may contribute to the sciatica, and it also helps to exclude sinister pathology, such as metastatic tumour involving the spinal vertebrae. The ESR will also exclude systemic disease.

Chemonucleolysis involves the intradiscal injection of a proteolytic enzyme, such as chymopapain, which dissolves disc material. Chymopapain was first isolated in 1941 and has been used intermittently since 1963 in clinical studies. There is a small risk of serious anaphylactic reaction following intradiscal injection. Although chymopapain dissolves the normal nucleus pulposus it has a high failure rate in the treatment of prolapsed disc, as it fails to affect the extruded disc material, and further nerve compression may occur following chemonucleolysis from the disc dissolving and collapsing, resulting in narrowing of the intervertebral neural foramen. The procedure is not recommended for use at this time.

Indications for surgery

Pain. The most common indication for surgery in patients with disc prolapse is pain in the following situations:

- Incapacitating pain despite 10 days of strict bed rest
- Continuing episodes of recurrent pain when mobilising despite adequate relief with bed rest. In this group of patients physiotherapy and a limited trial of a spinal brace might be tried, but they usually have only limited success.

Neurological deficit. A significant weakness or increasing amount of weakness is an indication for early investigation and surgery.

Central disc prolapse. Patients with bilateral sciatica or other features indicating a central disc prolapse, such as sphincter disturbance and diminished perineal sensation, should be investigated promptly. An acute central disc prolapse may lead to acute, severe, irreversible cauda equina compression and should be investigated and treated as an emergency.

Tumour. Surgery is indicated if the clinical features suggest that a tumour could be the cause of sciatica.

INVESTIGATIONS

Lumbar myelography (Fig. 13.3) is the time-honoured investigation for lumbar disc prolapse. The use of water soluble non-ionic contrast material

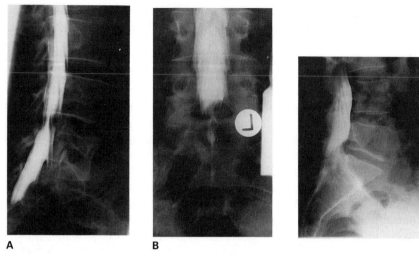

A   **B**

Fig. 13.3 Lumbar myelogram using water soluble contrast medium showing (A) posterolateral L4/5 disc proplapse and (B) complete block due to a large central L5/S1 disc protrusion.

avoids the risk of the postmyelogram arachnoiditis previously seen with the oil-based mediums. Although myelography is now much safer, there is a very small risk of reaction to the contrast medium, particularly epileptic seizures. Some patients suffer headaches following the myelogram. These are due to the lumbar puncture (Ch. 2) and/or the effects of the contrast material.

High quality CT scanning (Fig. 13.4) and MRI (Fig. 13.5) have largely superseded myelography for the diagnosis of lumbar disc prolapse.

Operative procedure for lumbar disc prolapse

The operation involves excision of the disc prolapse with decompression of the affected nerve root.

In the past the operation usually entailed a complete or partial laminectomy, identification of the compressed nerve root, its mobilisation off the disc prolapse and excision of the herniated disc. However, with improvements in instrumentation and magnification, e.g. the operating microscope, most disc prolapses can be excised with minimal disturbance to the normal bony anatomy and with the removal of only a small amount of bone, usually from the adjacent laminae on the side of the prolapse.

A full laminectomy may be necessary prior to the disc excision of a large central disc prolapse causing cauda equina compression.

A percutaneous lumbar discectomy to remove the nucleus pulposus is sometimes advocated for the 'bulging' lumbar disc. However, if the disc is 'bulging' the sciatica will nearly always settle with conservative treatment

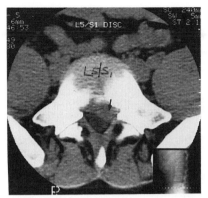
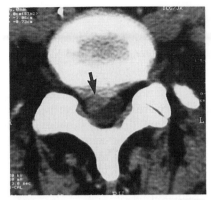

Fig. 13.4 CT scans of lumbar spine showing posterolateral disc prolapses.

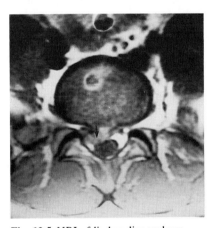
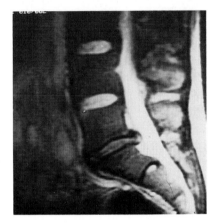

Fig. 13.5 MRI of limbar disc prolapse.

and surgery is not necessary. A percutaneous discectomy of the intradiscal contents will fail to relieve the sciatica if the disc has ruptured through the annulus, because it will not remove the herniated disc material causing the nerve root compression.

Postoperative mobilisation

Most patients commence walking the day after surgery and a gently graduated mobilising programme should be carefully explained to the patient, often with the help of a physiotherapist. Gentle back-strengthening exercises commence after 10 days and the patient should avoid prolonged periods of sitting, lifting and straining for the first 4 weeks. A graduated active exercise programme can commence after the first month.

Prognosis following surgery

The results following lumbar disc surgery are directly related to the accuracy of the pre-operative clinical evaluation. Excellent results can be achieved if:

- There is a good history of sciatica
- There are good signs of nerve root irritations
- The investigations show evidence of a herniated disc
- At surgery the nerve root is stretched by a disc prolapse
- The patient is well motivated.

If any of the above criteria are absent the results following surgery are disappointing.

Recurrent sciatica following surgery occurs in about 10% of cases and is usually due to further disc prolapse, either at the same level or at another level. The principles of management are similar to those described for the initial treatment of sciatica. Recurrent sciatica is occasionally due to adhesions developing around the nerve or intradural arachnoiditis. The treatment is conservative, with judicious use of bed rest followed by gentle mobilising exercises, simple analgesic medication and non-steroidal anti-inflammatory agents. Surgery to excise the adhesions is rarely successful in relieving the pain.

LUMBAR CANAL STENOSIS

The patient with lumbar canal stenosis usually complains of pain radiating diffusely into the legs, particularly when standing or walking. The pain may be a diffuse ache, or is sometimes described as having a 'burning' quality, it is usually relieved with sitting and patients often adopt a posture of bending the body forward when walking to help relieve the discomfort. The pain may be similar to that described by patients with vascular occlusive disease, although a key feature is the presence of pain when standing only.

On occasions there may be features of sciatica-like pain in association with the diffuse pain of lumbar canal stenosis due to entrapment of a nerve root by an osteophyte or within the 'lateral recess' of the canal.

The patient often complains of a subjective feeling of weakness and of a diffuse 'numbness' and 'tingling' radiating down the legs. Sphincter difficulties may occur if the stenosis is particularly severe.

Examination findings

The examination of the lower limbs and back often reveals little or no abnormality. Focal wasting may occur in the lower limbs if the compression is severe, and the ankle jerks may be depressed or absent. Definite sensory disturbance or weakness occur only in the most severe cases.

The peripheral pulses should be checked as the symptoms may mimic those due to peripheral vascular disease.

Pathology and anatomy

The stenosis of the lumbar canal may involve reduction of the sagittal diameter of the canal, narrowing of the 'lateral recess' and stenosis of the neural foramen. The pathology is frequently due to a combination of congenital canal stenosis and developmental pathology, such as lumbar spondylosis with hypertrophy of the facet joints and ligamentum flavum, osteophyte formation and thickening of the laminae causing further narrowing of the canal such that the space for the neural elements become compromised.

The most frequently affected levels are L4/5 and at L3/4. The lumbosacral level may be involved, but this is less common. The stenosis may also be related to a degenerative spondylolisthesis, particularly at the L4/5 level.

Management

The clinical diagnosis of lumbar canal stenosis is usually straightforward, but it should be confirmed by radiological investigations. A lumbar myelogram (Fig. 13.6) has been the usual method of diagnosis for lumbar disc prolapse, although high quality CT scanning (Fig. 13.7) and MRI are replacing the need for myelography. All these radiological studies demonstrate the canal stenosis. The myelogram will show marked indentation of the contrast column and, if the stenosis is severe, there may be a complete block to the flow of contrast.

The clinical features of lumbar canal stenosis do not respond favourably to conservative treatment and surgery is almost invariably successful in relieving the symptoms. The operation consists of a decompressive lumbar laminectomy extending over the whole region of the stenosis with decompression of the lumbar theca and nerve roots.

The patient can be mobilised promptly after the operation and a course of gently graduated active exercises prescribed, usually with the help of a physiotherapist.

BACK PAIN

Low back pain without leg pain or signs of nerve root compression is a common problem. The usual presentations are:

- Acute low back pain, often following minor trauma
- Chronic or recurrent low back pain.

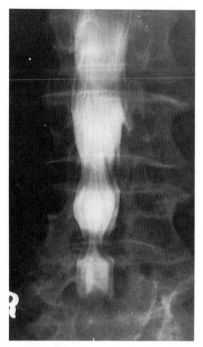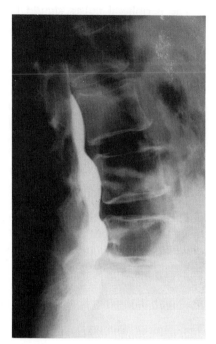

Fig. 13.6 Lumbar myelogram showing lumbar canal stenosis.

Acute sudden onset back pain, following a recognised episode of trauma, is usually due to soft tissue strain. If the injury has been severe it may have caused a fracture or disc herniation. The management of patients with an acute onset of back pain following trauma involves:

- History and examination to exclude symptoms and signs of nerve root compression
- Radiological evaluation to exclude fracture or disc herniation (if severe trauma)
- Conservative management with initial bed rest followed by gentle mobilisation and simple analgesic medication.

Most of the pain and stiffness should settle after a few days, although mild discomfort may linger for some weeks.

The more difficult problem is chronic or recurrent back pain, where the patient gives a history of less severe or even trivial trauma. In some cases no pathological cause will be found. The most common aetiology is due to degenerative disease which includes:

- Lumbar spondylosis
- Spondylolisthesis
- Degenerative disc disease.

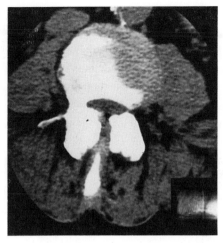

Fig. 13.7 CT scan of lumbar spine showing severe lumbar canal stenosis.

Other uncommon but important causes of low back pain which, in the early stages, may present without pain radiating into the legs or radicular signs, include:

- Spinal tumours (Ch. 15)
- Thoracic disc prolapse (Ch. 15)
- Spinal abscess (Ch. 15)
- Arteriovenous malformation (Ch. 15).

These serious but unusual causes may present with acute or chronic back pain but nearly always have other features, e.g. symptoms or signs of nerve root involvement, which would alert the clinician to the possibility of a more sinister basis for the back pain.

Intra-abdominal pathology should also be considered in patients presenting with back pain, especially:

- Pancreatic disease — pancreatitis or tumours
- Aortic aneurysm
- Renal disease — calculus, infection or tumour.

Lumbar spondylosis, a degenerative disease involving the vertebral column, is the most common demonstrable cause of low back pain and the arthritic process may involve any of the spinal joints and be associated with degenerative disc disease. Low back pain, without features of sciatica, is only rarely caused by disc prolapse, and then only if the prolapse is large and central.

Spondylolisthesis

Spondylolisthesis is a subluxation of one vertebral body on another, usually involving the L4 or L5 levels, and may be due to congenital defects involv-

Table 13.4   Classification of spondylolisthesis

Congenital	
Dysplastic	Congenital deficiency at superior facet of sacrum or inferior facet of 5th lumbar vertebra
Isthmic	Lesion in pars interarticularis
	Lytic fatigue fracture
	Elongated but intact pars
	Acute fracture
Degenerative	In adults, usually at L4/5; a cause of lumbar canal stenosis
Traumatic	
Pathological	Paget's disease, neoplastic, osteogenesis imperfecta and achondroplasia

ing the neural arch or to degenerative changes. Spondylolysis describes a defect in the pars interarticularis, often the precondition for spondylolisthesis.

Various classifications have been used to categorise spondylolisthesis, most subdivide the forms into those of congenital and degenerative origin (Table 13.4).

The congenital dysplastic variety results from congenital deficiencies at the superior facets of the sacrum or the inferior facets of the 5th lumbar vertebra. The lumbosacral junction is incapable of withstanding the truncal forces imposed by the erect stance and there is gradual forward slippage of the 5th vertebral body. This is frequently associated with spina bifida occulta of L5 or S1. The congenital isthmic category involves a defect of the pars interarticularis, either a lytic fatigue fracture or rarely, when the interarticularis fracture occurs following severe trauma.
A further subtype is when the pars is elongated but intact.

Degenerative spondylolisthesis, also known as pseudospondylolisthesis, results from severe localised arthritis of the facet (apophyseal joints) of the slipped vertebrae.

Radiological investigations, including plain X-rays and CT scan, will show the type of spondylolisthesis, the amount of slippage and the associated narrowing of the neural canals (Fig. 13.8).

Clinical presentation

The presenting features involve back pain and leg pain. The initial symptom is usually back pain, which may radiate into the buttocks, but patients often complain of a 'tight' feeling in the upper thighs. Symptomatic children and adolescents often have a gait disturbance, the so-called 'tight hamstring' syndrome.

The vertebral slippage may produce compression of the lumbar nerve roots in the neural foramen. This causes sciatica, the symptoms of which may be indistinguishable from those due to disc prolapse. Narrowing of the bony canal may result in clinical symptoms of 'lumbar canal stenosis'.

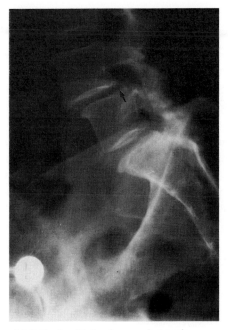

Fig. 13.8 Lumbar spondylolisthesis with lumbar canal stenosis.

Treatment

Children and adolescents. In the majority of children and adolescents symptomatic spondylolisthesis responds to conservative treatment. The following indications are guidelines for lumbar fusion:

- Pain unrelieved by conservative measures
- Progression of subluxation on serial radiological studies
- Subluxation of greater than 30%
- Tight hamstring gait.

The usual surgical procedure is a spinal fusion. Only rarely is a laminectomy necessary, and it should never be performed unless the spine is fused as there will be a progressive slip.

Adults. In most patients conservative therapy involving short periods of bed rest during exacerbations of discomfort, gentle mobilising exercises, simple analgesic medication and non-steroidal anti-inflammatory medication will be sufficient. If some pain persists following the bed rest a period with a properly fitted lumbar brace may be of value. The indications for laminectomy include:

- Symptomatic spinal canal stenosis (that is, symptoms of lumbar canal stenosis)

- Clinical features of nerve root compression (e.g. sciatica) unrelieved by conservative therapy.

A laminectomy decompresses the lumbar theca and nerve roots, usually with satisfactory relief of symptoms.

Spinal fusion, without laminectomy, is occasionally indicated and should be considered in patients with:

— Incapacitating low back pain unrelieved by conservative treatment, where the radiological findings show a relative absence of degenerative disease as a cause for the pain. This is an uncommon situation since, in most cases, it is not possible to identify that the spondylolisthesis is the sole cause of the back pain.
— Documented progressive subluxation. This is uncommon in adults but is a definite indication for spinal fusion.

Some surgeons prefer to combine a decompressive laminectomy with a spinal fusion, usually an intertransverse fusion between the transverse processes.

FURTHER READING

Hardy R W 1982 Lumbar disc disease, Seminars in Neurological Surgery. Raven Press, New York
Mixter W, Barr J 1934 Rupture of the intervertebral disc with involvement of the spinal canal. New England Journal of Medicine 211: 210–214
Sherman F C, Rosenthal R K, Hall J E 1979 Spine fusion for spondylolysis and spondylolisthesis in children. Spine 4: 59–67
Vierbiest H 1954 A radicular syndrome from developmental narrowing of the lumbar vertebral canal. Journal of Bone and Joint Surgery 36B: 230–237
Wiltse L L Newman P H, MacNab I 1976 Classification of spondylolysis and spondylolisthesis. Clinical Orthopaedics 177: 23–29

14. Cervical disc disease and cervical spondylosis

Cervical spine disorders predominantly cause neck pain and/or arm symptoms. Cervical disc prolapse and cervical spondylosis are the two common cervical spine disorders. Degenerative changes in the vertebral column are the basic underlying pathological processes in both these conditions. Although the two conditions may be distinct clinical entities, the shared common pathogenetic mechanism results in a spectrum of clinical presentation depending upon whether the degenerative disease has resulted primarily in disc rupture or cervical spondylosis. As in the lumbar region the critical clinical feature depends on whether there is nerve root entrapment causing arm pain and/or focal signs of neural compression in the upper limb. **Cervical cord compression** due to disc prolapse or cervical spondylosis is discussed in Chapter 15.

CERVICAL DISC PROLAPSE

In the 1934 report of their experiences with ruptured intervertebral discs, Mixter and Barr described four cases with cervical disc disease. Prolapse of an intervertebral disc is much less common in the cervical region than in the lumbar area. The disc herniation occurs most frequently at the C6/7 level and slightly less commonly at the C5/6 level. Disc herniation above these levels is much less common and occurs only infrequently at the C7/T1 level. The predominant frequency of disc prolapse at C6/7 and 5/6 is due to the force exerted at these levels which act as a fulcrum for the mobile spine and head.

Anatomy and pathology

The structure of the cervical disc is essentially the same as in the lumbar region and consists of an internal nucleus pulposus surrounded by the external fibrous lamina, the annulus fibrosus. The role of trauma in the degenerative process and disc herniation is not clear. It is probable that repetitive excessive stresses do exacerbate the normal ageing process and cause disc degeneration. Although it is frequently possible to identify some minor episode of trauma prior to the onset of an acute disc prolapse, a

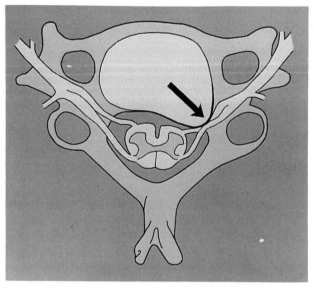

Fig. 14.1   Posterolateral cervical disc prolapse causing compression of the adjacent nerve root.

readily identifiable episode of more major trauma as the precipitating event is much less frequent.

The cervical disc prolapse is usually in the posterolateral direction, because the strong posterior longitudinal ligament prevents direct posterior herniation. The posterolateral disc herniation will cause compression on the adjacent nerve root as it enters and passes through the intervertebral neural foramen. Unlike the lumbar region, the nerves pass directly laterally from the cervical cord to their neural foramen, so that the herniation compresses the nerve at that level (Fig. 14.1). The arrangement of the cervical nerve roots and the relationship to the vertebral bodies differ from the lumbar region — the C1 nerve root leaves the spinal canal between the skull at the foramen magnum and the atlas, and the C8 root, for which there is no corresponding numbered vertebra, passes through the C7/T1 foramen. Consequently, a C5/6 disc prolapse will cause compression of the C6 nerve root, a C6/7 prolapse causes compression of the C7 nerve root and the C7/T1 disc prolapse causes compression of the C8 nerve root.

Occasionally a cervical disc may herniate directly posteriorly, causing compression of the adjacent cervical spinal cord (Ch. 15).

Clinical presentation

The characteristic presenting features of a patient with an acute cervical disc herniation consist of neck and arm pain and the neurological manifestations of cervical nerve root compression.

Although the pain usually begins in the cervical region it characteristically radiates into the periscapular area and shoulder and down the arm (brachial neuralgia). The neck pain commonly regresses while the radiating arm pain becomes more severe. It is usually described as a 'deep' 'boring' or 'aching' pain and the patient is usually severely distressed and debilitated by the discomfort. The distribution of the pain is widespread and conforms to scleratomes (segmental distribution to muscle and bone) rather than to dermatomes. The patient frequently complains of sensory disturbance, particularly numbness or tingling in the distribution of the dermatome affected. The location of the sensory disturbance is more useful than the pain as an indication of root level; thumb (and sometimes index finger) in C6 lesions, middle finger (and sometimes index finger) in C7 lesions, little and ring fingers in C8 lesions. The patient may notice weakness of the arm, particularly if the C7 root is affected as this causes weakness of elbow extension and the movement has only very little supply by other nerve roots (C8).

Examination features

Cervical spine movements will be restricted and the head is often held rigidly to one side, usually moderately flexed and tilted towards the side of the pain in some patients but occasionally away from it in others. Lateral tilt relaxes the roots on the side of the concavity but diminishes the intervertebral foraminae, flexion slightly separates the posterior part of the intervertebral space and lessens the tension in the prolapse. If the disc herniation is long-standing there may be wasting in the appropriate muscle group, particularly the triceps in a C7 root lesion. The patient is then examined for weakness in each of the muscle groups (Tables 14.1 and 14.2). Weakness of elbow extension and finger extension is most commonly caused

Table 14.1   Segmental innervation of upper limb musculature

C3,4	Trapezius; levator scapulae
C5	Rhomboids; deltoids; supraspinatus; infraspinatus; teres minor; biceps
C6	Serratus anterior; latissimus dorsi; subscapularis; teres major; pectoralis major (clavicular head); biceps; coracobrachialis; brachialis; brachioradialis; supinator; extensor carpi radialis longus
C7	Serratus anterior; latissimus dorsi; pectoralis major (sternal head); pectoralis minor; triceps; pronator teres; flexor carpi radialis; flexor digitorum superficialis; extensor carpi radialis longus; extensor carpi radialis brevis; extensor digitorum; extensor digiti minimi
C8	Pectoralis major (sternal head); pectoralis minor; triceps; flexor digitorum superficialis; flexor digitorum profundus; flexor pollicis longus; pronator quadratus; flexor carpi ulnaris; extensor carpi ulnaris; abductor pollicis longus; extensor pollicis longus; extensor pollicis brevis; extensor indicis; abductor pollicis brevis; flexor pollicis brevis; opponens pollicis
T1	Flexor digitorum profundus; intrinsic muscles of the hand (except abductor pollicis brevis; flexor pollicis brevis; opponens pollicis); hypothenar muscles

Table 14.2   Segmental innervation of upper limb joint movements

Shoulder	Abductors and lateral rotators	C5
	Adductors and medial rotators	C6, 7, 8
Elbow	Flexors	C5, 6
	Extensors	C7, 8
Forearm	Supinators	C6
	Pronators	C7, 8
Wrist	Flexors and extensors	C6, 7
Digits	Long flexors and extensors	C7, 8
Hand	Intrinsic muscles	C8, T1

by a C6/7 prolapse with compression of the C7 nerve root. Less commonly, disc herniation with compression of the C5 root will cause weakness of shoulder abduction, compression of the C6 root will cause mild weakness of elbow flexion and compression of C8 will cause weakness of the long flexor muscles.

The deep tendon reflexes provide objective evidence of nerve root compression in the following distribution:

- Biceps reflex   C5
- Brachioradialis (supinator) reflex   C6
- Triceps reflex   C7

Sensation should be tested in the arm and hand and the sensory loss will be characteristic for the nerve root involved (Fig. 14.2) although there may be some overlap.

A full neurological examination must be performed and particular care taken to assess the presence in the lower limbs of long tract signs, such as increased tone, a pyramidal pattern of weakness, hyper-reflexia or an upgoing plantar response. If there is a cervical disc herniation these features will indicate that it is compressing the spinal cord.

Summary of clinical features

Clinical localisation of disc prolapse is possible in most patients with brachial neuralgia due to cervical disc prolapse. The following features are typical (but not invariable) for disc herniation:

C6/C7 prolapsed intervertebral disc (C7 nerve root)

- Weakness of elbow extension
- Absent triceps jerk
- Numbness or tingling in the middle or index finger.

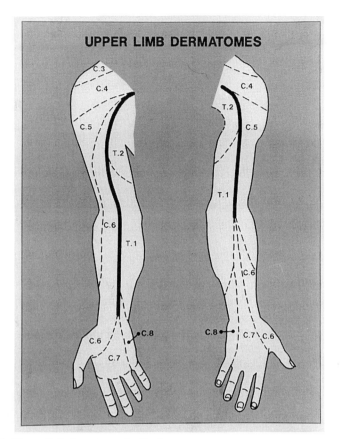

Fig. 14.2   Upper limb dermatome distribution.

C5/6 prolapsed intervertebral disc (C6 nerve root)

- Depressed supinator reflex
- Numbness or tingling in the thumb or index finger
- Occasionally mild weakness of elbow flexion.

C7/T1 prolapsed intervertebral disc (C8 nerve root)

- Weakness of long flexor muscles
- Diminished sensation in ring and little finger and on the medial border of the hand and forearm
- Triceps jerk may be depressed.

Differential diagnosis

The clinical features of an acute cervical disc prolapse, with severe neck and arm pain and commonly diminished sensation in the dermatome of the affected cervical root, is so characteristic that in the vast majority of cases the diagnosis is self-evident. The most common cause of radiating arm pain, other than acute prolapse, is spondylosis but, as has been indicated, disc prolapse and spondylosis are aspects of one continuing degenerative process and, in the cervical region, the distinction between them becomes blurred. Other unlikely but possible differential diagnoses include:

- Cervical nerve root compression by a spinal tumour (e.g. meningioma, neurofibroma) (Ch. 15)
- Thoracic outlet syndrome (Ch. 17)
- Pancoast's tumour infiltrating the roots of the brachial plexus
- Peripheral nerve entrapments, such as carpal tunnel syndrome, median nerve entrapment in the cubital fossa and tardy ulnar palsy (Ch. 17).

Management

Most patients with arm pain due to an acute soft cervical disc herniation achieve good pain relief with conservative treatment. This should include bed rest, a cervical collar, simple analgesic medication, non-steroidal anti-inflammatory medication and muscle relaxants. Manipulation of the neck is potentially hazardous and is contra-indicated.

The indications for further investigation and surgery are:

1. Pain
   (a) continuing severe arm pain for more than 10 days without benefit from conservative therapy
   (b) chronic or relapsing arm pain
2. Significant weakness in the upper limb that does not resolve with conservative therapy
3. Evidence of a central disc prolapse causing cord compression — this should be investigated urgently.

Radiological investigations

The cervical myelogram using water based non-ionic iodine contrast material is the most useful investigation for determining the presence and site of the disc herniation (Fig. 14.3). Computerised tomography scanning by itself is frequently not helpful but may be the preferred investigation if performed following intrathecal iodine contrast, because it will clearly demonstrate a disc herniation, and smaller volumes of intrathecal contrast are necessary than with myelography (Fig. 14.4).

Magnetic resonance imaging does not as yet have sufficient resolution to show posterolateral disc herniation, but improvements in the technique will inevitably improve its performance so that it will eventually become the most useful technique.

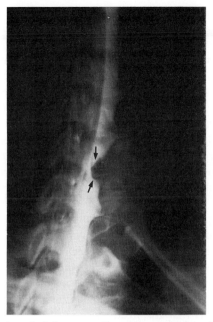

Fig. 14.3 Posterolateral cervical disc protrusion with compression of the cervical nerve root.

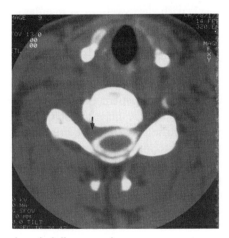

Fig. 14.4 Posterolateral cervical disc protrusion.

Operative procedure

The two most commonly performed operations for cervical disc prolapse are:

1. Cervical foramenotomy with excision of the disc prolapse
2. Anterior cervical discectomy, with or without subsequent fusion.

Cervical foramenotomy. This involves fenestration of the bone posteriorly, to provide direct access to the cervical nerve root, and disc prolapse. A small amount of bone from the lateral margins of the adjacent lamina and articular facets are removed to identify the nerve root in the foramen. Further bone can then be removed from around the nerve root to enlarge the neural canal. The nerve root is gently retracted and the disc herniation excised. The major advantages of the technique are that the nerve is directly decompressed both by removal of the disc herniation and by enlargement of the foramen, and cervical fusion is not necessary. The major disadvantage is the possibility of recurrent disc herniation, but this is very uncommon. In general, the results of the procedure are very satisfactory, with excellent relief of arm pain and, provided the nerve has not been irreparably damaged by long-standing disc herniation, return of full strength to the arm.

Anterior cervical discectomy. This involves an anterior approach to remove the cervical disc. Some surgeons perform formal fusion at the level using bone taken from the iliac crest or cadaver bone but, provided the disc has been completely removed, a formal fusion is usually not necessary as spontaneous fibrous or bony fusion will occur across the disc space. The major disadvantage is that the fusion will result in additional stress at the adjacent cervical levels, thereby rendering them more prone to degenerative disease.

An anterior approach with disc excision is mandatory for a central disc protrusion.

Postoperative care

Whatever approach is used, the patient is encouraged to mobilise the day after surgery. A soft cervical collar may be useful in the first week after a foramenotomy to minimise the neck pain. A firm collar is usually worn for the first 4–6 weeks after anterior discectomy, or until there is evidence of fusion.

The prognosis for pain relief following the operation is excellent provided the diagnosis has been accurate and the nerve decompressed.

CERVICAL SPONDYLOSIS

Cervical spondylosis is a degenerative arthritic process involving the cervical spine and affecting the intervertebral disc and zygapophyseal joints. Radiological findings of cervical spondylosis are present in 75% of people over 50 years of age who have no significant symptoms referable to the cervical spine.

Pathological changes

The degenerative process resulting in cervical spondylosis and its progression occur in most cases largely as a result of the inevitable stresses and traumas that occur to the cervical spine as a result of the normal activities of daily living. It is probable that the process is aggravated by repetitive or chronic trauma, as may occur in some occupations, and as a result of an episode of severe trauma.

The process principally involves the intervertebral discs and zygapophyseal joints. Reduced water content and fragmentation of the nuclear portion of the cervical discs are natural ageing processes. As the disc degenerates there is greater stress on the articular cartilages of the vertebral end plates and osteophytic spurs develop around the margins of the disintegrating end plates, projecting posteriorly into the spinal canal and anteriorly into the prevertebral space. The degenerative process involving the zygapophyseal joints will also lead to osteophyte formation. The intervertebral foramen may be narrowed by these osteophytes, so causing compression of the nerve root. The osteophyte formation that causes compression of the nerve in the neural foramen and which is seen around a bulging annulus, is sometimes called a 'hard disc protrusion', as distinct from the acute 'soft' cervical disc herniation.

The spondylitic process may cause narrowing of the spinal canal as a result of osteophyte formation, particularly the formation of hypertrophic bony ridges at the anterior intervertebral spaces of the spinal canal and hypertrophy of the ligamenta flava. This may result in compression of the underlying cord. Such compression is maximal during hyperextension of the neck and may cause cervical myelopathy (Ch. 15).

Presenting features

There are three major manifestations of cervical spondylosis, depending on whether there is compression of a cervical nerve root or the spinal cord:

1. Neck pain
2. Radiating arm pain
3. Cervical myelopathy (Ch. 15).

Neck pain. This is the most common clinical manifestation of cervical spondylosis and its onset may be precipitated by minor trauma. The pain usually settles over a period of a few days or weeks but frequently recurs and is associated with increasing stiffness of the neck.

Radiating arm pain. Brachial neuralgia (radiating arm pain) results from a nerve root being compressed in the neural foramen by osteophyte formation, with subsequent narrowing of the bony canal. The patient frequently has a history of intermittent neck pain as a result of cervical spondylosis for some months or years and the onset of the arm pain may be precipitated by an episode of minor trauma. The clinical features are similar to the neuralgia caused by an acute soft disc prolapse, in that the pain radiates diffusely into the periscapular area and shoulder, and into the upper limb in a sclerotome distribution. There may be other features of nerve root compression including numbness and tingling in the appropriate dermatome distribution, and weakness of the arm. Although the clinical features may be almost indistinguishable from those due to an acute soft disc prolapse, the process is usually not as acute and the patient often has a history of intermittent or chronic pain. Wasting of a muscle group in the appropriate nerve root distribution is more common because of the longer history, but the examination findings will otherwise be similar to those seen with an acute soft disc protrusion.

Cervical myelopathy. This may result from cervical spondylosis causing narrowing of the spinal canal with compression of the underlying spinal cord. The features of progressive weakness and sensory disability are described in Chapter 15.

Radiological findings

Plain cervical spine X-rays (Fig. 14.5) show:

- Narrowing of the disc space (the C5/C6 and C6/C7 levels are the most commonly affected)
- Osteophyte formation with encroachment into either the spinal canal or neural foramen
- Reduced mobility at positions of fusion and increased mobility at adjacent levels.

The indications for further radiological investigations depend on the clinical presentation. Although CT scan will clearly show the bony changes seen on the plain cervical spine X-rays, it is not indicated for the investigation of cervical spondylosis which is causing neck pain. Nerve root entrapment, causing arm pain, is best visualised by either a CT scan following intrathecal contrast or a cervical myelogram with water based non-ionic iodine contrast. The radiological assessment of cervical myelopathy is discussed in Chapter 15.

Differential diagnosis

Neck pain

There are numerous possible causes of neck pain, depending on the method of clinical presentation and the presence of neurological signs in the limbs. The most common cause of neck pain is a minor muscular or ligamentous strain which usually follows minor trauma. If there has been a major injury

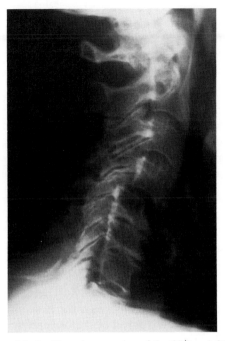

Fig. 14.5 Cervical spondylosis. There is narrowing of the C5/6 and C6/7 disc spaces, osteophyte formation and a subluxation at the C4/5 level.

then a fracture dislocation or acute disc herniation should be considered and excluded. Other rare causes of neck pain are spinal tumours or spinal abscess.

The other possible diagnoses in a patient presenting with arm pain are described earlier in the chapter.

Management

Neck pain due to cervical spondylosis

The pain usually resolves with simple conservative measures, including the use of non-steroidal anti-inflammatory medication and simple analgesics. During an acute episode the patient may be more comfortable in a soft cervical collar. As the pain subsides the patient should be encouraged to perform simple mobilising exercises which may be best undertaken with the supervision of a physiotherapist. If the episodes become frequent and severe the patient may need to consider a change of lifestyle, particularly work practices and recreational behaviour which might be aggravating the cervical spondylosis.

Arm pain

The symptoms frequently settle with the management described above. The indications for surgery are:

- Severe pain that does not settle with conservative treatment over 2–3 weeks
- Chronic or recurrent pain
- Progressive weakness in the arm which causes functional disability. The most frequently involved nerve root producing significant functional weakness is the C7 root, but the C8 or C5 roots may also result in functional disability as a result of long-standing root compression.

The choice of surgical procedure is similar to that for an acute soft disc prolapse. Cervical foramenotomy, with decompression of the nerve root, excision of the osteophytes and enlargement of the neural foramen, is an effective surgical technique. As the spondylitic process is often at multiple levels, two roots often need to be decompressed. Some surgeons favour an anterior approach and cervical discectomy. There is controversy over whether to excise the osteophyte, although the best results follow decompression of the nerve root by removal of the osteophyte extending into the neural foramen. As discussed previously, there is some debate as to whether it is necessary to perform a formal fusion following the disc excision.

Cervical myelopathy (see Ch. 15).

Further reading

Adams C B T, Logue V 1971 Studies in cervical spondylitic myelopathy: I. Movement of the cervical roots, dura and cord and their relationship to the course of the extrathecal roots. Brain 94: 557–568
Hoff J 1980 Cervical spondylosis. In: Wilson C B, Hoff J T (eds) Current surgical management of neurological disease. Churchill Livingstone, New York
Lees F, Aldren-Turner J W 1963 Natural history and prognosis of cervical spondylosis. British Medical Journal 2: 1607–1610
Lunsford L D, Bissonette D, Jannetta P J, Sheptak P E, Zorub D S 1980 Anterior surgery for cervical disc disease. Part I. Treatment of lateral cervical disc herniation 253 cases. Journal of Neurosurgery 53: 1–11
Martins A N 1976 Anterior cervical discectomy with and without interbody bone graft. Journal of Neurosurgery 44: 290–295

15. Spinal cord compression

Compression of the spinal cord is a common neurosurgical problem. Although the initial clinical manifestations vary considerably, if the condition is unrecognised and untreated the eventual outcome will inevitably be disabling paralysis and sphincter disturbance. Spinal cord compression requires early diagnosis and urgent treatment if these disastrous consequences are to be avoided.

The compression may occur at any position from the cervicomedullary junction to the conus medullaris. Although compression of the cauda equina is not strictly spinal cord compression, the pathophysiology and treatment is so similar that it is considered with cord compression.

Spinal trauma may also cause cord compression but will be discussed separately in the next chapter (Ch. 16).

Pathology

The spinal cord may be compressed by lesions situated:

- Extradurally   80%
- Intradural, extramedullary   15%
- Intramedullary   5%

The major groups of pathological causes are:

1. Tumour
   a. metastatic
   b. primary
2. Degenerative
   a. disc prolapse
   b. osteoporosis/spondylosis
3. Infection
   a. vertebral body
   b. disc space
   c. extradural
   d. intradural

4. Haematoma
   a. spontaneous (trauma)
   b. arteriovenous malformation
5. Developmental
   a. syrinx
   b. arteriovenous malformation
   c. arachnoid cyst.

Although there is a large range of possible causes of cord compression, in clinical practice the large majority are due to:

1. Extradural
   a. metastatic tumour
   b. extradural abscess
2. Intradural, extramedullary
   a. meningioma
   b. schwannoma
3. Intramedullary
   a. glioma (astrocytoma and ependymoma).

Table 15.1 shows a list of the possible causes of spinal cord compression and their primary positions.

Presenting features

There are two major presenting features that are the hallmarks of spinal cord compression:

1. Neurological deficit
2. Pain

There is considerable variation in the manner in which these two major features present, depending on:

- The site of the compression and the involvement of adjacent nerve roots
- The speed of the compression
- The pathological cause and the nature of the compressive lesion
- The involvement of the blood supply of the spinal cord.

Pain

Pain is a common early feature of cord compression and often precedes the onset of any neurological disturbance, sometimes by many months. Pain is due to:

— Involvement of local, pain-sensitive structures, such as the bone of the vertebral column. Pain in the back may also be caused by spasm of the erector spinae muscles.

Table 15.1   Spinal cord compression

Extradural
    Metastatic tumour
    Lymphoma
    Myeloma
    Leukaemia
    Primary vertebral body tumour
    Chordoma
    Disc prolapse
    Osteoporosis/spondylosis
    Extradural abscess
    Extradural haematoma

Intradural, extramedullary
    Meningioma
    Schwannoma
    Arteriovenous malformation
    Spinal seeding from intracranial tumour (medulloblastoma, ependymoma)

Intramedullary
    Glioma — ependymoma, astrocytoma
    Arteriovenous malformation, haematoma
    Abscess
    Metastatic tumour
    Syrinx
    Haemangioma

— Pain of spinal root origin due to involvement of the nerve root at the level of the compression. In cervical compression nerve root involvement will cause pain radiating into the upper limb in the distribution of the nerve root. Thoracic cord compression, with involvement of the thoracic nerve roots, will often be associated with pain radiating around the chest wall. This 'girdle' pain is an important feature associated with a lesion which may cause cord compression. Whereas back pain in general is a non-specific common symptom, usually associated with degenerative disease, 'girdle' pain should arouse the suspicion of an underlying sinister cause. The pain is often aggravated by coughing and straining.
— 'Central' pain due to spinal cord compression itself is an unpleasant diffuse dull ache, often with a 'burning' quality, and is frequently described with difficulty. It may involve a limb or side of the trunk, depending on the segment involved.

Flexion or extension of the neck may cause 'electric shock' or tingling radiating down through the body to the extremities of the limbs. This is called Lhermitte's sign, and is typically associated with cervical cord involvement, either by a compressive lesion or due to an inflammatory process.

Neurological deficit

The neurological features of spinal cord compression consist of:

- Progressive weakness
- Sensory disturbance
- Sphincter disturbance.

Motor impairment. The level of paralysis will depend on the position of the cord compression. Thoracic cord compression will result in a progressive paraparesis of the lower limbs and if the cervical cord is involved the upper limbs will also be affected. The compression of the corticospinal pathways will result in an upper motor neuron weakness with little or no wasting, increased tone, increased deep tendon reflexes and positive Babinski response. As the cord becomes more severely compressed a complete paraplegia will result. The weakness has an initial 'pyramidal' pattern, with the flexor movements being most severely affected whilst the extensor movements, e.g. hip extension, knee extension and plantar flexion, are relatively preserved.

As described in Chapter 1, the pattern of weakness may also be influenced by the position of the compressing lesion. The descending corticospinal pathways decussate at the level of the cervicomedullary junction so that lateral compression in the spinal cord will initially cause weakness, predominantly on the side of the compressing lesion.

The compressing mass will cause weakness of the nerve root segment at the involved level. In the cervical region this will result in a lower motor neuron weakness of the involved nerve roots in the upper limb, with the other associated features of focal wasting and depressed reflexes at that level. A mass below T1 in the thoracic area will cause no clinically demonstrable nerve root weakness. In the lumbar region involvement of the conus medullaris may produce a mixture of lower motor neuron features and upper motor neuron signs in the lower limbs.

Cauda equina compression produces a lower motor neuron pattern of weakness.

Sensory disturbance. A **sensory level** is the hallmark of spinal cord compression. In the thoracic region this will produce a sensory level to all modalities of sensation over the body or trunk, although there may be sparing of some modalities in the early stages of compression. A useful guide to remember is the T4 dermatome lies at the level of the nipple, the T7 at the xiphisternum and the T10 at the umbilicus. Careful examination will often reveal a band of minor hyperaesthesia at the level of the compression. If the compression is in the cervical area there will be sensory loss in the upper limb in the appropriate dermatomal pattern (Fig. 15.1).

Specific patterns of sensory loss will occur depending on the tracts within the cord that are initially involved. A laterally placed mass will initially cause a 'Brown-Séquard' syndrome. There will be contralateral impairment of pain and temperature sensation, with ipsilateral pyramidal weakness and

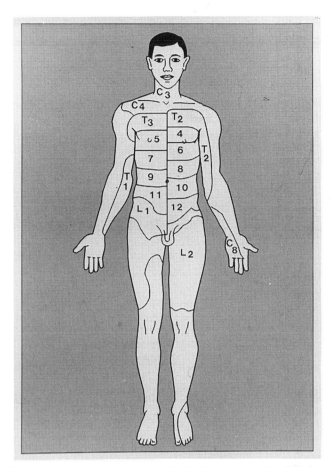

Fig. 15.1   Dermatomes of the trunk (thoracic) and adjacent cervical and lumbar areas. The sensory level will be a useful guide to the level of cord compression. (See also Figs. 13.2 and 14.2).

impairment of joint position sense, vibration and fine touch. This is due to the fibres of pain and temperature crossing to the opposite side of the spinal cord to ascend in the lateral spinothalamic tracts, whereas the fibres of proprioception ascend in the dorsal columns of the spinal cord and do not cross until they reach the low medullary region. Intrinsic lesions affecting the central cord in the cervicothoracic region and damaging the sensory neurons crossing to the lateral spinothalamic tract will initially cause a 'cape-like' distribution of thermoanalgesia, such as occurs in syringomyelia (Ch. 11, Fig. 11.3). The sacral fibres lie peripherally in the lateral spinothalamic tracts and so some degree of sacral sparing can occur, even with large intrinsic lesions. Analgesia affecting primarily the saddle area (buttocks and upper posterior thigh) occur particularly in cauda equina or conus medullaris lesion.

Sphincter involvement. Sphincter disturbance occurs following compression of the spinal cord, conus medullaris or cauda equina. The first symptom is difficulty in initiating micturition and this is followed by urinary retention, which is often relatively painless. Constipation and faecal incontinence will subsequently occur. The clinical signs include an enlarged, palpable bladder, diminished peri-anal sensation and decreased anal tone.

In summary the clinical features of spinal cord compression are:

- Pain — local and radicular
- Progressive weakness of the limbs
- Sensory disturbance — often a sensory level
- Sphincter disturbance.

Management

The general principles of management are similar whatever the cause of the cord compression. It is again emphasised that the investigations and treatment must be undertaken as a matter of urgency once the diagnosis is suspected, so as to reduce the possibility that the neurological deficit will progress or become permanent. **Spinal cord compression is a neurosurgical emergency.**

Radiological investigations

The radiological studies undertaken to confirm the diagnosis of spinal cord compression include:

- Plain spinal X-rays
- Myelography
- CT scan (with intrathecal contrast)
- MRI.

Spinal myelography, using water soluble, iodine based contrast agents injected intrathecally, has been the benchmark investigation for confirming the diagnosis and the level of spinal cord compression. The contrast is injected intrathecally in the lumbar region and the level of the compression can be identified. If there is a complete block to the flow of contrast it is often helpful to inject further contrast using a C1/2 puncture, so as to ascertain the upper level of the block. The pattern of 'block' on the myelogram will usually demonstrate whether the cord has been compressed by an extradural mass or an extramedullary intradural tumour, or whether the cord is swollen by an intramedullary lesion (Fig. 15.2).

The level should be marked on the skin and a further X-ray taken with a radio-opaque marker in place to aid surgical localisation.

Computerised tomography scanning at the level of the compression and just above and below the area will often help to further demonstrate the

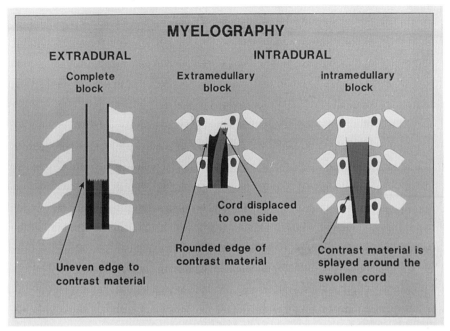

Fig. 15.2 Diagram of myelographic appearance due to extradural, intradural extramedullary, or intramedullary lesions.

nature and cause of the compression and give more detail about the adjacent bony structures.

Plain spinal X-rays are essential in patients with spinal cord compression. The important radiological features are:

- Focal bony destruction indicating a metastatic lesion, e.g. erosion of a pedicle, vertebral collapse
- Evidence of multiple destructive or sclerotic lesions, indicating multiple metastatic tumours
- Thinning of a pedicle and widening of the interpedicular distance, suggestive of long-standing intradural compression
- Scalloping of the posterior surface of the vertebral body, indicating long-standing intradural lesion
- Expansion of an intervertebral foramen on oblique X-rays, indicative of a neurofibroma.
- Destruction of a disc space suggestive of infection.

Magnetic resonance imaging is of considerable value in diagnosing the cause and position of spinal cord compression and, when more widely available, will probably replace myelography.

Other investigations

The other investigations performed in patients with spinal cord compression are:

- Further investigations to evaluate the extent of the disease and site of origin may be useful in patients with metastatic disease prior to surgery. However, these investigations should *not* delay the definitive treatment
- Many patients with malignant disease have a poor general medical condition and require cardiorespiratory and biochemical assessment prior to surgery.

Treatment

The standard treatment for spinal cord compression is urgent surgery, except in some cases of compression due to malignant tumour, in which treatment with high dose glucocorticosteroids and radiotherapy is indicated. This will be discussed further in the next section.

MALIGNANT SPINAL CORD COMPRESSION

By far the most common cause of spinal cord compression results from extradural compression by malignant tumours. The most common tumours are:

- Carcinoma of the lung
- Carcinoma of the breast
- Carcinoma of the prostate
- Carcinoma of the kidney
- Lymphoma
- Myeloma.

Less common tumours include leukaemias, carcinoma of the thyroid and primary sarcomas.

The thoracic region is by far the most commonly affected but metastases may occur at any site and are often multiple. The compression is due to the tumour itself or to vertebral collapse, or a combination of these.

The clinical features are basically as described in the previous section. The patient invariably complains of pain local to the involved region and a radicular girdle pain is frequently present. Although, in retrospect, minor symptoms of cord compression may have been present for a few weeks or even months, there is often a rapid neurological deterioration resulting in paralysis, sensory disturbance and sphincter difficulties.

Urgent investigation and treatment is essential if permanent severe disability (Figs. 15.3, 15.4 and 15.5) is to be avoided.

The standard treatment has been a decompressive laminectomy over the

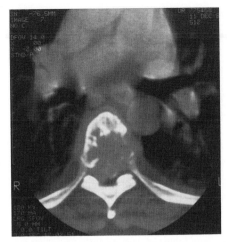

Fig. 15.3 Extensive destruction of vertebral body and adjacent neural arch with invasion into spinal canal by metastatic carcinoma.

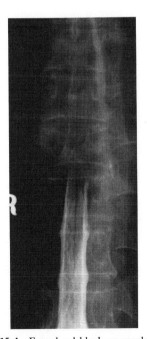 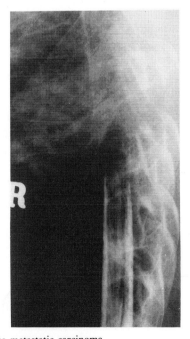

Fig. 15.4 Extradural block on myelogram due to metastatic carcinoma.

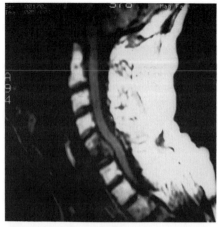

Fig. 15.5 MRI of metastatic tumour in cervical vertebral bodies and compression of spinal cord.

affected levels. The exposed tumour is resected as much as possible to relieve the cord compression. Glucocorticosteroids (e.g. dexamethasone) are often used to reduce local oedema of the spinal cord and the surgery is usually followed by radiotherapy.

The initial results following surgical decompression depend largely on the severity and length of time of the pre-operative compression. Patients with a complete paraplegia of more than 36 hours have a poor prognosis for neurological recovery.

Some studies have shown that urgent radiotherapy, with high dose glucocorticosteroids, may be effective in controlling the tumour causing spinal cord compression. The treatment must be commenced immediately following diagnosis and should be considered:

- If the patient has a known primary tumour that is radiosensitive (e.g. carcinoma of the prostate, lymphoma)
- If there is a partial incomplete neurological lesion that is only slowly progressive
- If sphincter function is retained.

This form of treatment is also particularly advantageous if the tumour is mostly anterior to the spinal cord because the compression from this type of lesion may not be satisfactorily relieved following a posterior decompressive laminectomy.

Conversely, radiotherapy as the primary form of treatment is not appropriate if:

- The tumour is known to be radioresistant
- The compression is primarily due to bone collapse rather than tumour mass

- The origin of the tumour is not known
- There is a rapidly progressive neurological deficit and/or sphincter disturbance.

In a small number of cases, the metastatic tumour will be localised to one or two vertebral bodies only and will be causing compression anterior to the spinal cord. In this situation a posterior decompressive laminectomy may not relieve the compression and may result in vertebral instability. Vertebral body resection, excision of the anterior tumour and reconstruction with fixation may be appropriate. However, this entails a very major operative procedure and may not be tolerated or indicated in debilitated patients with widespread metastatic tumour.

SCHWANNOMA (neurofibroma)

Schwannomas are the most common of the intrathecal tumours and may occur at any position. They arise invariably from the posterior nerve roots and grow slowly to compress the adjacent neural structures. Occasionally, the intrathecal tumour extends through the intervertebral foramen to form a 'dumbell' tumour and the tumour may rarely present as a mass in the thorax, neck or posterior abdominal wall.

The presenting features are those of a slowly growing tumour causing cord compression. Pain in a radicular distribution is the most common first symptom and is often present for several years. In the cervical region there may be evidence of long-standing neurological involvement of the cervical nerve root prior to the features of cord compression becoming apparent. There is frequently some degree of a Brown-Sequard syndrome due to the lateral position of the tumour.

The plain X-rays show radiological evidence of bone erosion and enlargement of the intervertebral foramen is typical (Fig. 15.6). A large tumour will erode the adjacent part of the vertebral body and there is frequently an increase in the interpedicular distance.

The myelogram and CT scan (following intrathecal contrast) will show an intradural tumour with cord compression (Fig. 15.7). The CT scan will also show the extraspinal extension. Magnetic resonance imaging (with gadolinium contrast) will replace myelography for the diagnosis of these lesions.

The treatment is surgical excision of the tumour. Access to the tumour is obtained by a laminectomy. If there is a large extraspinal extension it may be necessary to obtain additional exposure through the neck, chest or abdomen.

SPINAL MENINGIOMA

Spinal meningiomas occur particularly in middle-aged or elderly patients and show a marked female predominance. The thoracic region of the spinal

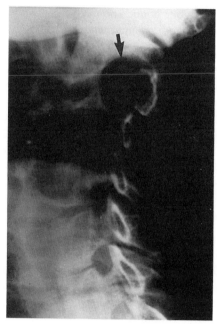

Fig. 15.6   Enlarged neural foramen due to schwannoma.

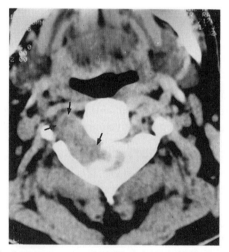

Fig. 15.7   'Dumbell' schwannoma extending through intervertebral neural foramen. The intrathecal contrast medium outlines the tumour in the spinal canal causing spinal cord compression.

cord is the most common site and they are invariably situated intradurally, causing marked compression of the adjacent cord.

The tumours grow extremely slowly and there is usually a long history of ill-defined back pain and a very slowly progressive paralysis prior to diagnosis.

The plain X-rays may show erosion of the pedicles due to long-standing intradural compression. Hyperostosis, which is frequently present in cranial meningiomas, does not occur in spinal meningiomas.

The diagnosis will be made using the radiological investigations mentioned earlier in the chapter. Magnetic resonance imaging with gadolinium contrast will give an accurate diagnosis of these tumours and, when more readily available, will replace myelography (Fig. 15.8).

The treatment of spinal meningioma is resection of the tumour and the involved dura. The tumour often lies lateral to the cord and, following the excision, there is an excellent chance of neurological improvement, even when there is substantial neurological disability at the time of diagnosis. Occasionally, the tumour lies directly anterior to the spinal cord and resection without further injury to the cord in these circumstances is difficult.

INTRAMEDULLARY TUMOURS

Intrinsic intramedullary tumours are uncommon and much less frequent than the extradural or intradural extramedullary tumours mentioned previously. The tumours usually present in the 3rd and 4th decades although they may occur at any age. The two most common tumours of the spinal cord are:

1. Ependymoma
2. Astrocytoma.

Ependymomas comprise about 60% of intrinsic spinal tumours and the majority of these arise from the filum terminale, causing compression of the cauda equina. Most of these tumours have a 'myxopapillary' appearance.

Astrocytomas of the spinal cord may occur at any level and frequently initially have a low grade histological appearance.

Presenting features

The presenting features of the tumours depend on the level of cord involved. The ependymomas arising in the filum terminale will cause features of cauda equina compression. There is often a history of low back and leg pain, progressive weakness in the legs (often with radicular features), sensory loss over the saddle area and eventually sphincter disturbance.

Spinal rigidity and pain are common features in patients with intrinsic spinal cord tumours, particularly in children, and there is a progressive paralysis and sensory loss. A 'cuirasse' (cape-like) pattern of sensory loss

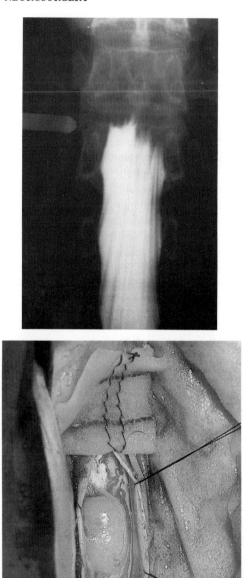

Fig. 15.8   (A) Intradural extramedullary block on myelogram due to meningioma. (B) Meningioma with severe compression of adjacent spinal cord.

may be seen initially but there is invariably progression to involve all lower segments below the level of the tumour. Tumour expansion and involvement of the anterior horn cells may produce a lower motor neuron weakness and wasting of the corresponding muscle groups, but long tract involvement causes upper motor neuron weakness below the level of the lesion.

The progression of the spinal cord involvement will depend on the histological nature of the tumour. Although the tumours are initially low grade, they may evolve into a more aggressive morphology.

Radiology

The plain X-rays will show expansion of the spinal canal with increase of the interpedicular distance through several segments, scalloping of the vertebral bodies and sometimes thinning of the neural arches. Imaging of the spinal cord will show expansion of the cord and no evidence of extrinsic compression. A syrinx is frequently associated with an intramedullary tumour (Fig. 15.9).

Treatment

It is often possible to obtain a complete macroscopic excision of an ependymoma arising from the filum terminale which is causing compression of the cauda equina. Meticulous microsurgical techniques are necessary to dissect the tumour from the nerve roots. In some ependymomas of the spinal cord it is possible to obtain a plane of cleavage and perform a partial or even complete resection. However, it is not possible to resect astrocytomas of the cord and surgery is usually restricted to obtaining a

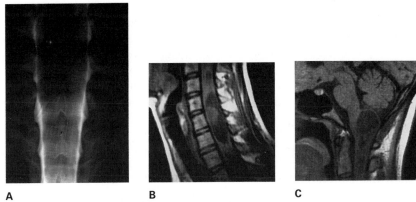

A   B   C

Fig. 15.9 Cervical cord intramedullary ependymoma in a 24 year old female. (A) Myelogram shows typical features of intramedullary tumour with 'splaying' of contrast around the expanded cervical cord. (B) MRI shows the tumour and the associated syrinx cavity extending up into the medulla.

diagnosis by biopsy, aspiration of cyst cavities and exclusion of other possible rare resectable lesions. Radiotherapy is usually administered.

The prognosis is good if an ependymoma can be resected. However, although patients with astrocytomas may have prolonged survival there is frequently progressive tumour growth resulting in permanent, severe neurological disability. Death will result if the tumour extends into the high cervical level or brain stem.

INTERVERTEBRAL DISC PROLAPSE

Intervertebral disc herniation is a common cause of cervical nerve root compression causing arm pain (Ch. 14) and lumbar nerve root compression causing sciatica (Ch. 13). The nerve root compression results from posterolateral disc herniation. Occasionally, the disc may prolapse directly posteriorly (centrally) causing compression of the spinal cord in the cervical or thoracic region and cauda equina in the lumbar region (Ch. 13).

Cervical disc prolapse

Central posterior cervical disc herniation causes a rapidly progressive paralysis with upper motor neuron features below the level of the compression and lower motor neuron features at the level of the compression. There is frequently a preceding history of some neck discomfort and occasionally brachial neuralgia. However, the patient usually presents following the sudden onset of severe neck and arm pain with rapidly progressive paralysis.

Plain X-rays may show only narrowing of a disc space. Myelography will show an anterior compression at the level of a disc space which is usually either C5/6 or C6/7. The lesion will also be well demonstrated by either CT scan (with intrathecal contrast) or MRI (Fig. 15.10).

Urgent surgery is necessary to relieve the compression. The disc is excised by an anterior approach which involves removing the disc at that level and, using microsurgical techniques, excising the disc fragments which have usually prolapsed through the posterior longitudinal ligament. It is sometimes necessary to drill away the adjacent margins of the vertebral body to obtain adequate exposure and a formal vertebral fusion may be necessary.

Thoracic disc prolapse

A central posterior thoracic disc prolapse is less common. It usually occurs in males, predominantly between the ages of 30 and 55, and usually occurs below the T8 level.

The thoracic disc protrusion is usually a consequence of disc degeneration. The thoracic spinal canal is small and there is very little space between the disc and the thoracic cord. In addition, the circulation to the low thoracic region is a 'water shed' and the region is often largely supplied by

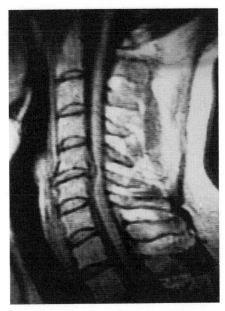

Fig. 15.10   MRI of cervical disc prolapse causing spinal cord compression.

a single unilateral radicular vessel — the artery of Adamkiewicz — which arises usually between T8 and L2, particularly on the left side.

The most common presenting symptom is poorly localised back pain related to the degenerative disc disease and stretching of the pain sensitive posterior longitudinal ligament. There are often features of radicular involvement with girdle pain. The neurological features of thoracic cord compression may progress rapidly or proceed only slowly.

There are numerous possible differential diagnoses for thoracic disc prolapse. It is extremely difficult to exclude spinal degenerative disease as the cause when back pain is the only symptom and there are no neurological signs. The clinical picture associated with the neurological deficit could be due to any other cause of spinal cord compression, as well as to multiple sclerosis.

The plain X-rays show disc space narrowing and there is often evidence of calcified disc material either in the intervertebral space or within the canal. Disc space calcification is highly suggestive of thoracic disc herniation and is present in up to 70% of cases, as opposed to an incidence of less than 4% in the normal population. Myelography will show an anterior compression at the level of the disc space. Computerised tomography scanning, following intrathecal contrast, is helpful in confirming the diagnosis. As with other causes of spinal cord compression the diagnosis can be made with MRI (Fig. 15.11).

It is essential that an accurate pre-operative diagnosis is made because

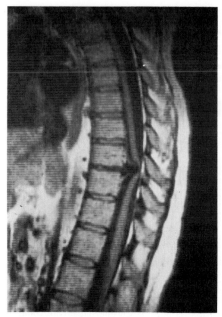

Fig. 15.11 MRI of thoracic disc prolapse causing spiral cord compression.

treatment involves excision of the disc protrusion by an anterior or antero-lateral approach. The disc herniation should not be resected using a laminectomy for access because the protrusion lies in front of the spinal cord and any manipulation of the thoracic cord will inevitably result in devastating neurological consequences. The usual surgical approach is to perform a costotransversectomy at the involved level, reflect the pleura and excise the disc and disc prolapse from in front of the dura without any manipulation of the cord.

SPINAL ABSCESS

Spinal epidural abscess is a rare condition requiring urgent treatment. The abscess usually occurs in the low thoracic or thoracolumbar region and is due either to haematogenous spread from obvious distant or occult infection or to direct spread from the adjacent vertebral column, particularly the pedicle or neural arch. Osteomyelitis of the body of the vertebrae is less likely to infect the extradural space because there is no loose, anterior, fatty areolar tissue and the posterior longitudinal ligament helps to restrain the intraspinal spread of infection.

The most common organism is *Staphylococcus aureus* but other causative organisms include streptococci, pneumococci and *Pseudomonas* species.

Spinal cord compression is due to inflammatory swelling and pus. Involvement of the extradural spinal veins causes thrombophlebitis which can spread into the veins of the spinal cord and the radicular arteries may develop an arteritis and thrombosis. Consequently, the cord is not only compressed by the abscess itself, but it is also at risk from infarction due to venous and arterial thrombosis.

The presenting features consist of:

- Severe local spinal pain
- Neurological signs of a rapidly progressive spinal cord compression
- Constitutional features of infection such as high fever, sweating and tachycardia.

Lumbar puncture for myelography should be performed carefully if a spinal extradural abscess is suspected and aspiration of the extradural space should be undertaken before the subarachnoid space is entered. If pus is obtained from the needle it should be advanced no further, to avoid the risk of meningitis. If there is no pus in the extradural space at the level of lumbar puncture the needle can be advanced into the subarachnoid space and the myelogram can proceed. Not infrequently, the CSF contains an increased protein and sometimes a mild polymorphonuclear pleocytosis.

Treatment consists of urgent laminectomy and complete evacuation of the extradural abscess. The patient should be started on high dose antibiotics.

Subdural spinal abscesses. These are rare. Some are associated with congenital dermal sinuses and others are a consequence of haematogenous spread from sepsis at a different site.

The clinical presenting features are similar to those of spinal extradural abscess and meningitis is more likely to occur.

Intramedullary abscesses. These result from haematogenous spread, a penetrating injury or in association with a congenital dermal sinus. They are rare and the patients present with features of rapidly progressive spinal cord involvement.

SPINAL TUBERCULOSIS (Pott's disease)

Although spinal tuberculosis is uncommon in western countries it is still relatively prevalent in some Asian regions and in South America. The osteomyelitis affects two or more adjacent vertebral bodies and destroys the intervening disc space.

Spinal cord compression occurs as an early feature due to tuberculous granulation tissue and pus, extruded sequestrae and fragments of intervertebral disc and vertebral collapse. Alternatively, the compression may be a late manifestation resulting from the cord being distorted over the apex of an angular kyphos.

Treatment involves the use of antituberculous chemotherapy. If there is progressive cord compression the abscess, granulation tissue and diseased bone may be excised by an anterolateral approach with access by a costotransversectomy or a more extensive vertebral resection.

SPINAL ARTERIOVENOUS MALFORMATION

Although spinal vascular malformations only occasionally cause actual compression of the spinal cord, the presenting features are those of primary spinal cord involvement and may mimic a compressive lesion.

There are numerous morphological and pathological classifications of spinal vascular malformations. Arteriovenous malformations (AVM) constitute the most common type of vascular anomaly and occur with a frequency of approximately 4% of all primary spinal tumours. They are much more frequent in males, occurring four times more frequently than in females. Other uncommon morphological types include telangiectasia (capillary angiomas), cavernous malformations and venous malformations composed entirely of veins.

The gross appearance of the spinal AVM is highly variable. The malformation may be a simple arteriovenous fistula involving a single coiled vessel and resulting in a fistulous communication or, at the other extreme, it may be the so-called 'juvenile' type, in which there are multiple, large feeding arteries supplying an extensive dilated vascular mass that may fill the spinal canal and permeate throughout the cord. This is the type most frequently seen in children. The so-called 'glomus' type consists of single or multiple vessels converging on a highly localised vascular plexus which is drained by one or more arteriolised veins.

The malformations may occur at any level and involve not only the surface of the cord but frequently have an intramedullary component.

A major type of spinal AVM involves the 'nidus' of the malformation being embedded in the dura covering the nerve root, and the intradural malformation being the dilated arterialised veins of the dural nidus. This type of malformation was only recognised in the 1970s and it is probably the most common form. It is confined to the thoracolumbar and sacral regions and in nearly all cases there is a solitary feeding vessel supplying the nidus of malformation in the dura. Nearly all cases occur in elderly men.

Presenting features

The clinical manifestations of AVM involving the spinal cord may be due to a number of mechanisms:

- A steal phenomenon. It is possible that the malformation steals blood from the normal neural tissue and that this shunt causes local spinal cord hypoxia
- Thrombosis, which may cause catastrophic symptoms
- Compression or, more appropriately, a pulsatile compression, probably plays only a small role
- Chronic increase of venous pressure, which could explain the progressive myelomalacia
- Haemorrhage.

The presenting features include:

1. Back pain and root pain
2. Progressive neurological disability involving:
   a. paresis
   b. sensory disturbance
   c. sphincter dysfunction
   d. impotence
3. A sudden catastrophic neurological event due either to haemorrhage within the cord or thrombosis
4. Subarachnoid haemorrhage.

Pain is a common feature. Most patients present with a progressive neurological loss which, in half of the cases, is intermittent and recurrent.

About 15% of patients present with subarachnoid haemorrhage. The diagnosis is obvious when the haemorrhage is accompanied by paraplegia or quadriplegia. However, there may not be any obvious associated cord manifestations and the diagnosis of spinal subarachnoid haemorrhage may be difficult. The onset of subarachnoid haemorrhage associated with sudden severe back pain is strongly indicative of an AVM of the spinal cord.

Investigations

Myelography may show the tortuous vessels which will also be seen on CT scan following intrathecal iodine contrast. The exact nature of the malformation can only be determined by highly selective spinal angiography (Fig. 15.12). The technique, requiring considerable expertise, has been facilitated by the use of digital subtraction angiography. Magnetic resonance imaging will facilitate the diagnosis of these lesions.

Treatment

The previous surgical technique of stripping the malformation from the surface of the cord has now been largely replaced by the recognition that the majority of these angiographic intradural malformations are merely the arterialised dilated veins of the dural AVM. All that is necessary is to excise the dural nidus or obliterate the arterialised draining vein from the nidus. It is not necessary to 'strip away' the intradural component covering the cord.

The surgical treatment of the true intradural AVM, which often has a major intramedullary component, is fraught with hazard. The surgical technique involves accurate identification of the draining vessels at the level of the malformation and meticulous microsurgical dissection to preserve the normal cord tissue. The large, intramedullary, juvenile type malformations are frequently inoperable because an attempted surgical excision would inevitably result in devastating consequences. In the future it may be possible

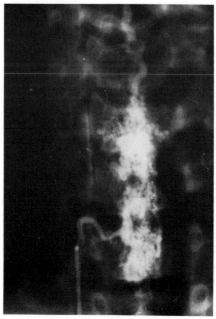

Fig. 15.12   Spinal angiogram of arteriovenous malformation and major feeding vessel.

to combine angiographic embolisation of these malformations with surgical excision.

CERVICAL MYELOPATHY

Cervical myelopathy results from cervical cord compression due to a narrow, cervical, vertebral canal. The constriction of the canal enclosing the cervical cord is due to:

- Congenital narrowing
- Cervical spondylosis involving hypertrophy of the facet joints and osteophyte formation
- Hypertrophy of the ligamenta flava
- Bulging (or prolapse) of a cervical disc
- Excessive mobility, usually associated with cervical spondylosis.
  The myelopathy results from:
- Direct pressure on the spinal cord
- Ischaemia of the cord due to compression and obstruction of small vessels within the cord, or to compression of the feeding radicular arteries within the intervertebral foramen.

The morphological changes within the cord include:

- Degeneration and loss of nerve cells, cavitation and proliferation of glia within the grey matter
- Demyelination of the lateral and posterior columns
- Wallerian degeneration in ascending tracts above and descending tracts below the compression
- Proliferation of small blood vessels with thickening of the vessel walls
- The anterior columns are rarely affected.

Clinical features

There is frequently a long history of slowly progressive disability, although it is not unusual for the neurological disability to deteriorate rapidly, particularly following an injury.

The presenting features are pain and neurological disturbance attributable to cervical cord involvement.

Neck pain. This is not due to the cervical myelopathy itself but may occur as part of the degenerative disease of the cervical spine. Narrowing of a neural foramen may result in entrapment of a cervical nerve root causing brachial neuralgia. This is discussed in Chapter 14.

Muscular weakness. This is the most common initial symptom and usually occurs earlier in the lower limbs. The patient initially notices clumsiness involving the hands and fingers, particularly in fine skilled movements, and dragging or shuffling of the feet. According to the level and extent of the cord lesion the signs in the upper limbs will be predominantly of a lower or upper motor neuron type and there will be a spastic paraparesis of the lower limbs.

Depending on the level of the compression there may be wasting of the suboccipital spinal muscles, shoulder girdle muscles and biceps and triceps. Fasciculation may be present but is usually not severe. The deep tendon reflexes in the upper limbs will be depressed at, or exaggerated below, the level of compression corresponding with the presence of lower motor neuron and upper motor neuron damage, respectively. The supinator (brachioradialis) reflex may be of value in localising the level. If it is absent, but the reflex evokes flexion of the digits and sometimes the biceps or triceps, this is regarded as evidence of a lesion restricted to the C6 segment (the inverted supinator reflex).

The lower limbs will show upper motor neuron changes due to corticospinal tract involvement with increased tone, a pyramidal pattern of weakness, exaggerated reflexes and upgoing plantar responses.

Sensory symptoms. These frequently occur as diffuse numbness and paraesthesiae in the hands and fingers. Severe sensory loss is unusual in spondolytic myelopathy, but an entirely normal sensory examination is also rare. The sensory changes may be limited to the upper limb and may involve a dermatomal pattern if a particular nerve root is being compressed. Posterior column involvement will be reflected by a loss of joint position sense and vibration.

The major differential diagnoses are:

- Spinal tumour
- Multiple sclerosis
- Motor neuron disease (particularly if only minor sensory changes)
- Syringomyelia (Ch. 11)
- Subacute combined degeneration of the cord.

Radiological investigations

The plain X-rays of the cervical spine may show a narrow vertebral canal which may be either congenital and/or due to spondolytic degenerative disease and osteophyte formation. Flexion–extension views testing the mobility of the cervical spine may show excessive movement of the vertebrae.

Although a CT scan without intrathecal contrast may confirm the narrow canal, it is necessary to perform either cervical myelography followed by a CT scan, or MRI for better identification of the osteophyte or disc encroachment into the spinal canal and for a definitive demonstration of cord compression.

Myelography will show the level of the compression, the extent of the vertebral levels over which the compression is occurring and whether it is predominantly in front of or behind the cord. These are critical issues, required in the planning of surgery. The same features can be shown with MRI (Fig. 15.13). An additional benefit of magnetic resonance imaging is that it may show myelomalacia (high signal within the cord) indicating a poorer prognosis.

Treatment

Surgery is definitely indicated for clinically progressive or moderate or severe myelopathy. There is some controversy over the indications for the surgery in patients with a mild, non-progressive myelopathy because these patients will often improve with conservative treatment, including rest in a cervical collar. However, surgery is usually advisable, and is definitely indicated if there is marked compression of the cervical cord because these patients may suffer a severe cord injury resulting in quadriparesis or quadriplegia following even a minor injury to the cervical region, such as a jolt or 'whiplash' type of injury. A further reason for advising early surgery is that the neurological deficit may not improve following an operation, due to irreversible changes within the cervical cord, so that it is preferable that the condition be arrested in its early stage.

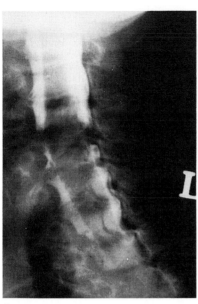
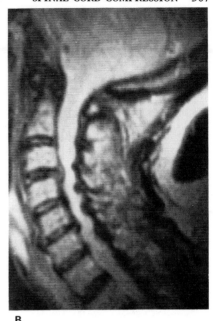

A **B**

Fig. 15.13 Cervical canal stenosis. (A) Severe cervical canal stenosis with incomplete block on myelogram. (B) MRI of cervical canal stenosis.

The type of surgical procedure performed will depend upon:

- The extent of the compression
- The number of vertebral levels involved
- Whether the compression is predominantly in front of or behind the cord
- The presence of cervical instability.

A decompressive cervical laminectomy is the preferred operation if there is a narrow canal over a number of levels and if there is significant posterior compression, usually from hypertrophied ligamenta flava.

If the compression is predominantly anterior to the cord at one or two levels, usually due to an osteophyte or disc bulge, an anterior approach with excision of the compressive lesion and anterior cervical fusion is preferred.

Whatever surgical procedure is used extreme care must be taken in removing the compression to avoid further injury to the highly sensitive cervical cord.

As indicated previously, surgery should arrest the progress of the cervical myelopathy and only in a minority of patients will there be marked improvement of neurological function following the operation. A small percentage of patients who have severe neurological impairment and evidence of myelomalacia on MRI may have further neurological deterioration following surgery.

FURTHER READING

Hulme A 1960 A surgical approach to thoracic intervertebral disc protrusion. Journal of Neurology, Neurosurgery and Psychiatry 23: 133–137

Logue V 1979 Angiomas of the spinal cord: Review of the pathogenesis, clinical features and results of surgery. Journal of Neurology, Neurosurgery and Psychiatry 42: 1–11

Mack P 1979 Spinal metastases: Current status and recommended guidelines for management. Neurosurgery 5: 726–746

Malis L I 1978 Intramedullary spinal cord tumours. Clinical Neurosurgery 254: 512–540

Rosenblum B, Oldfield E, Doppman J L, Di Chiro G 1987 Spinal arteriovenous malformations: a comparison of dural arteriovenous fistulas and intradural arteriovenous malformations in 81 patients. Journal of Neurosurgery 67: 795–802

Simeone F A, Rashbaum R 1977 Transthoracic disc excision. In: Schymidek H H, Sweet W H (eds) Current techniques in operative neurosurgery. Grune and Stratton, New York, pp 324–333

Solero C L, Fonari M, Giombini S, Lasio G, Oliveri G, Cimino C, Pluchino F 1989 Spinal meningiomas: review of 174 operated cases. Neurosurgery 25: 240–252

Stein B M 1979 Surgery of intramedullary spinal cord tumours. Clinical Neurosurgery 26: 529–542

Stein B M 1985 Spinal intradural tumours. In: Wilkins R H, Rengachery S S (eds) Neurosurgery. McGraw Hill, New York, pp 1048–1061

Sundaresan N, Galicich J H, Chu F C H, Huvos A G 1979 Spinal chordomas. Journal of Neurosurgery 50: 312–319

Symon L, Kuyama H, Kendall B 1984 Dural arteriovenous malformations of the spine. Journal of Neurosurgery 60: 238–247

16. Spinal injuries

Trauma to the spinal column occurs at an incidence of approximately 2–5/100 000 population. Although the majority of spinal injuries do not affect the cord or spinal roots, about 10% will result in quadriplegia.

Adolescent and young adult males are the most commonly affected group. Most of the serious spinal cord injuries are a consequence of road traffic accidents although there are other, major causes of quadriplegia, for example water sports, especially diving into shallow water, and injuries following ski-ing accidents.

MECHANISMS OF INJURIES

Although severe disruption of the vertebral column usually causes serious neurological damage it is not always possible to correlate the degree of bone damage with spinal cord injury. Minor vertebral column disruption does not usually cause neurological deficit, but occasionally may be associated with severe neurological injury. The mechanism of injury will determine the type of vertebral injury and neurological damage.

Trauma may damage the spinal cord by direct compression by bone, ligament or disc, interruption of the vascular supply and/or traction.

The X-rays taken following a spinal cord injury show the vertebral alignment at that time but do not necessarily indicate the amount of disruption that may have occurred at the moment of injury, or the degree of ligamentous damage. In general the injuries can be classified by mechanism of the trauma.

Cervical spine

Flexion and flexion–rotation injuries

This is the most frequent type of injury to the cervical spine; C5/6 is the most common site. Usually, one or both of the posterior facets are subluxed or dislocated and may be locked in this position. There is extensive posterior ligamentous damage and these injuries are usually unstable. The spinal cord may be compressed and distracted, sustaining both direct damage and vas-

309

cular impairment from involvement of the anastomotic segmental vessels or feeders.

Compression injuries

The vertebral body is decreased in height and may be comminuted with the posterior aspect of the body encroaching upon the spinal canal. C5/6 is the most common level for this fracture. These injuries are usually stable because the posterior bony elements and longitudinal ligaments are intact. When combined with a rotation force in flexion, the 'tear-drop' fracture may occur with separation of a small antero-inferior fragment. About half of the cord injuries cause complete neurological deficit below the level of the lesion, the remainder being incomplete with the most damage to the anterior aspect of the cord.

Hyperextension injuries

These injuries are most common in the older age groups and in patients with degenerative spinal canal stenosis. Bony injury is often not demonstrated and the major damage is to the anterior longitudinal ligament secondary to hyperextension. Most of the injuries result in incomplete cord damage resulting from compression of the cord between the degenerative body and disc anteriorly and the hypertrophic ligamentum flavum protruding posteriorly. The injuries are nearly always stable and central cervical cord syndrome is the most common neurological impairment.

Thoracolumbar spine

Flexion rotation injuries

These injuries occur most frequently at the T12/L1 level and result in anterior dislocation of the T12 on the L1 vertebral body. There is usually disruption of the posterior longitudinal ligament and posterior bony elements. The inferior vertebral body often sustains an anterior superior wedge fracture and compression. These are unstable injuries which usually result in complete neurological deficit of either the spinal cord, conus or cauda equina.

Compression injuries

These injuries are common and the vertebral body is decreased in height. They are usually stable injuries and neurological damage is uncommon.

Hyperextension injury

This is a very uncommon mechanism of injury at the thoracolumbar spine. It involves rupture of the anterior longitudinal ligament, rupture of the intervertebral disc and fracture through the involved vertebral body anteriorly. The injuries are unstable and usually cause severe cord injury.

Open injuries

These may result from stab injuries or gunshot wounds resulting in cord damage due to the blast injury, vascular damage and/or cord penetration by the missile or bony fragments.

TYPES OF NEUROLOGICAL IMPAIRMENT

Immediately after a severe cord injury there is a state of diminished excitability of the isolated spinal cord. This is referred to as 'spinal shock' or 'altered reflex activity'. The transient depression in the segments caudal to the cord lesion is due to sudden withdrawal of a predominantly facilitating or excitatory influence from supraspinal centres. There is an areflexic flaccid paralysis. The duration of spinal shock varies, minimal reflex activity may appear within a period of 3–4 days or may be delayed up to 6–8 weeks, the average duration being 3–4 weeks.

The spinal cord injury is caused by:

- The direct force applied to the cord
- Ischaemia due to vascular injury
- Secondary haemorrhage in and around the cord.

The degree of neurological injury will be determined by the extent and severity of these mechanisms.

Complete lesions

The most severe consequence of spinal trauma is complete transverse myelopathy, in which all neurological function is absent below the level of the lesion, causing either a paraplegia or quadriplegia, depending on the level. There will also be impairment of autonomic function including bladder and bowel.

Motor deficit

Injuries to the spinal cord will result in upper motor neuron paralysis characterised by loss of voluntary function, increased muscle tone and hyper-reflexia. Injuries to the lumbar spine causing cauda equina injuries result in lower motor neuron paralysis characterised by reduced muscle tone, wasting and loss of reflexes. A combination of upper and lower motor neuron lesions result from a thoracolumbar injury involving the conus medullaris and cauda equina.

Sensory deficit

In complete lesions the afferent long tracts carrying the various sensory modalities are interrupted at the level of the lesion, abolishing sensory appreciation of pain, temperature, touch, position and tactile discrimination below the lesion. Visceral sensation is also lost. Sensation may decrease over a few spinal segments before being lost altogether. Occasionally there is a level of abnormally increased sensation, hyperaesthesia and hyperalgesia at or just below the lesion.

Autonomic deficit

Vasomotor control. Cervical and high thoracic lesions above the sympathetic outflow at T5 may cause hypotension. Interruption of the sympathetic splanchnic vasomotor control will initially cause a severe postural hypotension as a result of impaired venous return.

Temperature control. The patient with a complete spinal lesion will not have satisfactory thermal regulation as there will be impairment of the autonomic mechanisms for vasoconstriction and vasodilatation.

Sphincter disturbance

There is impairment of bowel and bladder control, this is discussed later.

Incomplete lesions

Anterior cervical spinal cord

Acute **anterior cervical spinal cord syndrome** is due to compression of the anterior aspect of the cord. This causes damage to the corticospinal and spinothalamic tracts, with motor paralysis below the level of the lesion and loss of pain, temperature and touch sensation but relative preservation of light touch, proprioception and position sense, which are carried in the posterior columns. The exact pathophysiological process causing this syndrome has not been precisely defined and it may be due either to stretch applied by the attachment of the dentate ligaments at the equatorial plane of the cord or to ischaemic injury from compromise of the anterior spinal artery which supplies the anterior two-thirds of the cord.

Central spinal cord

Acute **central spinal cord syndrome** is usually due to a hyperextension of the cervical spine with compression of the spinal cord between the degenerative intervertebral disc anteriorly and the thickened ligamentum flavum posteriorly. The cord damage is located centrally, with the most severe injury to the more centrally lying cervical tracts which supply the upper limbs. There is a disproportionate weakness in the upper limbs below the level of the lesion in comparison with the lower extremities. Sensory loss is usually minimal although this is variable and frequently occurs in no specific pattern.

Brown-Séquard syndrome

The **Brown-Séquard syndrome** results from hemisection of the spinal cord (Ch. 1) as from a stab wound, although it infrequently follows a blunt injury. There is paralysis of the limbs below the level of the lesion with loss of pain, temperature and touch on the opposite side of the body. The posterior columns will be interrupted ipsilaterally but as some fibres cross there is not a great deficit.

Spinal cord concussion

There may be a transient loss of function from concussion of the spinal cord. The exact pathological processes involved in spinal cord concussion are not clear but they are probably similar to those occurring in cerebral concussion, resulting in temporary impairment of neuronal function. Recovery usually begins within 6 hours and should be detected within 48 hours.

MANAGEMENT OF SPINAL INJURIES

As with head injuries, there is little that can be done to repair the damage caused by the initial injury and therefore the major efforts are directed towards prevention of further spinal cord injury and the complications resulting from the neurological damage. The general principles of management are:

- Prevention of further injury to the spinal cord
- Reduction and stabilisation of bony injuries
- Prevention of complications resulting from spinal cord injury
- Rehabilitation.

Initial treatment

The first aid management of patients with injuries to the spinal column and spinal cord requires the utmost caution in turning and lifting the patient. The spine must be handled with great care to avoid inflicting additional damage. Before moving the patient sufficient help should be available to provide horizontal stability and longitudinal traction. Spinal flexion must be avoided. A temporary collar should be applied if the injury is to the cervical spine. An assessment should be made for other injuries to the chest, abdomen or limbs.

Hypotension and hypoventilation immediately following an acute traumatic spinal cord injury may not only be life-threatening but may also increase the extent of neurological impairment. Resuscitation techniques may need to be modified to ensure that the spine remains stable. Respiratory insufficiency may require oxygen therapy and ventilatory assistance. Loss of sympathetic tone may result in peripheral vasodilatation with peripheral vascular pooling and hypotension. Treatment will include the use of intravascular volume expanders, α-adrenergic stimulators, intravenous atropine and occasionally the use of a transvenous pacemaker. There must be careful attention to the body temperature — the spinal patient is poikilothermic and will tend to assume the temperature of the environment. Body temperature must be preserved in cold weather and the patient must not be overheated in warm weather. A nasogastric tube should be passed to avoid problems associated with vomiting due to gastric stasis and paralytic ileus. A urinary catheter should be passed to prevent the complications of bladder overdistension, although intermittent catheterisation may become preferable later. Prophylaxis for deep vein thrombosis and subsequent pulmonary embolus should be commenced as soon as possible using minidose heparin (5000 subcutaneously twice daily). Some centres also favour using various types of compression stockings on the lower limbs.

Radiological investigations

Plain cervical spine X-rays and CT scan will show the bone injuries and MRI is helpful in showing the associated cord pathology (Fig. 16.1). If a cervical spine injury is suspected but the plain X-ray and CT scan show no abnormality, the X-rays should be *carefully* repeated in flexion and extension to exclude instability due to ligamentous damage.

Spinal reduction and stabilisation

As soon as the systemic parameters have been stabilised, attention should be directed to alignment and stabilisation of the spine. The use of skeletal traction for the restoration and/or maintenance of the normal alignment of the spinal column is a time-honoured and effective treatment. There are various types of cervical traction devices. The spring loaded tongs have become popular because of their ease of application and maintenance. The usual practice is to apply weight to the traction device to a maximum of 5 lb (2.25 kg) for each level below the occiput (e. g. C6 = 30 lb (13.6 kg)). It is usual to commence with 10 lb (4.5 kg) and, under X-ray or fluoroscopic control, gradually add weights up to the maximum if necessary. Extreme care should be taken to avoid distraction at the fracture site, the

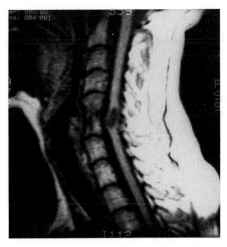

Fig. 16.1   MRI of spinal injury showing the bone damage and cord injury.

traction on the underlying cord may worsen the neurological injury. Reduction of facet dislocations may be more difficult and require more weight for the traction. Some advocate manipulation of the neck under fluoroscopic control while weight is being applied to accomplish reduction of locked facets. In Australia and Europe, cervical traction under general anaesthesia has been used for closed reduction of some fracture dislocations but this has not been popular in the United States. Open surgery may be necessary to reduce the fracture — subluxation with overriding and locked facet joints.

Following reduction the position may be maintained with skeletal traction or halo immobilisation.

Injuries of the thoracolumbar spine can usually be managed conservatively by postural reduction in bed. The correct posture must be maintained during positioning on the side, as well as on the back; this is achieved by the appropriate placement of bolsters and pillows by a turning team.

Indications for surgical intervention

There has been considerable controversy over surgical intervention in patients with spinal cord injuries. The damage to the spinal cord occurs principally at the time of the injury and it is not surprising that there has been no evidence to show improved neurological function from acute operative decompression of the spine. The following are the general indications for surgical intervention:

1. Progression of neurological deficit is an absolute indication. It requires emergency intervention if a compressive lesion is demonstrated by either MRI or CT scan.

2. Patients who have a partial neurological injury, with preservation of some distal neurological function, and who fail to improve should have further radiological assessment. Surgery could be considered if this shows persisting extrinsic compression of the spinal cord within the canal (particularly from a herniated cervical disc), a depressed fractured lamina or an osteophytic bar, although removal of the compression may not result in any neurological improvement.
3. An open injury from a gunshot or stab wound should be explored to remove foreign particles, elevate bone spicules and, if possible, repair the dura.
4. The most common indication for operative intervention is to stabilise the spine. This is usually undertaken:
   a. if there is gross instability, particularly in the presence of an incomplete neurological lesion
   b. if it has not been possible to reduce locked facets by closed reduction — posterior reduction and fusion is appropriate
   c. operative procedures to stabilise the unstable cervical spine and so avoid prolonged bed rest are favoured by some.

Other treatments for spinal cord injury

Numerous pharmacological agents have been investigated in experimental laboratory models but as yet there has been no controlled clinical study to show the usefulness of these agents in spinal cord injury. The treatments include glucocorticoids, diuretics, local hypothermia, barbiturates and endogenous opiate agonists. Although there is no proven benefit, some spinal units still use glucocorticoids and osmotic diuretics for the treatment of oedema.

Further management

Following reduction and immobilisation of the fractures the principles of the continuing care involve the avoidance of potential complications in patients who are paraplegic or quadriplegic and early rehabilitation, which commences as soon as the injury is stabilised.

General care

Careful attention to the general condition and metabolic state is essential following the injury; patients frequently develop a negative nitrogen balance and may become anaemic. Urinary tract or other infections will aggravate the metabolic disorders. The patients and their relatives will require skilled counselling and emotional support during the treatment and rehabilitation period.

Skin care

Meticulous attention to pressure will avoid the development of pressure sores which would seriously complicate the recovery and rehabilitation of the patient.

Gastrointestinal complications

Paralytic ileus occurs in acute spinal cord paralysis and, if unrecognised, the patient is at risk from vomiting and inhalation. A nasogastric tube should be passed in the initial management of the patient. Acute gastric dilatation may also develop and is also treated by nasogastric suction. In 3–5% of patients with acute spinal cord injuries acute peptic ulceration occurs.

Bladder care

Urinary tract problems are a major cause of potential morbidity and mortality. During the period of spinal shock, the areflexic, flaccid paralysis below the level of the lesion includes bladder function. The patient will develop acute retention with overflow incontinence and a catheter is required. Reflex activity returns in upper motor neuron lesions as the phase of spinal shock passes. The spinal micturitional reflex arc is intact in a lesion above the conus and an autonomic type of bladder results. The bladder will empty involuntarily as it fills with urine. The capacity may be less than normal, but there is good voiding pressure capacity. There is no sensation of bladder fullness. In a lower motor neuron lesion the spinal micturitional reflex is interrupted and an autonomous bladder results. Bladder function is governed by a myogenic stretch reflex inherent in the detrusor fibres themselves. This type of dysfunction is characterised by a linear increase in intravesicle pressure, with filling until capacity is reached. Urine may then flow past the sphincter by overflow incontinence. In a mixed upper and lower motor neuron lesion, such as with a conus medullaris and cauda equina injury, it is possible to have a flaccid lower motor neuron detrusor and a spastic sphincter, as well as the reverse.

The principles of management of the bladder consist of maintaining proper bladder drainage to prevent dilatation of the upper urinary tract and renal impairment and the treatment of urinary tract infections. A catheter is passed initially and bladder training is commenced after the period of spinal shock. The details of bladder training and management depend on whether the neurogenic bladder has resulted from an upper or a lower motor neuron lesion and on the results of a cystometrogram showing the intravesical volume pressure relationship.

Limb care

It is essential that the paralysed limbs should be put through their full range of movements regularly. Physiotherapy, in particular, is essential to prevent contractures as the tone returns and spasticity develops.

SPECIAL CERVICAL SPINE INJURIES

Jefferson's fracture

Jefferson described bilateral fractures of the posterior arch of the atlas from a direct vertical blow to the head in four patients. The mechanism of the fracture is due to the head pressing down on the spinal column and the atlas being squeezed between the occipital condyles above and the axis below. The grooves for the vertebral artery are the sites where the arches of the atlas are weakest and when fractures occur at this site bursting fragments are displaced outwards.

Fractures of the odontoid process

A fracture of the odontoid process may occur at the tip, through the base of the dens or at the base and extend into the adjacent C2 vertebral body. The fractures that occur at the base of the dens are the most common and may cause disruption of the blood supply to the dens, resulting in nonunion of the fracture.

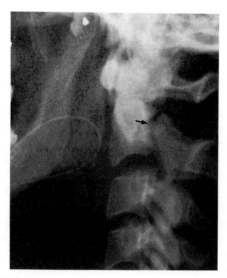

Fig. 16.2 Hangman's fracture

Many of the odontoid fractures can be treated by immobilisation in a firm brace or halo for 4 months. If there is non-union and instability a posterior C1/2 fusion will be necessary. Transoral internal fixation of the odontoid fracture has been advocated but is probably rarely indicated.

Hangman's fracture (Fig. 16.2)

This fracture is the avulsion of the laminar arches of C2 with dislocation of the C2 vertebral body on C3. It is the characteristic lesion resulting from judicial hanging.

FURTHER READING

Harris P, Karmi M Z, McClemont E, Matlhiko D, Paul K S 1980 The prognosis of patients sustaining severe cervical spine injury (C2–C7 inclusive). Paraplegia 18: 324–330
Heiden J S, Weiss M H, Rosenberg W, Apuzzo M L J, Kurze T 1975 Management of cervical spinal cord trauma in Southern California. Journal of Neurosurgery 43: 732–736
Norrell H 1978 The treatment of unstable fractures and dislocations. Clinical Neurosurgery 25: 193–208
Norrell H 1980 The early management of spinal injuries. Clinical Neurosurgery 27: 385–400
Sherk H H 1978 Fractures of the atlas and odontoid process. Orthopaedic Clinics of North America 9: 973–984
Wood-Jones F 1913 The ideal lesion produced by judicial hanging. Lancet i: 533

17. Peripheral nerve entrapments, injuries and tumours

Peripheral nerves may be trapped, compressed or injured at any position along their course, although there are certain regions where they are especially vulnerable. Nerve entrapments occur particularly where the peripheral nerve passes through a tunnel formed by ligaments, bone and/or muscle. Traumatic injury to the nerve occurs when it is either relatively superficial and exposed or lying adjacent to bone, where it may be directly injured by the jagged, fractured ends of the bone.

PERIPHERAL NERVE ENTRAPMENT

Entrapment neuropathies occur when nerves pass near joints. In this position they are particularly vulnerable to compression:

- Due to bone and joint disorders in the region
- Because they frequently pass under a tendinous arch
- Movement of the adjacent joint may exacerbate any compression.

Less common forms of entrapment neuropathy may lie at a distance from a joint. Table 17.1 shows a list of the common and less frequent entrapment

Table 17.1 Entrapment neuropathies

Median nerve
   Carpal tunnel syndrome★
   Supracondylar entrapment
   Cubital fossa entrapment
   Anterior interosseus nerve entrapment

Ulnar nerve
   Tardy ulnar palsy★
   Deep branch of ulnar nerve

Radial nerve — posterior interosseus nerve

Suprascapular nerve

Meralgia paraesthetica — lateral femoral cutaneous nerve of thigh

Sciatic nerve

Tarsal tunnel syndrome

Thoracic outlet syndrome★

★The more common entrapment neuropathies.

neuropathies. Although thoracic outlet syndrome does not cause compression of a peripheral nerve, it will be considered in this chapter because the clinical features may mimic peripheral nerve entrapment and because the pathophysiology is similar to compression of a peripheral nerve.

Carpal tunnel syndrome

This is by far the most common nerve entrapment, women are affected four times more often than men.

The carpal tunnel is a fibro-osseous tunnel on the palmar surface of the wrist (Fig. 17.1). The dorsal and lateral walls consist of the carpal bones, which form a crescentic trough. A tunnel is made by the fibrous flexor retinaculum (transverse carpal ligament) which is attached medially to the pisiform and hook of the hamate and laterally to the tuberosity of the scaphoid and crest of the trapezium. The contents of the tunnel are the median nerve and the flexor tendons of the flexor digitorum superficialis, flexor digitorum profundis and flexor pollicis longus.

Although the features of carpal tunnel syndrome may present at any stage throughout the adult years, the initial symptoms often occur in women during pregnancy and in both sexes when they are performing unusually strenuous work with their hands. There are a number of systemic conditions

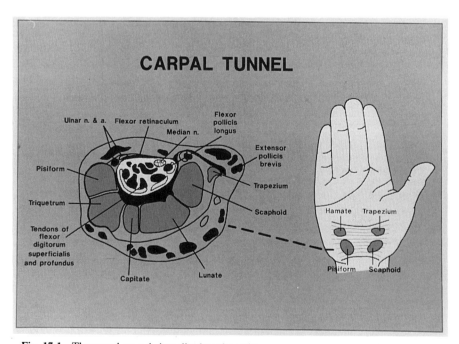

Fig. 17.1 The carpal tunnel, just distal to the wrist.

which are associated with, and may predispose to, carpal tunnel syndrome. These include:

- Pregnancy and lactation
- Contraceptive pill
- Rheumatoid arthritis
- Myxoedema
- Acromegaly.

Any local condition that will decrease the size of the carpal tunnel will also predispose to carpal tunnel syndrome. Such conditions include a ganglion, tenosynovitis, unreduced fractures or dislocations of the wrist or carpal bones and any local arthritis.

The principal clinical features of carpal tunnel syndrome are:

- Pain
- Numbness
- Tingling.

The pain, which may be described as burning or aching, is frequently felt throughout the whole hand and not just in the lateral three digits. There is often a diffuse radiation of pain up the forearm to the elbow and occasionally into the upper arm. The symptoms are worse at night, and on waking the patient has to shake the hand to obtain any relief. The pain is also aggravated by activity of the hand.

Although the numbness and tingling is principally in the lateral three and a half fingers, in the distribution of the median nerve, the patient frequently complains of more diffuse sensory loss throughout the fingers. This symptom is also worse at night and with activity.

The patient frequently complains that the hand feels 'clumsy', but with no specific weakness.

There are often only minimal signs of median nerve entrapment at the wrist. The Tinel sign may be elicited by tapping over the median nerve but its presence or absence has little diagnostic value.

If the compression has been prolonged and severe there may be signs of median nerve dysfunction, including:

- Wasting of the thenar muscle
- Weakness of muscles innervated by the distal median nerve, especially abductor pollicis brevis
- Diminished sensation over the distribution of the median nerve in the hand.

Some patients, particularly the elderly or diabetic, may present with only minor discomfort but rapid wasting, weakness and numbness in the hand.

The clinical diagnosis can be confirmed by electromyographic examination (EMG). The earliest feature of carpal syndrome is prolonged sensory latency and the sensory evoked response may show a diminished amplitude and is often absent. The distal motor latency may also be prolonged. Needle examination may show loss of motor units and presence of denervation potentials in the thenar muscles.

Treatment

Surgery is a simple and effective method of relieving the compression and curing the symptoms. However, conservative treatment is appropriate if:

- The symptoms are mild or intermittent
- There is a reversible underlying precipitating condition such as pregnancy or oral contraceptive pill.

Conservative treatment includes the use of a wrist splint, particularly at night, and non-steroidal anti-inflammatory medication. Corticosteroid injection into the carpal tunnel is sometimes advocated but, at best, this offers only temporary relief and may damage the median nerve.

The operation involves the division of the flexor retinaculum through a curvilinear incision made in the palm of the hand extending from the distal wrist crease and exposing the whole of the flexor retinaculum in the hand. The operation can be performed under general anaesthetic, regional anaesthesia or local anaesthesia, with or without a tourniquet. It is essential to divide the whole of the retinaculum and to avoid damage to the recurrent branch of the median nerve that innervates the thenar muscles. Although this important nerve usually arises distally, from the median nerve on the radial side in the carpal tunnel, it is common for it to have an anomalous origin and course before entering the thenar muscles.

Although some surgeons advocate postoperative immobilisation of the hand it is preferable to encourage movement of the upper limb, including the fingers and wrist, to avoid stiffness of the joints.

Other median nerve entrapments

The median nerve may occasionally be compressed at other sites, particularly:

- In the cubital fossa
- Under a supracondylar process of the humerus and Struther's ligament.

Cubital fossa

The median nerve may occasionally be compressed in the region of the cubital fossa:

- Under the bicipital aponeurosis
- As it passes between the two heads of pronator teres muscle

• As it passes under the fibrotendinous arch of the origin of flexor digitorum superficialis muscle.

It is not usually possible to differentiate the exact cause of the compression prior to exploration. The symptoms are similar and have an insidious onset. There is usually a vague pain in the forearm with increasing weakness of the hand and numbness in the thumb and index finger. The clinical findings are of weakness of the median nerve-innervated muscles, especially the flexor pollicis longus, the radial half of the flexor digitorum profundis and the thenar muscles, and of numbness in the distribution of the median nerve.

Although the symptoms may resolve with conservative treatment, which should include rest of the limb and avoidance of heavy work, it is usually necessary to explore the nerve and relieve the compression.

Compression of the median nerve under a supracondylar process of the humerus is rare. A fibrous ligament (Struther's ligament) extends from the anomalous bony process arising from the anteromedial surface of the humerus — the supracondylar process — to the region of the medial epicondyle and forms a fibro-osseous foramen through which the median nerve and brachial artery pass. The clinical features are of progressive median nerve palsy, particularly with pronator weakness, which distinguishes this syndrome from more distal median nerve entrapment. Surgery consists of excision of Struther's ligament and removal of the bony spur.

Ulnar nerve entrapment at the elbow

The ulnar nerve runs behind the medial epicondyle of the humerus. It enters the forearm through a fibro-osseous tunnel formed by the aponeurotic attachment of the two heads of flexor carpi ulnaris, which span from the median epicondyle of the humerus to the olecranon process of the ulnar, forming the cubital tunnel (Fig. 17.2). The ligament tightens during flexion of the elbow and the volume of the cubital tunnel decreases with increasing pressure over the underlying nerve. Injuries in the region producing deformity of the elbow predispose to compression, although the features of ulnar nerve entrapment do not usually appear for some years. This delay in the appearance of symptoms led to the term 'tardy ulnar palsy'.

In most cases there is no particular predisposing cause. In a minority there are underlying factors which predispose to nerve entrapment, including lengthy periods of bed rest from coma or major illness and poor positioning of the upper limbs during long operations causing prolonged pressure on the nerve, arthritis of the elbow, ganglion cysts of the elbow joint and direct trauma.

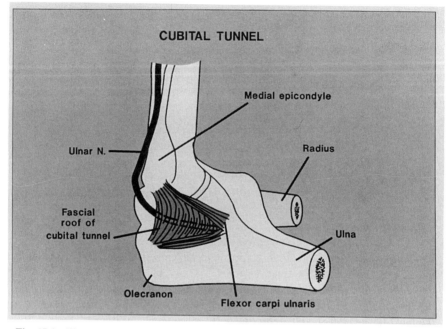

CUBITAL TUNNEL

Medial epicondyle

Ulnar N.

Radius

Fascial
roof of
cubital tunnel

Ulna

Olecranon

Flexor carpi ulnaris

Fig. 17.2   The ulnar nerve passing behind the medial epicondyle of the humerus and through the cubital tunnel.

The clinical features consist of:

- Paraesthesia and numbness in the ring and little fingers of the hand and the adjacent medial border of the hand
- Wasting of the ulnar innervated muscles of the hand (particularly the hypothenar eminence and interossei muscles)
- Weakness.

The most common initial presenting feature is paraesthesia in the ring and little fingers and the adjacent ulnar border of the hand. The patient may complain of a painful 'burning' or 'aching' in the forearm and/or the hand, but pain is usually not a prominent symptom. There will be progressive clumsiness of the hand with impairment of fine movements.

In advanced cases there will be wasting of the ulnar innervated muscles, particularly noticeable will be the hypothenar eminence and dorsal interossei. Entrapment of the ulnar nerve will lead to weakness of the muscles of the hypothenar eminence, the interossei, the two medial lumbricals, the adductor pollicis, the flexor digitorum profundus (ring and little fingers) and the flexor carpi ulnaris. Paralysis of the small muscles of the hand causes 'claw hand', this posture being produced by the unopposed action of the antagonists of the paralysed muscles. Since the interossei cause flexion of the fingers at the metacarpophalangeal joints and extension at the interphalangeal joints, when these muscles are paralysed the opposite posture is maintained by the long flexors and extensors, which cause flexion at the interphalangeal joints and hyperextension at the metacarpophalangeal joints. This is most pronounced in the ring and little fingers as the two radial lumbricals, innervated by the median nerve, compensate to some degree for the impaired action of the interossei on the index and middle fingers. Froment's sign is demonstrated by asking the patient to grasp a piece of cardboard between the index finger and thumb against resistance. There will be flexion of the interphalangeal joint of the thumb because the median innervated flexor pollicis longus is used, rather than the weakened adductor pollicis. The sensory disturbance will be in the little finger and medial half of the ring finger and medial border of the hand.

The diagnosis will be confirmed by nerve conduction studies. The conduction velocity in the ulnar nerve across the elbow is slowed, the amplitude of the motor response in the abductor digiti minimi is decreased and the sensory latency is prolonged. Needle examination of the ulnar innervated muscles will show reduction in the voluntary motor unit action potentials.

Treatment

Conservative treatment may be tried if the clinical features are minor and not progressive. It should include the advice to avoid pressure on the nerve at the elbow during reading, sitting or lying and to cease heavy work with the arms. Non-steroidal anti-inflammatory medication may be helpful.

Surgery is indicated if there are progressive symptoms or signs and if there is any wasting or weakness. The surgical procedure must release the nerve from compression and prevent further damage to the nerve from flexion and extension movement of the elbow. The surgical techniques have included:

- Neurolysis
- Medial epicondylectomy
- Transposition of the nerve.

The nerve is explored through a curvilinear incision centred just behind the medial epicondyle. The dense fascia over the nerve, forming the roof of the cubital tunnel, is divided, extending from the medial intermuscular septum above to where the nerve runs between the two heads of the flexor carpi ulnaris below. If the elbow is then flexed it will be noted that the nerve is usually trapped behind the medial epicondyle, so that it is further traumatised during movement of the elbow, despite the bridge of fibrous tissue being divided. Excision of the medial epicondyle through a subperiosteal resection of the condyle allows the nerve to move freely during a full range of movement of the elbow. Transposition of the nerve is not usually necessary and is not recommended.

Ulnar nerve compression at the wrist

The ulnar nerve may occasionally be trapped and compressed at the wrist and the clinical features of this compression depend on the exact position of the entrapment.

The deep branch of the ulnar nerve may be compressed at the pisohamate hiatus. The condition can sometimes arise spontaneously, but there is usually a history of injury, often of a heavy and repetitive type. Most of the patients are men and it classically occurs in those using heavy jack hammers, wire cutting shears and in motor cyclists, where there is repetitive trauma over the ulnar aspect of the hand. There is marked wasting and weakness of the hand muscles innervated by the ulnar nerve. Flexor carpi ulnaris and the medial half of the flexor digitorum profundis are not impaired. Although there is often spontaneous improvement after the trauma is ceased, surgery may be necessary to relieve the compression.

Less commonly, the ulnar nerve is compressed at the wrist a little more proximally in 'Guyon's canal' which is an oblique fibro-osseous tunnel that lies within the proximal part of the hypothenar eminence. The roof of the tunnel is formed by the palmar fascia and palmaris brevis muscle. The floor is formed by the flexor retinaculum and the pisohamate ligament. The terminal part of the tendon of flexor carpi ulnaris and the pisiform bone form the medial wall. The distal part of the lateral wall is formed by the curved ulnar surface of the hook of the hamate. The canal contains the ulnar nerve and ulnar artery. In the middle of the canal the ulnar nerve divides into the superficial and deep branches. The superficial branch continues distally and supplies a small branch to the palmaris brevis muscle and sensation to the medial half of the ring finger and little finger. The deep motor branch passes laterally around the hook of the hamate and under the pisohamate hiatus, a fibrotendinous arch.

Compression in Guyon's canal, often by a ganglion, leads to features similar to the more distal compression of the deep branch of the ulnar nerve, as well as to sensory loss and involvement of the palmaris brevis muscle. Sensation is retained on the dorsal aspect of the hand, as the distal branch of the ulnar nerve arises proximal to the wrist. The symptoms may resolve with conservative therapy but surgical decompression is often required.

Suprascapular nerve entrapment

The suprascapular nerve is occasionally compressed in the suprascapular notch under the suprascapular ligament.

There is an occasional acute, precipitating traumatic event, although there is usually no readily identifiable prior injury. The earliest presenting features are deep pain around the suprascapular region and shoulder. The frequent clinical finding is marked atrophy of the supra-and infraspinatus muscles. There is often weakness of external rotation of the arm.

The major differential diagnosis is a rotator cuff injury of the shoulder. Nerve conduction studies will aid in the diagnosis. Section of the suprascapular liagment usually satisfactorily relieves the compression and provides good symptomatic relief.

Posterior interrosseous nerve entrapment

The radial nerve divides into two terminal branches — the superficial radial nerve and the posterior interosseous nerve, which supplies extensor carpi radialis brevis and the supinator muscles before it passes under a tough fibrotendinous ring at the origin of the supinator muscle. The posterior interosseous nerve traverses the supinator muscle, winds around the lateral side of the radius and emerges on the dorsal aspect of the forearm, where it supplies the extensor muscles of the wrist and fingers. The usual site of entrapment is at the origin of the supinator muscle under the fibrotendinous ring (arcade of Frohse), although other adjacent skeletal abnormalities may also cause a traumatic neuritis in the region.

The clinical presentation involves an inability to extend the fingers at the metacarpophalangeal joints (finger drop). There is not usually any wrist drop because the extensor carpi radialis longus is supplied by the radial nerve proximal to its terminal branching.

If symptoms do not improve spontaneously with conservative therapy exploration and division of the compressing band is necessary.

Thoracic outlet syndrome

Thoracic outlet syndrome is an entrapment neuropathy of the brachial plexus at the root of the neck. Numerous upper limb pain problems are frequently and erroneously attributed to compression at the thoracic outlet. Although the brachial plexus may be trapped at the cervicobrachial junction, it is a relatively uncommon cause of upper limb symptoms.

The neurovascular bundle, consisting of the roots and trunks of the brachial plexus and the subclavian artery (Fig. 17.3) emerge from the neck into the axilla through a slit or triangle with a narrow base bounded anteriorly by the scalenus anterior, posteriorly by the scalenus medius and inferiorly by the first rib.

Historically, a cervical rib was thought to be the cause of compression of the neurovascular bundle. However, in the majority of patients the symptoms are due to a compressive fibrous band, continuous with the medial edge of scalenus medius which extends from an elongated transverse process of C7 (a 'forme fruste' of a cervical rib) to the first rib and produces its symptoms by compression of the brachial plexus, particularly the lower trunk.

The presenting features may be due to either neural or vascular compression and the features of either one of these will usually predominate. If

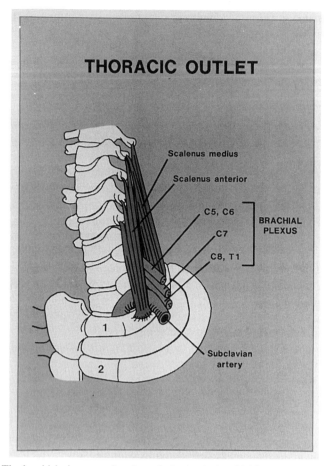

Fig. 17.3 The brachial plexus passing through the cervicobrachial junction.

there is a cervical rib the patient may present with vascular features of increasing pallor and coldness of the hand which, if variable in intensity, may simulate Raynaud's syndrome. The clinical features of neural compression are usually gradual and are more likely to occur with a fibrous band than a full cervical rib. The major presenting features are:

- Arm pain
- Motor weakness and sensory loss caused by compression of the lower trunk of the brachial plexus.

The syndrome occurs typically in young to middle-aged females and the pain may be diffuse or in the distribution of the lower trunk of the brachial plexus. Atrophy may be present in the thenar and hypothenar eminence and other intrinsic hand muscles and weakness may involve not only the small muscles of the hand but sometimes the long flexors, particularly on the ulnar side of the forearm. There may be diminished sensation in the distribution of the C8 and T1 dermatomes.

Plain X-rays may show the characteristic elongated transverse process of C7. Nerve conduction studies and electromyography may help with the diagnosis.

Surgery should only be performed if there is unequivocal clinical evidence of neural entrapment. As indicated earlier the condition has often been erroneously diagnosed as the cause of non-specific arm pain. If there are objective neurological signs of entrapment the surgical procedure is division of the fibrous band or, in the case of a cervical rib excision, of the bone, to relieve compression. These procedures are best performed through a supraclavicular approach using magnification to identify and protect the neural structures. A transaxillary approach is also used to remove a cervical rib.

Lower limb entrapment neuropathies

Entrapment neuropathies of the lower limb are uncommon.

Meralgia paraesthetica

Meralgia paraesthetica results from entrapment of the lateral cutaneous nerve of the thigh beneath the inguinal ligament, just medial to the anterior superior iliac spine. At this position the nerve passes between two roots of attachment of the inguinal ligament to the iliac bone and there is a sharp angulation of the nerve as it passes from the iliac fossa into the thigh.

Prolonged standing or walking and an obese pendulous anterior abdominal wall accentuates the downward pull on the inguinal ligament and may predispose to entrapment of the nerve. The syndrome is most frequently seen in middle-aged, overweight men, and also in young army recruits during strenuous training.

The principal symptom is a painful dysaesthesia in the anterolateral aspect of the thigh. The patient often describes the sensation as 'burning', 'pins and needles' or 'prickling' which may be accentuated by standing up straight and relieved by flexion of the hip.

The only neurological sign is diminished sensation over the anterolateral aspect of the thigh in the distribution of the lateral cutaneous nerve of the thigh.

The symptoms may only be minor and the patient may be satisfied with reassurance. The unpleasant features may resolve with conservative treatment, which should include weight reduction in an obese patient. Surgery may be necessary if the symptoms are debilitating. This involves decompression of the nerve or, if that fails, division of the nerve.

Tarsal tunnel syndrome

The tarsal tunnel is the counterpart of the carpal tunnel of the wrist and is located posterior and inferior to the medial malleolus. The flexor retinaculum extends from the medial malleolus above to the medial tubercle of the os calcis below. The posterior tibial nerve, a terminal branch of the sciatic nerve, enters the foot through the tarsal tunnel with the posterior tibial vessels and the tendons of the tibialis posterior, flexor digitorum longus and flexor hallicus longus muscles.

Men and women are equally affected. The principal symptoms are pain, numbness and tingling along the plantar aspect of the foot and toes.

Electrodiagnostic studies will help confirm the diagnosis. Operation involves division of the retinaculum and decompression of the nerve, usually with excellent results.

Sciatic nerve palsy

A sciatic nerve pressure palsy typically occurs in patients following a prolonged period of unconsciousness and is most frequently seen after drug overdose. It is not a true entrapment neuropathy but rather a direct pressure palsy.

Common peroneal (lateral popliteal) nerve palsy

Entrapment of the common peroneal nerve may occur rarely as it winds around the neck of the fibula deep to the peroneus longus muscle, resulting in a foot drop. More commonly, paralysis of the nerve will occur as a result of direct trauma in this superficial vulnerable position.

ACUTE NERVE INJURIES

Peripheral nerve anatomy

The axon projects from the cell body (the perikaryon) and is surrounded by a basement membrane and myelin sheath. The axon is covered by the **endoneurium**, the innermost layer of connective tissue, and a number of axons are grouped together in a bundle called a fascicle, which is invested by a further connective tissue sheath called the **perineurium**. A peripheral nerve consists of a group of fascicles covered by an outermost layer of connective tissue, the **epineurium**. The nerve fibres can be classified according to their diameter and function. The nerve conduction velocity is proportional to the square root of the fibre diameter. The largest myelinated axons which produce the most rapidly conducting potential are known as A fibres, which can be further subdivided into alpha, beta, gamma and delta, based on their size and conduction velocity. The smaller, slower conducting B fibres are mostly responsible for autonomic conduction and the unmyelinated C fibres have the slowest conduction.

Classification of nerve injuries

There is no single classification system that can describe all the many variations of nerve injury. Most systems attempt to correlate the degree of injury with symptoms, pathology and prognosis. In 1943, Seddon introduced a classification of nerve injuries based on three main types of nerve fibre injury and whether there is continuity of the nerve (Table 17.2).

Neurotmesis. This is the most severe injury in which the nerve has been completely divided and complete distal wallerian degeneration occurs. There is complete loss of motor, sensory and autonomic function. Electrical studies will show absence of voluntary muscle potentials and evidence of denervation after 2–3 weeks.

Although the term neurotmesis implies a cutting of the nerve, the term is also used when the epineurium of the nerve is still in continuity but the axons have been so destroyed and replaced by scar tissue that spontaneous regeneration is impossible. The most common injuries to cause neurotmesis are laceration and a missile injury, but it can also result from other types of trauma including a crush or traction injury.

If the nerve has been completely divided, axonal regeneration causes a neuroma to form in the proximal stump.

Axonotmesis. This is characterised by complete interruption of the axons and their myelin sheaths, although the encapsulating tissue, the epineurium and perineurium, are preserved. Spontaneous regeneration will occur because the intact endoneurial sheaths guide the regenerating fibres to their distal connections. There is complete and immediate loss of motor, sensory and autonomic function distal to the lesion with an EMG picture similar to that of neurotmesis. Regeneration occurs at a rate of 1–2 mm per day, so that the time of recovery will depend on the distance between a lesion and the end organ and on the age of the patient.

The major types of injuries causing an axonotmesis include compression, traction, missile and ischaemia.

Neurapraxia. The mildest form of injury, neurapraxia is akin to a transient 'concussion' of the nerve. There is a temporary loss of function, which is reversible within hours to months of the injury (the average is 6–8 weeks). If there is a complete, initial loss of function, neurapraxia cannot be distinguished from the more serious type of injury but will be recognised only in retrospect when recovery of function has occurred sooner than would be possible following Wallerian degeneration. There is frequently greater involvement of motor than sensory function with autonomic function being retained.

Table 17.2 Classification of nerve injuries (Seddon)

	Neurotmesis	Axonotmesis	Neurapraxia
Pathological			
Anatomical continuity	May be lost	Preserved	Preserved
Essential damage	Complete disorganisation Schwann sheaths preserved	Nerve fibres interrupted of larger fibres, no degeneration of axons	Selective demyelination
Clinical			
Motor paralysis	Complete	Complete	Complete
Muscle atrophy	Progressive	Progressive	Very little
Sensory paralysis	Complete	Complete	Usually much sparing
Autonomic paralysis	Complete	Complete	Usually much sparing
Electrical phenomena			
Reaction of degeneration	Present	Present	Present
Nerve conduction distal to the lesion	Absent	Absent	Preserved
Motor-unit action potentials	Absent	Absent	Absent
Fibrillation	Present	Present	Occasionally detectable
Recovery			
Surgical repair	Essential	Not necessary	Not necessary
Rate of recovery	1–2 mm/day after repair	1–2 mm/day	Rapid; days or weeks
March of recovery	According to order of innervation	According to order of innervation	No order
Quality	Always imperfect	Perfect	Perfect

Adapted from Seddon. Reproduced with permission.

Causes of peripheral nerve injury

The type of trauma will determine the nature of the injury to the nerve. In practice there are numerous possibilities, but these can be grouped into the major types:

— **Lacerations** cause neurotmesis with complete or partial division of the nerve. The usual injury results from a knife wound, laceration by glass or extensive contusion of the area with a chainsaw.
— **Missile injuries** may cause the spectrum of nerve injury from complete disruption of the nerve to a mild neurapraxia. If the brachial plexus is injured a variety of these injury types may occur to various parts of the plexus.
— **Traction** and **stretch** trauma may also result in either complete disruption of the nerve or, if minor, a neurapraxia. This type of mechanism is particularly responsible for brachial plexus injuries following motor bike accidents, radial or perineal nerve injuries. It is a common mechanism of nerve injuries associated with skeletal fractures.
— **Fractures** or fracture dislocation may cause nerve injuries when the adjacent nerve is either compressed by the displaced bone fragments, causing injury by stretch or ischaemia or, less commonly, severed by the jagged edge of the bone. Axonotmesis is the most common type of injury.
— **Compression ischaemia** may produce a neurapraxia in mild cases or, if prolonged and severe, axonotmesis or neurotmesis. It is the cause of the pressure palsies following improper application of a tourniquet or the 'Saturday night palsy' in which the radial nerve has been compressed against the humerus. Increased pressure in a closed fascial compartment, as can occur following a musculoskeletal injury, may cause ischaemic damage to a peripheral nerve and delay in treatment will result in severe ischaemic damage to the nerves and muscles resulting in paralysis and contraction deformities, such as in Volkmann's ischaemic contracture.
— **Injection** injury results from either direct trauma by the needle or the toxic effect of the agent injected. As would be expected, the sciatic and radial nerves are the most commonly affected.
— **Electrical** and **burn** injuries are uncommon causes of serious peripheral nerve damage.

Management of nerve injuries

The basis of the management depends on a precise assessment of the damage that has been done to the nerve. The types of injuries vary considerably from an isolated single nerve lesion to a complex nerve injury in a patient with multiple trauma. The following are the general guidelines for management:

1. Determination of the exact nerve involved by:
   a. the clinical deficit
   b. the position of the injury
2. Assessment of the type of nerve damaged by the mechanism of the injury
3. If a neurapraxia or axonotmesis is suspected on clinical grounds there is no specific surgical treatment for the nerve but physiotherapy should commence as soon as possible to prevent stiffness of the joints and contractures
4. Immediate or early exploration of the nerve should be undertaken in the following situations:
   a. if it is highly probable that the type of injury (e.g. laceration) will have caused the nerve to be severed
   b. if the nerve injury has been caused by a displaced fracture that needs reduction by open surgery exploration of the nerve can be carried out at the same time. The operative procedure involves identification of the nerve and relieving any compression. If the nerve has been severed the nerve ends should be isolated and continuity restored by either direct suture or inserting a nerve graft. Some surgeons advocate performing a graft as a secondary procedure only, and delaying this until the wound has healed and the risk of infection has subsided
5. Delayed exploration of the nerve will be indicated if the clinical and EMG findings indicate failure of regeneration of the nerve beyond the time expected. That is, if the injury has resulted in a neurotmesis rather than an axonotmesis or neurapraxia.

Brachial plexus injury

The mechanisms of injury are the same as for any peripheral nerve. Birth injuries usually have one of three patterns:

1. Erb's palsy due to damage to the upper trunk of the brachial plexus
2. Klumpke's paralysis due to damage to the lower trunk of the brachial plexus (C8 and T1), resulting from the arm being held up while traction was applied to the body during a breach delivery
3. Paralysis of the whole arm as a result of severe birth trauma.

In adolescents and adults the most common cause is severe traction on the brachial plexus resulting from violent trauma, most frequently a motor bike or motor vehicle accident. The trauma may result in damage to any part of the plexus, but severe axial traction may result in tearing of the arachnoid and dura with nerve root avulsion.

The management involves determination of the exact neurological injury, and particularly the part of the brachial plexus involved. A Horner's syndrome is useful evidence for avulsion of the nerve roots from the spinal cord.

A myelogram or CT scan/myelogram may show the pseudomeningocele, which is characteristic of nerve root avulsion. Magnetic resonance imaging will probably replace these investigations in the future.

Electrical studies rarely add any new diagnostic information concerning the neurological damage but they do provide useful baseline studies for future comparison. It is reasonable to obtain these studies 8 weeks after the injury.

There is controversy concerning the exact indications for surgical intervention for closed brachial plexus injuries in adults. Obviously, if the injury is partial and improving there is no indication for surgery and supportive management, including intensive physiotherapy and mobilisation of the joints, should be commenced as soon as possible. Similarly, there is no place for surgery if there is clinical or radiological evidence of nerve root avulsion from the cord. In general there is little benefit from exploration of the plexus in closed injuries, although some surgeons do advocate exploration approximately 4 months after the injury if clinical electrical evidence shows the lesion to be complete.

Pain following nerve injuries

A number of pain problems occur specifically after nerve injuries. These include:

- Causalgia (Ch. 20)
- Phantom limb pains (Ch. 20)
- Irritative nerve lesions — neuroma
- Brachial plexus trauma pain.

Phantom limb pain and causalgia are described in more detail in Chapter 20. Causalagia occurs rarely. It is a burning pain that follows a partial or minor nerve injury and is relieved by sympathectomy. Phantom limb pain may occur following a traumatic amputation of a limb or after the surgical amputation for tumours or peripheral vascular disease.

There is a diffuse range of pain problems following peripheral nerve injuries that is broadly termed 'irritative nerve lesions'. The pathological cause of the pain is often not evident, although in some cases a neuroma may be demonstrable and the pain is relieved following excision.

A particularly severe form of pain following nerve injury occurs after brachial plexus trauma. The onset of the pain is frequently delayed by some weeks or months and the pain is described as having both deep and superficial components. The deep pain is continuous and is described as an 'ache' throughout the affected limb. The superficial 'burning' pain is particularly severe distally in the limb and is associated with a hyperpathia. The skin is usually dry and cool and hyperthermia and sweating are uncommon.

The management of these pain problems involves an assessment of the particular pain pattern and the underlying pathological cause. In general, treatment consists of simple conservative measures, including supportive care and simple analgesic medication. If a neuroma is thought to be the cause of the pain it should be excised. The pain from brachial plexus injuries is notoriously difficult to treat and is often unresponsive to conservative therapies. The dorsal root entry zone (DREZ) operation has been moderately successful in controlling the pain in a significant percentage of these patients. The operation involves ablation of the dorsal root entry zone over the involved segments by thermocoagulation. There is a small risk of further damage to the cord by the procedure but most patients are willing to accept this because of the severity of the pain.

PERIPHERAL NERVE TUMOURS

The classification and nomenclature of peripheral nerve tumours has been confusing, mainly due to disagreements as to the embryological origin of the various tumours. Peripheral nerve tumours may arise from the nerve sheath or be of neuronal origin. The nerve sheath tumours may be neuro-ectodermal or mesodermal in origin, the neuronal tumours arise from the neuro-ectoderm.

The nerve sheath tumours originating from the neuro-ectoderm may arise from the Schwann cells, which form the axonal myelin, or from the perineurial cells. Those of mesodermal origin arise from the fibrocytes that lie in the endoneurium and throughout the nerve sheath. The neuronal or nerve cell tumours nearly always arise in the ganglia of the autonomic nervous system.

The more common peripheral nerve tumours are shown in Table 17.3.

Table 17.3 Peripheral nerve tumours

Benign tumours
  Schwannoma
  Neurofibroma
    cutaneous neurofibroma
    intraneural (plexiform) neurofibroma

Malignant tumours
  Malignant schwannoma
  Nerve sheath fibrosarcoma (neurofibrosarcoma)

Non-neoplastic
  Morton's neuroma
  Traumatic neuroma

Benign tumours

Schwannoma

Schwannomas may arise from intracranial nerves (Ch. 7) or intraspinal nerves (Ch. 15). The extraspinal schwannomas may arise from motor, sensory or autonomic nerves and are usually encountered as solitary lesions in adults. They may be associated with von Recklinghausen's neurofibromatosis. They are sometimes classed together with neurofibromas as 'benign nerve sheath tumours'. They are discrete, smooth and sometimes lobulated; they originate focally in a fascicle. As they grow the discrete mass deflects the other fascicles over its surface. Malignant transformation is rare.

As in other schwannomas there are two distinct architectural patterns, Antoni A and B. The histological features of Antoni A typically consist of strands and whorls of closely packed spindle cells with elongated, darkly staining nuclei. The nuclei show a tendency to aggregate and often show striking pallisading. The type B consists of loosely arranged stellate cells and a spongy meshwork of vacuolated cells.

Benign schwannomas are usually asymptomatic and most patients present with a painful lump or local tenderness if the tumours are superficial. Occasionally, the benign tumours may present with pain or neurological disturbance, particularly if they arise in an enclosed space such as the carpal or tarsal tunnel. Most of the tumours arise in the head, neck and extremities.

The treatment involves tumour resection and, using microsurgical techniques, preservation of nerve function.

Neurofibroma

Cutaneous neurofibromas. Originating from small peripheral nerves in the dermis, cutaneous neurofibromas enlarge to elevate the skin into a soft, hemispheric or pedunculated mass. Cutaneous neurofibromas may be a component of Von Recklinghausen's disease (Fig. 17.4), but most occur independently of this disorder. Their location usually permits complete excision.

Intraneural neurofibromas. Less common than the cutaneous variety, intraneural neurofibromas usually arise from larger nerves, have a frequent association with Von Recklinghausen's disease and have a potential for malignant transformation. They commonly occur in the cervical, brachial or lumbosacral plexus. The tumour is formed by an intraneural proliferation of Schwann cells and is usually a diffuse transformation of long segments of nerves and their branches. This plexiform neurofibroma is pathognomonic for Von Recklinghausen's disease. A focal solitary lesion is rare.

The nerve containing the plexiform neurofibroma has a macroscopic appearance similar to rope, with the enlarged fascicles forming the braids of the rope.

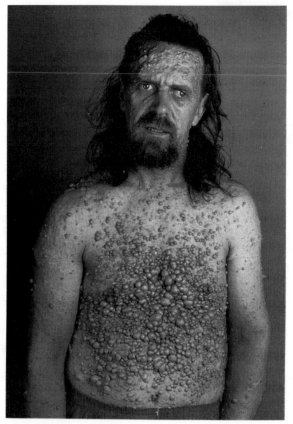

Fig. 17.4 Numerous cutaneous neurofibromatoma in a patient with Von Recklinghausen's disease. Other cutaneous features include café au lait spots and fibromas. The neurological features of Von Recklinghausen's may involve bilateral acoustic schwannomas, multiple meningiomas and gliomas and flexiform neurofibromas.

The surgical treatment provides a dilemma. Approximately 10% may undergo malignant transformation, but radical resection will usually result in serious neurological impairment. In general, an initial partial resection, with preservation of neurological function, should be attempted. The patient should be observed closely and if there is evidence of malignant transformation a radical resection should be performed.

Malignant tumours

Malignant tumours of peripheral nerves can arise spontaneously in a normal nerve from Schwann cells of neuro-ectodermal origin or fibrocytes of mesodermal origin, or in a plexiform neurofibroma of Von Recklinghausen's disease. The tumours are classified as either malignant schwannoma or a nerve sheath fibrosarcoma. Sometimes, more overt mesenchymal characteristics such as osteoid, chondroid and rhabdomyoblasts are contained in malignant peripheral nerve neoplasms.

The patient usually presents with an enlarging painful mass with a progressive neurological disturbance in the distribution of the nerve involved.

The tumour presents macroscopically as a lobulated, fusiform enlargement of the nerve that may extend over a long length, both proximal and distal to the major mass. The surrounding tissues are compressed and histological examination may show microscopic invasion.

Surgery will entail a radical resection provided there is no evidence of widespread metastases.

Non-neoplastic tumours

Morton's neuroma is a reactive fibrosis associated with degeneration of a nerve. It occurs predominantly in women in the plantar digital nerve between the heads of the 3rd and 4th metatarsals. The patient presents with pain and, macroscopically, the lesion is a discrete enlargement of the neurovascular bundle. The 'neuroma' can be excised simply and the problem cured.

Traumatic neuromas appear macroscopically as a fusiform enlargement of the nerve or, if there has been transection of the nerve, as a bulbous expansion of the proximal stump.

A painful neuroma can be excised. This is particularly appropriate if a nerve block proximal to the neuroma gives total pain relief.

The treatment of a neuroma of a nerve in continuity is more difficult when there is retained nerve function. Neurolysis, with division of the epineurium, may relieve the pain. Occasionally excision of the neuroma in continuity and resuture of the nerve may be necessary.

FURTHER READING

Brain W R, Wright A D, Wilkinson M 1947 Spontaneous compression of both median nerves in a carpal tunnel. Six cases treated surgically. Lancet i: 277–282
Burger P C, Vogel F S 1982 Surgical pathology of the nervous system and its coverings, 2nd edn. John Wiley, New York
Ebeling P, Gilliat T R W, Thomas P K 1960 A clinical and electrical study of ulnar nerve lesions in the hand. Journal of Neurology, Neurosurgery and Psychiatry 23: 1–8
Kline D G, Judice D J 1983 Operative management of selected brachial plexus lesions. Journal of Neurosurgery 58: 631–649
Pang D, Wessel H B 1988 Thoracic outlet syndrome. Neurosurgery 22: 105–121
Seddon H 1975 Surgical disorders of the peripheral nerves, 2nd edn. Churchill Livingstone, London
Sunderland S 1978 Nerves and nerve injuries. Churchill Livingstone, Edinburgh

18. Facial pain and hemifacial spasm

Facial pain may result from local pathology involving the face, mouth, jaw, temporomandibular joint, paranasal sinuses or salivary glands, or it may be due to distinct pain disorders such as trigeminal neuralgia, glossopharyngeal neuralgia and postherpetic neuralgia. These specific pain entities are relatively uncommon but the clinical manifestations are stereotyped so that a diagnosis should be apparent.

TRIGEMINAL NEURALGIA

Trigeminal neuralgia consists of excruciating paroxysmal pain, which lasts for seconds to minutes, in the distribution of the 5th cranial nerve. It was described by Avincenni 900 years ago and the term 'tic douloureux' was applied by André in 1756. Charles Bell demonstrated the anatomical basis for sensation in the face in the 1820s and distinguished the sensory component of the trigeminal nerve from the motor function of the facial nerve and consequently defined an anatomical basis for trigeminal neuralgia. It is estimated that it occurs in about one in every 70 000 people.

Aetiology

There is controversy concerning the precise aetiology of trigeminal neuralgia. The microvascular compression theory is popular and postulates that the 5th cranial nerve is compressed at the brain stem junction by a vascular loop. In 1934, Dandy first proposed that trigeminal neuralgia was caused by the nerve being compressed and distorted by the superior cerebellar artery, and this theory of microvascular decompression was extended by Gardner, at the Cleveland Clinic, to form the basis of hemifacial spasm with pressure on the 7th cranial nerve. The concept has been popularised by Jannetta, who proposed that trigeminal neuralgia is the result of compression of the root entry zone, which is a junctional area between the central and peripheral myelin on the nerve adjacent to the brain stem. However, others suggest that the pain is due to central dysfunction in the brain stem in structures related to the nucleus of the 5th nerve.

Trigeminal neuralgia may occasionally present as a symptom of multiple sclerosis, which should therefore be considered as a cause in patients under 40 years of age.

In approximately 3% of cases there may be a mass, such as a meningioma, epidermoid or arteriovenous malformation, in the posterior fossa. This mass distorts the nerve and produces pain similar to trigeminal neuralgia.

Clinical features

The main clinical feature is the sudden, severe pain that lasts for a moment and then goes, leaving nothing behind — except the fear of its return. Shaving, talking, eating, washing or even a cold wind may disturb the skin and trigger a paroxysm of pain which is so severe that the patient is immobilised in agony.

The particular characteristics of trigeminal neuralgia are:

- The pain is strictly limited to one or more branches of the trigeminal nerve. It most commonly affects the 2nd and/or 3rd division
- The pain is sudden and short-lived, usually lasting seconds, or at the most, minutes
- The pain is frequently provoked by light mechanical stimuli within the trigeminal area. In particular, it is often 'triggered' by touching the side of the face, or is brought on by facial movement, such as chewing. These patients are often unable to shave and they shield their faces when outside in the wind
- There is no detectable abnormality of trigeminal nerve function.

The incidence of trigeminal neuralgia reaches its maximum between the ages of 50 and 70 years, is very rare below the age of 25 and uncommon under the age of 40. The pain affects the territory of the 2nd and 3rd divisions of the trigeminal nerve with equal frequency, and may involve both territories simultaneously. The area of the 1st division of the trigeminal nerve is involved less frequently. In about 5% of cases the neuralgia affects both sides of the face, but not usually simultaneously so that each bout of pain remains strictly unilateral. Bilateral trigeminal neuralgia occurs more commonly in patients with multiple sclerosis.

Remissions of the pain are frequent and may last for months or even years; occasionally complete freedom from the pain occurs.

There are no physical signs. The patient may present with a scarf shielding the head and will talk from the corner of the mouth so as not to precipitate a spasm of pain. If the pain has been very severe the patient may be emaciated and dehydrated from being unable to eat or drink and the face may be dirty and unshaven from fear of precipitating an attack of pain.

Investigations

A CT scan of the brain should be performed to exclude a mass in the cerebellopontine angle in the posterior fossa.

Differential diagnosis

The pain of trigeminal neuralgia is characteristic but must be differentiated from:

- Atypical facial pain
- Pain of dental origin, such as malocclusion or dental abscess
- Pain from the temporomandibular joint
- Postherpetic neuralgia
- Migrainous neuralgia (cluster headache).

Treatment

Management of a patient with trigeminal neuralgia may involve the use of a number of treatment modalities including:

- Drugs
- Local procedures on peripheral branches of the trigeminal nerve
- Percutaneous procedures involving the trigeminal ganglion or the retrogasserian rootlets
- Posterior fossa craniotomy procedures.

Drugs

Carbamazepine (Tegretol®) initially relieves the pain in the great majority of patients although doses of 200 mg tablets up to 4–5 times a day are often necessary for adequate pain control. However, the patients frequently have a relapse of pain and need further treatment. In addition, many patients are unable to tolerate the side-effects of carbamazepine which occur at the doses necessary to control the discomfort. The most frequent adverse reactions are dizziness, drowsiness, unsteadiness, nausea and vomiting. Haemopoietic complications due to bone marrow depression occur rarely. Other drugs that can be tried include phenytoin, baclofen and clonazepam, although they are not as effective.

Procedures involving peripheral branches of the trigeminal nerve

Infra-orbital or supra-orbital nerve section may be performed in the un-common situation of the pain being localised to the area in the distribution of these nerves. However, the pain frequently recurs and these procedures should probably be limited to the elderly frail patient.

Percutaneous thermocoagulation

Percutaneous thermocoagulation of the retrogasserian rootlets or ganglion of the trigeminal neuralgia can result in analgesia in selected areas of the trigeminal distribution. In this procedure a needle is passed percutaneously, under X-ray control, through the foramen ovale into the ganglion and nerve roots just behind the ganglion in Meckel's cave. The nerve rootlets and ganglion are stimulated with a radiofrequency current, which results in a differential loss of pain sensation but retention of light touch sensation. Alternatively, glycerol may be injected into Meckel's cave so as to bathe the retrogasserian nerve rootlets. Although these procedures have a high initial success in relieving pain, they may produce facial numbness and the trigeminal neuralgia frequently recurs. The procedures may be repeated when the pain recurs or alternative treatments may be considered.

Posterior fossa craniotomy procedures

Total or partial trigeminal nerve section. Trigeminal root section, either by a posterior fossa craniotomy or middle cranial fossa approach (Frazier's operation) used to be a common procedure for trigeminal neuralgia but is now almost obsolete. Section of the nerve results in facial numbness and the morbidity may be quite disabling, particularly if the ophthalmic division supplying the cornea is affected. However, a partial section of the posterior half of the nerve causes only relatively minor disturbance of facial sensation and may result in lasting pain relief for trigeminal neuralgia involving the 2nd and/or 3rd divisions. An uncommon, but feared, disabling complication of nerve section is a painful dysaesthesia of the face, 'anaesthesia dolorosa', for which there is no treatment. Anaesthesia dolorosa only rarely results from percutaneous radiofrequency rhizotomy.

Microvascular decompression.   This is now the procedure of choice. The operation is performed via a small retrosigmoid posterior fossa craniotomy using the operating microscope. The vessel, most commonly the superior cerebellar artery, is dissected away from the 5th cranial nerve at the brain stem entry junction and the nerve is then shielded from the vessel by a small patch of sponge. Over 90% of patients have an initial complete relief of pain, although about 15% have some relapse of trigeminal neuralgia over the next 5 years.

Summary of treatment

There are a number of methods of treating trigeminal neuralgia and the treatment chosen will frequently depend on the patient's preference when the various options are explained. In general, carbamazepine is used first. If the medication is not tolerated, or when the pain relapses, the main choice is between a radiofrequency percutaneous rhizotomy or a posterior fossa craniotomy and microvascular decompression. Unless the patient is elderly and frail, microvascular decompression is the preferred option, as it has the greatest chance of producing permanent relief of pain with no facial numbness.

GLOSSOPHARYNGEAL NEURALGIA

Glossopharyngeal neuralgia is much less common than trigeminal neuralgia, there being approximately one case for every 50 of trigeminal neuralgia. It was first defined as a clinical entity by Harris in 1921. It is characterised by intense attacks of pain in the distribution of the glossopharyngeal nerve and the auricular and pharyngeal branches of the vagus nerve.

Aetiology

The precise cause of glossopharyngeal neuralgia is unclear, although Janetta proposed the theory of microvascular compression of the 9th nerve, as for trigeminal neuralgia and the 5th cranial nerve.

Presenting features

The patients present with attacks of severe pain involving the throat, tongue or ear. The pain may start anywhere in the territory of the glossopharyngeal nerve or auricular and pharyngeal branch of the vagus nerve. The tonsil, root of the tongue and ear are common sites and the pain often extends into the base of the jaw and the neck. At times the pain may be confined to the throat and occasionally only the ear is involved. In some patients the pain involves the area of the mandibular division of the trigeminal nerve, which may lead to a wrong diagnosis.

The attacks are frequently induced by talking, swallowing or chewing, and consequently, in severe cases, the patient may become cachectic. Occasionally, an episode of throat pain precipitated by swallowing may be associated with bradycardia, hypotension and syncope.

Differential diagnosis

The distribution of the pain will distinguish glossopharyngeal neuralgia from trigeminal neuralgia. Geniculate neuralgia, described by Hunt, is rare and involves the sensory component of the facial nerve (nervus intermedius). Geniculate neuralgia has two major forms affecting either the ear, with secondary radiation into the deep structures of the face, or pain involving primarily the deep facial structures.

Treatment

Patients with glossopharyngeal neuralgia may derive benefit from treatment with carbamazepine, although with less effect than for trigeminal neuralgia. However, surgery for glossopharyngeal neuralgia is straightforward and effective. The operation involves a small posterior fossa craniotomy with section of the 9th nerve and upper 10% of the fibres of the vagus nerve. The sensory loss resulting from these nerve sections results in no disability.

POSTHERPETIC NEURALGIA

Herpes zoster may involve the distribution of the trigeminal nerve, particularly the ophthalmic division. In a manner similar to shingles involving the trunk or limbs, postherpetic neuralgia occurs more frequently in elderly patients. The pain, usually in the distribution of the ophthalmic division, is severe, constant and unremitting, and is described as 'burning' or a 'crawling' sensation under the skin.

The diagnosis is usually obvious by the herpetic rash. Occasionally, however, the rash may be minor and barely noticeable.

There is no surgical treatment for postherpetic neuralgia of the trigeminal nerve and sensory root section is of no benefit. Carbamazepine may alleviate some of the discomfort, although unfortunately its benefit is usually limited.

There is some evidence that the use of steroids and acyclovir in the patients presenting with herpes zoster may reduce the risk of postherpetic neuralgia.

ATYPICAL FACIAL PAIN

Facial pain which has no pathological basis is relatively common and most frequently affects middle-aged females. The pain presents a diagnostic problem which can often only be solved after underlying pathology has been excluded by clinical and radiological investigations.

The pain is usually situated in the central portions of the face or cheek and is described as boring, dull or aching. The lancinating paroxysms of pain characteristic of trigeminal neuralgia and glossopharyngeal neuralgia are absent. Dental malocclusion and pain from the temporomandibular joint, Costen's syndrome, should be excluded.

HEMIFACIAL SPASM

Hemifacial spasm is a facial disorder that is not painful, but its proposed aetiology is so similar to trigeminal neuralgia that it is best described in this chapter. The condition is characterised by unilateral spasms of the facial muscles supplied by the facial nerve.

Aetiology

The aetiology is similar to that proposed for trigeminal neuralgia and the microvascular compression theory postulates that the 7th cranial nerve is compressed at the brain stem junction by a vascular loop, usually an artery. Gardner advocated this theory in the 1960s and it has been popularised by Jannetta who proposed that, as for trigeminal neuralgia and the 5th cranial nerve, hemifacial spasm is due to pulsatile compression at the root exit zone of the 7th cranial nerve, which is a junctional area between the central and peripheral myelin where the 7th nerve leaves the brain stem. Very uncommonly, hemifacial spasm is associated with a compressive mass such as an epidermoid, aneurysm or meningioma. Occasionally, hemifacial spasm and trigeminal neuralgia may co-exist in the same patient.

Clinical features

The onset of hemifacial spasm usually commences in middle or old age and there is a slight female predominance. The spasms usually commence around the orbicularis oculi muscles and subsequently spread down the face to involve the other facial muscles innervated by the facial nerve. The spasms are episodic and are frequently precipitated by emotional distress, chewing, talking or laughing. The condition causes the patient considerable social embarrassment and the spasms of the orbicularis oculi result in eye closure, making driving difficult.

In contrast to trigeminal neuralgia, where there is no clinical evidence of 5th cranial nerve dysfunction, there is frequently minor facial weakness between the episodes of spasm. Otherwise, there are no neurological findings.

Management

The diagnosis is self-evident, with the spasms being located on one side of the face. In the very early stages, hemifacial spasm needs to be differentiated from simple blepharospasm, but this is confined to the muscles around the eye and is usually bilateral.

A CT scan should be performed to exclude the unlikely possibility of a posterior fossa mass lesion causing the condition.

There is currently no effective medical treatment, although injections of botulin toxin into the branches of the nerve peripherally are being tried, with limited, transient success.

At present, the only effective treatment is surgical and the operation is a microvascular decompression of the 7th cranial nerve. However, as the condition is benign and painless the principal indication for operation is social embarrassment. In many patients the hemifacial spasm is so annoying and socially distressing that they are keen to proceed with an operation, bearing in mind its possible risks. Surgery is definitely inappropriate if the patient is not troubled by the spasm.

The microvascular decompression is performed through a small posterior fossa craniotomy and, using the operating microscope, the vessel compressing the 7th nerve at the brain stem junction is carefully mobilised away. The nerve is then protected from the vessel by a small patch of sponge. The operation is usually highly effective in relieving the spasm. There is a small risk of unilateral hearing loss due to the proximity of the 8th nerve and its blood supply. As the operation involves a craniotomy, often in elderly patients, there is a small risk of serious complication, mostly as a result of cerebrovascular complications. This possibility should temper an obvious enthusiasm for an effective operation.

FURTHER READING

Adams C B T 1989 Microvascular compression, an alternative view and hypothesis. Journal of Neurosurgery 57: 1–12

Apfelbaum R I 1983 Surgery for tic douloureux. Clinical Neurosurgery 31: 351–368

Burchiel K J, Steege T D, Howe J F, Loeser J D 1981 Comparison of percutaneous radiofrequency gangliolysis and microvascular decompression for the surgical management of tic douloureux. Neurosurgery 9: 111–119

Dandy W E 1929 An operation for the cure of tic douloureux: partial section of the sensory root at the pons. Archives of Surgery 18: 687–734

Dandy W E 1934 Concerning the cause of trigeminal neuralgia. American Journal of Surgery 24: 447–455

Gardner W J 1962 Concerning the mechanism of trigeminal neuralgia and hemifacial spasm. Journal of Neurosurgery 19: 947–948

Jannetta P J, Abbasy M, Maroon J C, Ramos F M, Albin M S 1977 Aetiology and definitive microsurgical treatment of hemifacial spasm: operative techniques and results in 47 patients. Journal of Neurosurgery 47: 321–328

Jannetta P J 1980 Neurovascular compression in cranial nerve and systemic disease. Annals of Surgery 192: 518–525

Stookey B, Ransohoff J 1959 Trigeminal neuralgia: its history and treatment. Charles C Thomas, Springfield

19. Pain — neurosurgical management

Pain is the most common symptom in patients presenting to a neurosurgeon, in fact it is often the only symptom that the patient will complain of. The features of the pain are often characteristic of the particular underlying disease; these features include:

- Mode of onset
- Pattern of the pain — continuous or intermittent
- Duration
- Position of the pain
- Quality of the pain
- Features that alleviate or exacerbate the pain.

There are three major clinical groups of pain problems:
1. Benign specific pain syndromes
2. Benign nonspecific pain syndromes
3. Cancer pain.

MECHANISMS OF PAIN

There is no 'pain centre' in the brain — such a concept would be quite inadequate to account for the complexity of pain. There are three major psychological–anatomical–physiological components to pain which aid in the understanding of the mechanisms of pain and in treating patients. These are:

1. Sensory–discriminative
2. Motivational–affective
3. Cognitive–evaluative.

Melzack and Casey proposed that each of these components are subserved by physiologically specialised systems in the brain.

Sensory – discriminative dimension

The sensory–discriminative dimension involves the spatial, temporal and magnitude properties of pain and is subserved mostly by neospinothalamic

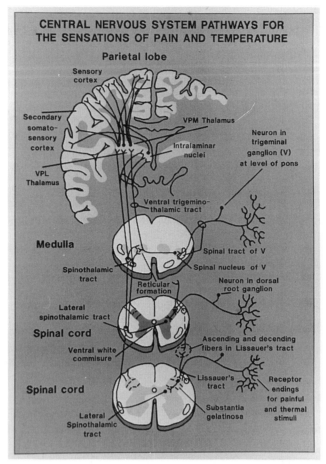

Fig. 19.1 Pathways that mediate pain and temperature (Adapted from Gilman and Newman, 1987. Published with permission).

projections to the ventrobasal thalamus and then to the somatosensory cortex (Fig. 19.1). The pain pathways are described in Chapter 1. The receptors for pain consist of unencapsulated endings of peripheral nerves. The neural responses are mediated through the myelinated A delta and unmyelinated C fibres. Pain may be felt as two waves, separated by a very short interval. The first is sharp and localised, with conduction along group A fibres. The second wave, which is rather diffuse and more disagreeable, depends on the slower conduction of group C fibres. The cell bodies are in the dorsal root ganglia. Their axons traverse the dorsal roots and enter the dorsolateral fasciculus (tract of Lissauer) of the spinal cord, in which ascending and descending branches travel for one or two segments. These fibres, which give off many collateral branches in their short course, terminate in the substantia gelatinosa of the dorsal grey horn. The substantia gelatinosa consists of golgi type II neurons whose axons are either confined to the nucleus or run for short distances in the tract of Lissauer, connecting adjacent regions of the substantia gelatinosa. Axons of the tract cells in the chief nucleus of the dorsal horn cross the midline in the ventral commissure and then course rostrally in the lateral spinothalamic tract. Fibres are continually being added to the ventromedial aspect of the lateral spinothalamic tract. At the upper cervical levels fibres from the sacral segments are dorsolateral, followed by fibres from lumbar and thoracic segments, while fibres from the cervical segments are in the ventromedial position. The fibres ascend through the brain stem, supplying inputs to the reticular formation and the superior colliculus, before terminating in the nuclei of the thalamus, particularly the intralaminar, ventral posterolateral (VPL) and posterior nuclear complex. There is a somatotopic representation of the opposite side of the body in the lateral portion of the thalamic nucleus. Tertiary neurons then project to the primary and secondary sensory area in the cerebral cortex.

Pain fibres from the head enter the pons through the sensory root of the trigeminal nerve and turn caudally in the trigeminal spinal tract, the spinal tract of V, which extends to the upper cervical levels. Terminals of the spinal tract of V form synapses in the adjacent nucleus, the spinal nucleus of V. Axons of the spinal nucleus of V cross to the opposite side and ascend as the ventral trigeminothalamic tract to the ventral posteromedial nucleus (VPM) of the thalamus, as well as to the intralaminar nuclei. The fibres then pass to the somatosensory cortex. There is a spatial arrangement of fibres in the sensory root and spinal tract corresponding to the divisions of the trigeminal nerve. Ophthalmic fibres in the sensory root are dorsal, mandibular fibres are ventral and the maxillary fibres between these. Because of rotation of fibres as they enter the pons, the mandibular fibres are dorsal and the ophthalmic fibres ventral in the trigeminal spinal tract. The dorsal part of the spinal trigeminal tract includes pain and temperature fibres from the facial, glossopharyngeal and vagus nerves, which may supply areas of the external ear, lining of the auditory canal, tympanic membrane, posterior tongue, pharynx and larynx.

Motivational — affective dimension

The motivational–affective dimension component of pain is involved with the aversive quality of pain, which provides the unique, distinctly unpleasant component to the sensory experience. The brain stem reticular formation and the limbic system, which receive projections from the spinoreticular and paleospinothalamic components of the somatosensory pathways, play an important role in the motivational affective dimension.

Cognitive–evaluative dimension

The cognitive–evaluative dimension relates to the person's understanding of pain as regards their intellectual, social and cultural background. Cognitive activities such as cultural values, anxiety, attention and suggestion all have a profound effect on the pain experience. Cognitive functions are able to act selectively on sensory processing or motivational mechanisms and there is evidence that the sensory input is evaluated and modified before it activates the discriminative or motivational systems. Men wounded in battle may feel little pain from the wound but may complain bitterly about a seemingly trivial medical procedure such as intramuscular injection or venepuncture. The neural mechanisms that perform these complex functions must conduct rapidly to the cortex so that the somatosensory information has the opportunity to undergo further analysis, interact with other sensory inputs and activate previous memory stores. Melzack and Wall proposed that dorsal column and dorsolateral projection pathways act as a 'feed forward' limb of this loop. The frontal cortex may play a particularly significant role.

Theories of pain mechanisms

There have been numerous theories of pain mechanisms over the past few centuries. In 1644, Descartes described a 'specificity' theory, in which he conceived that the pain system was a direct channel from the skin to the brain. There are numerous other theories which have concentrated on one or more of the various dimensions of pain and tried to explain these in a single process. The '**gate control theory**', proposed by Melzack and Wall in 1965, is a useful concept of the mechanism of pain. Although some of the details have been disproved, the proposal that afferent stimulation can influence pain perception is accepted. The theory proposes that neural mechanisms in the dorsal column of the spinal cord act like a 'gate', which can either increase or decrease the flow of nerve impulses from the periphery to the central nervous system. The input from the sensory nerve fibres can be modulated by the gate before evoking the perception of pain and the person's response. The relative activity of the large diameter A-beta fibres and the smaller diameter of the A-delta and C fibres influence the gate to either increase or decrease the sensory transmission (Fig. 19.2).

To this proposed mechanism of pain can be added the central pathways that relate to the three major dimensions of pain. In addition, the midline raphe nuclei of the brain stem have connections with the periventricular and periaqueductal areas and their axons descend to the spinal cord through the dorsolateral fasciculus. These axons terminate in the dorsal horn, where they modify the responses to painful stimuli. Opioid peptides (endorphins) are the neurotransmitters involved in these mechanisms.

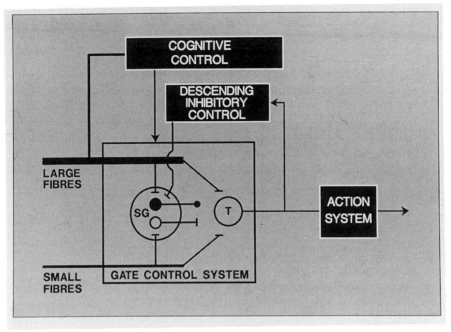

Fig. 19.2   The gate control theory of pain as proposed by Melzack and Wall. Excitatory (white circle) and inhibitory (black circle) links extend from the substantial gelatinosa (SG) to the transmission cells (T) as well as descending inhibitory control from the brain stem systems. All connections are excitatory except the inhibitory link from SG to T. The round knob at the end of the inhibitory link implies that its action may be presynaptic, postsynaptic or both. (From Melzack and Wall, 1985. Reproduced with permission).

BENIGN SPECIFIC PAIN SYNDROMES

There are numerous benign pain syndromes that have a specific, well recognised pathological disorder. The more common syndromes presenting in neurological and neurosurgical practice are:

- Head pain. Headache due to raised intracranial pressure, dural irritation, migraine or occipital neuralgia
- Facial pain due to trigeminal neuralgia, disorders of the temporomandibular joint or sinusitis
- Upper limb pain, most commonly due to cervical nerve root compression from a cervical disc prolapse, carpal tunnel syndrome or thoracic outlet syndrome
- Pain involving the trunk in a dermatome distribution due to thoracic nerve root inflammation or compression, due to shingles (herpes zoster) or tumour
- Lower limb pain due to sciatica or lumbar canal stenosis.

These clinical problems are discussed in the relevant chapters. The treatment is specific and, in general, effective. The success of the treatment depends on an accurate diagnosis and appropriate management.

There are two uncommon specific benign pain syndromes that present to neurosurgeons, causalgia and phantom limb pain. These pain problems have perplexed neuroscientists and neurosurgeons as to the aetiology of the pain and its treatment.

Causalgia

Causalgia is a rare pain condition that usually follows an injury of a major nerve; it has the following characteristics:

- It is severe and persistent
- It has a burning unpleasant quality
- It spreads beyond the territory of the injured nerve or nerves
- It is aggravated by physical and emotional stimuli.

The pain usually involves the hand or foot but may spread through the affected limb. Because use of the extremities is avoided, stiffness develops and there are frequently 'trophic' changes, with the skin becoming thin and shiny. There is usually an exaggerated response to any form of cutaneous stimulus. A sympathectomy almost invariably relieves the pain, although the mechanism for this is not understood.

Phantom limb pain

Phantom limb pain is the perception of a painful sensation in an extremity that has been amputated.

Virtually all amputees have phantom sensations but only a small percentage have disabling pain in the phantom limb. Pain in the stump of the limb due to local factors is common and must be differentiated from true phantom limb pain, although they may be related.

The cause of phantom limb pain is unknown. It may develop immediately after the injury or at any stage up to some years later. The pain may result from deafferentation of the dorsal horn neurons and more rostral structures, although environmental and affective factors do play a role in the patient's pain behaviour and influence the disability.

The management of this problem is particularly difficult. It involves a careful assessment of the environmental and psychological factors that may affect the patient. Numerous treatments have been tried, including various types of physical therapies, analgesic medication, antidepressants, minor tranquilisers, anticonvulsants (carbamazepine) and psychological treatments including hypnotherapy and psychotherapy.

Many neurosurgical ablative procedures, such as cordotomy, dorsal rhizotomy, neurectomy and sympathectomy, have been tried without success.

The dorsal root entry zone (DREZ) operation has been used with some initial success in the treatment of phantom pain. The operation involves destruction of the zone where the dorsal root fibres enter into the spinal cord, usually by thermocoagulation.

BENIGN NON-SPECIFIC PAIN SYNDROMES

Patients with chronic pain that does not have an underlying specific pathological cause are frequently referred to a neurosurgeon for assessment and management. The pain problems may involve any region of the body but there are a number of particularly common types of clinical presentation:

- The head — headache
- Face — atypical facial pain
- Upper limb — non-specific arm pain
- Spine — non-specific neck, thoracic or low back pain
- Lower limb — diffuse leg pain.

Many of the patients who present may have a structural, organic basis for a component of the pain problem, but the clinical manifestations are far more extensive than can be explained by any pathological changes that can be demonstrated either by clinical or radiological findings. In some cases the presenting pain problem may just be a marked exaggeration of a true organic problem. In others, the presenting features will bear no relationship at all to any recognised clinical abnormality. Detailed questioning may reveal that the patient 'gains' from the pain and that this gain may be either psychological or involving definite material benefit for the patient. Unfortunately, pending litigation is a real and often powerful conscious or subconscious motive for the continuation or exaggeration of symptoms.

Management

The management of these patients generally involves:
— Exclusion of an organic basis for the complaint. This will involve detailed history and examination and radiological investigations. It is absolutely vital that the clinician should objectively assess the patient thoroughly. Patients with neurological disorders will often present with atypical clinical manifestations early in the disease process. It is wise, and very helpful, to reassess the patient at a subsequent examination to be certain there is not an organic basis for the presenting complaint. It is important not just to dismiss a patient as being disagreeable, eccentric or having an odd personality, as they may also have an organic problem which may or may not bear relationship to their underlying personality trait.
— The clinician should assess the possibility of any psychological origins for the pain and the social background of the patient. Reassurance is

often all that is necessary. For example, frequently a patient may present with chronic headaches and, if it becomes apparent that a friend or relative died recently from a brain tumour, all the patient requires is reassurance that they do not have a tumour. Unfortunately many of the problems are not this simple and more detailed counselling or psychiatric advice may be necessary.

— Maintain a positive mental attitude. Chronic, non-specific benign pain problems are debilitating for the patient and the various doctors involved. It is all too easy just to dismiss the patient and hope the problem will fade away as the patient disappears from sight. The patient has often sought numerous opinions and usually has a negative attitude about himself, his pain and the medical profession. It is helpful if the doctor can give positive advice, reassure the patient there is no serious underlying disease, encourage a positive mental attitude and be optimistic that the pain should resolve.

— Never use addictive medications. In particular it is essential never to resort to the use of narcotic analgesia, as this will inevitably make a difficult problem disastrous.

CANCER PAIN

The successful relief of pain in a patient suffering from cancer is one of the major challenges of neurosurgery. For many patients the diagnosis of cancer is not only associated with an enormous sense of grief and anxiety, but their greatest fear is that they will suffer severe pain during the illness. The two common misconceptions are that all cancer is painful and that cancer pain cannot be relieved. It is essential that the patients are reassured early in their illness that any pain they develop will be relieved.

The basic principles of the management of cancer pain are:

- Explanation, reassurance and counselling
- Modification of the pathological process. Bone metastases are the main cause of pain in the majority of patients with carcinoma of the kidney, thyroid and in multiple myeloma. Modification of the pathology by surgery (e.g. oöphorectomy for carcinoma of the breast, orchidectomy for carcinoma of the prostate), radiotherapy, chemotherapy or hormonal treatment should be considered in consultation with an oncologist
- Elevation of the pain threshhold. Reduction of anxiety and improvement of a depressed mood will help to elevate the pain threshhold. Considerable benefit may result from admission to hospital or a specialised unit (palliative care unit or hospice unit), even for a short time. Adequate assessment and control of pain may

permit patients to return home. A feeling of security leads to reduced anxiety which can lessen pain and improve other symptoms

- Appropriate analgesic medication
- Neurosurgical techniques.

Pharmacological agents in cancer pain management

There is a concept of an 'analgesic ladder', which involves moving from weak to strong analgesic drugs, with appropriate adjuvant therapy when necessary, until pain is controlled. These adjuvants, or co-analgesics, which may include anti-emetics, antidepressants and corticosteroids, can be of great value in potentiating the primary analgesics. However, they may at the same time compound the side-effects, either by interfering with the pharmacology of the primary analgesics or by exacerbating a primary side-effect, such as sedation, of these analgesics.

The first choice is aspirin or an aspirin-like drug. These drugs provide excellent analgesic, anti-inflammatory and antipyretic effects. An alternative to aspirin is paracetamol, which has a similar antipyretic and analgesic activity but only a weak anti-inflammatory effect. The major advantage of both these drugs is their freedom from unwanted side-effects, such as those exerted by the opiates on the central nervous system. They are particularly active in the treatment of bone pain but they also have powerful analgesic activity on other organs. Aspirin's well known side-effect on the gastro-intestinal tract may diminish its use in some situations but enteric coated aspirin may be of assistance in patients who have gastric intolerance to soluble aspirin. It is important to appreciate that soluble aspirin has a maximum duration of analgesic action of only 3–4 hours and consequently it must be given strictly every 4 hours in appropriate dosage. The usual method of administration is to administer the aspirin every 4 hours in a dose below that which will produce toxicity, which is usually heralded by ringing in the ears. Paracetamol is usually commenced at a dose of 500 mg – 1 g every 4 hours and is increased as necessary. However, at doses of more than 12 gm in 24 hours the incidence of hepatic toxicity increases precipitously.

Codeine phosphate is a popular, short-acting, mild narcotic which may be useful in pain not adequately controlled by simple analgesics.

The aim of the use of narcotic analgesics is to control the pain with a minimum of side-effects, preferably by the oral route. The narcotic should be 'titrated' to a dose that will alleviate the pain. Morphine is the most common narcotic drug. Oral morphine is very satisfactory, provided the dose is carefully adjusted to suit the individual patient. Its oral bio-availability is approximately one-third that of the parenteral use and this must be taken into consideration when changing patients from one route to the other. Oral medication should be a regular 4-hourly dose.

There are numerous other narcotic preparations that may be administered either orally, parenterally or via a suppository and which may be useful in the individual patient to control pain. The major disadvantage of oral or parenteral narcotic medication are the side-effects, particularly drowsiness and nausea. There are now longer-acting forms of slow release oral morphine that can be administered twice daily, these may be preferable if they are available.

Neurosurgical techniques for pain control

Neurosurgical procedures will interfere with one or more of the psychological–anatomical–physiological pathways described previously (Table 19.1). Although, in general, neurosurgical procedures are only performed when the patient has continuing unrelieved pain despite the best medical treatment, some techniques are simple and are worth undertaking so that the dose of analgesia can be diminished.

The major neurosurgical techniques are:

- Nerve section. This is the time-honoured neurosurgical tool, although it has only a limited place in the control of cancer pain. Occasionally it may be of use when the tumour infiltrates a peripheral nerve. Section of the cranial nerves in the posterior fossa may relieve the pain of an infiltrating head and neck tumour, although these patients are often severely debilitated and the necessary multiple nerve section may further increase the morbidity.
- Spinal cordotomy. Cordotomy involves section of the lateral spinothalamic tract and can be performed either by open operation or percutaneously at the Cl/2 level. Although a high cervical cordotomy may initially control the pain in the upper limb the effect is often

Table 19.1 Neurosurgical procedures for cancer pain

Nerve section
  Cranial nerves
  Peripheral nerves

Cordotomy
  Open
  Closed

Sympathectomy

Cerebral procedures
  Deep brain stimulation
  Thalamotomy
  Leucotomy

Opiate administration
  Epidural
  Intrathecal (lumbar, subarachnoid)
  Intraventricular

transient. Unfortunately it has only a limited place in the control of cancer pain, as it will control pain satisfactorily on only one side of the body, usually in the lower limb. Unfortunately, it is rare for cancer pain to be this well localised. Bilateral cordotomy has a high morbidity and will not control pain if it is diffuse.

— Sympathectomy. A percutaneous chemical or surgical sympathectomy is a potent method of relieving pancreatic pain due to carcinoma but it is disappointing for benign pancreatic pain.

— Intracerebral procedures. Cerebral procedures, such as deep brain stimulation, thalamotomy and leucotomy, are now only rarely indicated in the control of cancer pain.

— Subarachnoid opiate administration. Most cancer pain can be effectively controlled with oral or suppository administration of opiates. The lumbar intradural subarachnoid administration of morphine has revolutionised the treatment of patients with terminal cancer pain and has dramatically altered the management of those patients whose pain is unrelieved by oral or suppository administration or who do not tolerate the side-effects of the high doses of narcotics necessary to control the pain. The technique allows very small doses of narcotic to be given directly into the subarachnoid space and avoids many of the unpleasant side-effects of high dose narcotic administration. Opiate receptors have been identified in the brain and spinal cord. The receptor density is high in the periventricular structures such as the amygdala, caudate, putamen, medial thalamus and habenular, in the peri-aqueduct grey matter and in the floor of the 4th ventricle. The greatest concentration of receptors in the spinal cord is in the substantia gelatinosa. These receptors are the likely synaptic site of action for local terminals, which release endogenous compounds with actions similar to opioid alkaloids (endorphins), as well as for the injected subarachnoid morphine.

The basic technique of lumbar intradural opiate administration involves the insertion of a catheter into the subarachnoid space of the lumbar theca. The catheter is threaded subcutaneously to the anterior abdominal or chest wall, where it is connected to a subcutaneous reservoir. The morphine can be injected directly into the reservoir, using meticulous sterile technique because of the risk of infection. Alternatively, infusion pumps can be implanted subcutaneously, filled with morphine and joined to the spinal catheter. Their major disadvantage is the expense of the pump.

Injection of morphine through the lumbar catheter will result in pain relief in most sites of the body, although it is less successful for pain involving the head, neck and upper limbs. In these situations an intraventricular catheter, with a subcutaneous reservoir, can be inserted for morphine administration.

There is a small risk of respiratory depression and the patient should be observed closely following the initial doses. If a subcutaneous reservoir is implanted the treatment regime usually commences with 0.5 mg morphine twice daily. The patient should fill in a pain chart which will document the level of pain throughout the day; the intrathecal morphine can be increased as necessary. The pain is usually satisfactorily controlled with a dose of morphine of between 1 and 10 mg/day. Supplementary oral narcotic or non-narcotic medication can also be used.

The major complications are infection of the catheter, which may lead to meningitis, and blockage of the catheter.

FURTHER READING

Gilman S, Newman S W 1987 Manter and Gatz's Essentials of clinical neuroanatomy and Neuropathology, 7th edn. F A Davis, Philadelphia

Melzack R 1973 The puzzle of pain. Basic Books, New York

Melzack R, Wall P D 1965 Pain mechanisms: a new series. Science 150: 971–979

Melzack R, Wall P D 1985 In: Wilkins R H, Rengachary S S (eds) Gate control theory in neurosurgery. McGraw Hill, New York, ch. 304, pp 2317–2319

Nashold B S, Ostdahrl H 1979 Dorsal root entry zone lesions for pain relief. Journal of Neurosurgery 51: 59–69

White J C, Sweet W H 1969 Pain and the neurosurgeon. Charles C Thomas, Illinois

Yaksh T L 1987 Opioid receptor systems and the endorphins. A review of their spinal organisation. Journal of Neurosurgery 67: 157–176

20. Movement disorders — neurosurgical aspects

Involuntary movement disorders are related to diseases of the extrapyramidal system, in particular the basal ganglia and their connections. The lesions are usually diffuse, affecting both the nuclear connections and communicating pathways, and involve disorders of the delicate balance of neurotransmitter substances. The pharmacological basis of movement disorders is generally a result of a chemical imbalance between two or more opposing neurotransmitter systems. The major basal ganglion neurotransmitters identified include dopamine, norepinephrine, gamma-aminobutyric acid, serotonin, acetylcholine and glutamic acid.

ANATOMICAL OVERVIEW

The basal ganglia, and their connections, form the anatomical substrate for most of the movement disorders, although the exact abnormality may not be clearly defined.

The corpus striatum is the major centre in the complex extrapyramidal motor system and is composed of:

- The globus pallidus (paleostriatum)
- The caudate nucleus and putamen (the neostriatum).

The putamen and globus pallidus together form the lentiform nucleus.

The complex interconnections between the basal ganglia nuclei, the red nucleus, the cerebellar outflow tracts, the brain stem reticular formation and the motor cortex are shown in Figures 20.1 and 20.2. There are two interconnecting pathways of particular importance to the neurosurgical management of movement disorders:

1. The corpus striatum neurons project to the globus pallidus and subsequently to the ventral anterior nucleus of the thalamus by:
   a. the lenticular fasciculus which passes rostral to the subthalamic nucleus
   b. the ansa lenticularis passing below the subthalamic nucleus.
   The majority of the fibres of the lenticular fasciculus and the ansa lenticularis merge in Forel's field H, enter the thalamic fasciculus

(Forel's field H1) and project rostrally and dorsally into the ventral anterior and ventral lateral thalamic nuclei. Fibres from the thalamus pass to the supplementary motor cortex. The circuit is completed by cortical neurons projecting to the caudate nucleus, then to the putamen and on to the globus pallidus (Fig. 20.1).

2. A circuit links the cerebellum to the thalamus via the dentate nucleus and red nucleus, and these fibres then pass to the primary and secondary motor cortex. Neurons descend from the cortex to the nuclei in the pontine reticular formation which project to the cortex of the cerebellum (Fig. 20.2).

Neurosurgical lesions to control movement disorders have been made:

- In the ansa lenticularis (ansotomy)
- In the globus pallidus (pallidotomy)

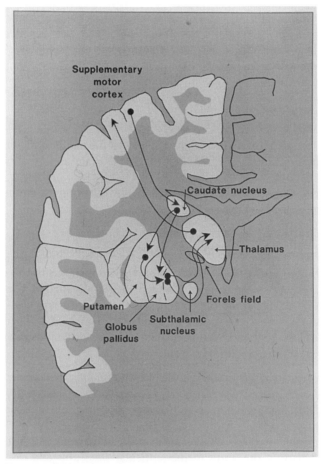

Fig. 20.1 Extrapyramidal pathway for movement showing Forel's field and relationship to basal ganglia and thalamus described in text.

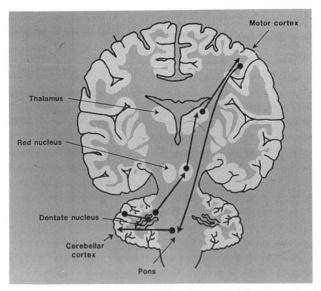

Fig. 20.2 Dentatorubrothalamic extrapyramidal pathway which is adjacent to that shown in Figure 20. 1.

- In Forel's field
- In the ventrolateral nucleus of the thalamus (thalamotomy)
- In the dentate nucleus (dentatotomy).

INVOLUNTARY MOVEMENT DISORDERS

Parkinson's disease

Parkinson's syndrome was described by James Parkinson in 1817 in *An Essay on the Shaking Palsy* and was recognised as an extrapyramidal disorder by Kinnier Wilson in 1912. The principle pathological disorder is a depletion of dopamine stores in the cells of the substantia nigra and neostriatum.

Parkinson's syndrome has a number of possible causes, of which idiopathic Parkinson's disease is the most common (Table 20.1). Parkinson's disease following encephalitis lethargica is now rare, although it may occur during the course of degenerative disorders such as Alzheimer's disease.

The essential clinical features are:

— A coarse tremor (4–8 Hz) which usually begins unilaterally in the upper limbs but eventually spreads to all limbs. Movement of the fingers occurs at the metacarpophalangeal joints and may be combined with movements of the thumb, the 'pill rolling' movement.
—Rigidity. When tested by passive movement the muscles may yield to tension in a series of jerks — cog wheel rigidity — although the

Table 20.1 Differential diagnosis of Parkinson's syndrome

Degenerative
   Idiopathic parkinsonism, adult and juvenile forms
   Striatonigral degeneration
   Shy–Drager syndrome
   Olivopontocerebellar degeneration
   Supranuclear palsy
   Parkinson–ALS–dementia complex

Infectious
   Postencephalitic parkinsonism
   Creutzfeldt–Jakob disease

Toxic
   Heavy metals (manganese)

Drugs
   Phenothiazines
   Butyrophenones
   Rauwolfia alkaloids
   α-methyldopa

Vascular
   Stroke
   Carbon monoxide

Neoplasm

Metabolic
   Hypoparathyroidism
   Wilson's disease

Taken from Olanow. Reproduced with permission

    increased muscle rigidity is sometimes smooth and is called 'plastic' or 'lead pipe' rigidity.
— Bradykinesia. The impairment of movement, consisting of difficulty in initiating movement (akinesia) and slowness with which it is performed (bradykinesia), is the most disabling feature of Parkinson's disease. In general, the movements which are carried out by the small muscles are the most affected. Consequently, early in the disease the patient shows weakness of ocular movements and facial movements, resulting in the 'mask-like' facies, and there is impairment of mastication and articulation. Swinging the arms when walking is diminished early and as the disease progresses the gait becomes severely impaired. The slowness is most severe on initiating movements and the patient may 'freeze'.
— Other abnormalities include dementia, which occurs in a third of parkinsonian patients, seborrhoea, sialorrhoea and gastrointestinal problems.

Management

L-dopa therapy revolutionised the treatment of Parkinson's disease and dramatically decreased the need for stereotactic surgery. Most patients are managed with medical therapy and are not referred to the neurosurgeon. However, stereotactic surgery does have a limited place in the treatment of Parkinson's disease.

Tremor responds best to stereotactic surgery, rigidity less and brady-kinesia least of all. However, bradykinesia responds best to l-dopa treat-ment; and the tremor least well. Consequently, medical management is the best form of therapy for what is usually the most disabling symptom. How-ever, if tremor is the most disabling symptom, and particularly if it is unilateral, surgery should be considered if there is a failure to respond to medical management. Bradykinesia is rarely an indication for stereotactic surgery, as the response to such surgery is poor.

The stereotactic lesion is made in Forel's field or the ventrolateral nucleus of the thalamus.

Essential tremor

Benign, or 'essential', familial tremor often has a familial basis, frequently commences before the age of 30 and may be fine and rapid or slower and coarse. It is characteristically an 'action tremor', as it tends to be increased by voluntary movement and emotion. The patient frequently notes that it may be improved following drinking alcohol. The usual medication includes propanolol and/or diazepam.

Stereotactic surgery may be considered if the tremor is not improved with medication and if the patient is disabled by the symptoms; significant im-provement has been reported in 70–80% of cases.

Tremor secondary to neurological degenerative diseases such as multiple sclerosis, cerebrovascular disease, encephalitis or trauma responds less favourably to surgery.

Cerebral palsy

The two components of cerebral palsy that may be helped by neurosurgical intervention are:

- The choreo-athetoid movements
- Spasticity.

Chorea is characterised by rapid, jerky, irrelevant, asymmetrical move-ments of the limbs and trunk. **Athetosis** is a relatively slow movement with a sinuous or writhing character. These two movements frequently co-exist in cerebral palsy, together with other features which may include combi-nations of spasticity, rigidity, dystonia, ataxia and tremor.

Cerebral palsy patients with choreo-athetosis and/or spasticity, who are not severely disabled by the other features of cerebral palsy and who do not have severe mental retardation, may be considered for stereotactic surgery.

Lesions are made in the ventrolateral thalamus or in Forel's field for choreo-athetosis, and in the dentate nucleus for spasticity. The lesions frequently need to be bilateral. Although initial significant improvement is reported in over 70% of cases in some series, the effect diminishes with time.

Chronic stimulation of the cerebellum using implanted electrodes has been advocated for the treatment of spasticity in cerebral palsy but there is no convincing evidence of significant benefit at this stage.

Hemiballismus

This movement disorder is characterised by violent, irregular, jerky movements of one side of the body, these arise primarily from the shoulder. The anatomical basis is a lesion of the subthalamic nucleus contralateral to the abnormal movement. It usually results from vascular disease but occasionally occurs in multiple sclerosis. It is an uncommon complication of stereotactic surgery resulting from the inadvertent involvement of the subthalamic nucleus during the production of a lesion in the thalamus.

The condition often settles spontaneously and drug treatment is ineffective. Stereotactic surgery is of benefit in over half the patients and the usual target is the ventrolateral nucleus of the thalamus or Forel's field.

Dystonia

Dystonia is an abnormal posture produced by spasms of muscles and/or exaggerated muscle tone. Dystonia may be generalised, as in dystonia muscularum deformans, or restricted to specific muscle groups. Spasmodic torticollis is sometimes regarded as a partial form of torsion dystonia and is discussed in the next section.

Symptomatic dystonia may occur in many neurological disorders including cerebral palsy, infantile hemiplegia, Wilson's disease and intoxication with phenothiazines. Idiopathic torsion dystonia is inherited as an autosomal recessive trait in Ashkenazi Jews and as an autosomal dominant disorder in non-Jewish populations, but many cases are sporadic. The onset usually occurs in childhood or adolescence and is often initially manifest as a spasmodic plantar flexion of the feet. The involuntary movements in the upper limbs consist of rotation or torsion and are associated with torsion movements of the vertebral column, particularly in the lumbar region. Medical treatment, including L-dopa, haloperidol, carbamazepine and anticholinergic therapy, is usually of little benefit. Stereotactic surgery produces some benefit in over half the patients. The procedure involves bilateral stereotactic lesions in the ventrolateral nucleus or Forel's field.

Spasmodic torticollis

Spasmodic torticollis is characterised by a clonic or tonic contraction of the cervical muscles which produces rotation of the head and neck, this may be sustained or spasmodic. Retrocollis is a similar disorder in which the neck is distended.

The aetiology of this unusual condition has not been clearly defined. Although in some cases the condition may be hysterical, it is evident that torticollis may be due to organic disease of the nervous system and some regard it as a limited form of torsion dystonia. It has been noted as a sequel of encephalitis lethargica or as part of other extrapyramidal syndromes. The microvascular compression theory, similar to that for trigeminal neuralgia and hemifacial spasm but with compression of the spinal accessory nerve or nerves, has been proposed, but as yet there is no evidence to substantiate this possibility.

The clinical manifestations include a rotation of the head and neck by contraction of the cervical muscles. The contraction of the sternocleidomastoid, trapezius and splenius muscles is evident on examination, although the deep muscles of the neck are also involved. Rotation may occur with or without lateral flexion. The contraction may be chronic, with repeated jerks, or predominantly tonic with a sustained posture. Retrocollis is due to bilateral contraction of the splenius and trapezius.

Management

The distinction between hysterical torticollis and torticollis of an organic origin may be difficult. Treatment should include psychotherapy and minor tranquillizers if it is thought that the torticollis has a hysterical basis.

EMG studies may help to evaluate the exact muscles involved in producing the torticollis. Tetrabenazine is occasionally successful if there is an organic basis but it may produce drug-induced parkinsonism. There are a number of surgical operations, which include:

- Division of the accessory nerves and the anterior roots of C1–3
- Myotomy, particularly section of the dominant sternocleidomastoid muscle
- Various stereotactic procedures
- Microvascular decompression of the spinal accessory nerve or nerves.

Intradural section of one or both accessory nerves and of the anterior upper cervical roots is the most commonly performed procedure. The anterior roots of C1–3 are usually divided on the passive side and C1–4 on the dominant side. The operation has been reported as producing satisfactory results in up to 80% of patients, although the general experience of most surgeons indicates a lower success rate. It is a major operative procedure with a significant risk of morbidity, particularly dysphagia, and a low risk of mortality.

FURTHER READING

Bucy P C 1951 The surgical treatment of extrapyramidal diseases. Journal of Neurology, Neurosurgery and Psychiatry 14: 108–115

Burke R E, Fahn S 1981 Movement disorders. In: Appel S H (ed) Current neurology. John Wiley, New York, pp 92–137

Cooper I S 1969 Involuntary movement disorders. Hoeber, New York

Dandy W E 1930 An operation for treatment of spasmodic torticollis. Archives of Neurology 20: 1021–1032

Gildenberg P L, Tasker R R 1982 Spasmodic torticollis. Contemporary Neurosurgery 4(6): 1–7

Hamby W B, Schiffer S 1969 Spasmodic torticollis: results after cervical rhizotomy in 50 cases. Journal of Neurosurgery 31: 323–326

Hoehn M M, Yahr M D 1967 Parkinsonism: onset, progression and mortality. Neurology 17: 427–442

Kelly P J, Gillingham F J 1980 The long term results of stereotactic surgery and L-dopa therapy in patients with Parkinson's disease: A 10 year follow-up study. Journal of Neurosurgery 53: 332–337

Lundsford L D 1988 Modern stereotactic neurosurgery. Martinus Nijhoff, Boston

Marsden C D, Harrison M J G 1974 Idiopathic torsion dystonia (dystonia muscularum deformans): A review of 42 patients. Brain 97: 793–810

Olanow C W 1981 Current concepts in the management of movement disorders. Clinical Neurosurgery 28: 137–170

Parkinson J 1817 An essay on the shaking palsy. Sherwood Neely and Jones, London

Rasmussen T, Marino R Jr 1979 Functional neurosurgery. Raven Press, New York

21. Epilepsy and its neurosurgical aspects

Christine Kilpatrick

Epilepsy is a common neurological disorder occurring in 1% of the population with approximately 1 in 50 having a single seizure at some stage in their lives. Epilepsy is defined as a tendency to have recurrent seizures, and a single seizure, therefore, does not comprise epilepsy.

An epileptic seizure may be described as a transient derangement of the nervous system due to a sudden, excessive and disorderly discharge of cerebral neurons. This was the postulation of Hughlings Jackson, the eminent British neurologist, and to the present time this remains the accepted mechanism. The electrical discharges result in a diversity of clinical manifestations ranging from the dramatic clinical event of a tonic–clonic, or grand mal, seizure, to a brief episode of loss of awareness with minimal motor involvement, characteristic of an absence, or petit mal, seizure.

In general, neurosurgical practice involves the management of epilepsy:

- When an epileptic seizure is the presenting symptom of an underlying intracranial lesion such as a brain tumour
- As a complication of head injury or intracranial surgery
- In the surgical management of patients with intractable epilepsy, in particular the management of temporal lobe epilepsy.

CLASSIFICATION OF SEIZURES AND EPILEPSIES

It is important to distinguish between types of seizures and types of epilepsies, the former being the symptom and the latter being the syndrome or disease. The task of finding a satisfactory classification of epileptic phenomena is one which has exercised the minds of experts over many decades. The earliest classification was published by Hughlings Jackson and Gower during the late 19th century and the modern classification, of both seizures and epilepsies, was proposed in 1970 by the International League Against Epilepsy and revised most recently in 1989.

Classification of seizures

Table 21.1 summarises the now accepted international classification of epileptic seizures. Although the classification shown in the table is simplified,

Table 21.1 Classification of seizures

Generalised
Tonic–clonic (grand mal)
Absence (petit mal)
Myoclonic
Tonic
Atonic
Partial (focal)
Simple partial seizure — without impairment of conscious state
Complex partial seizure — impairment of conscious state
Partial seizure secondarily generalised
Unclassifiable

it aims to be a simple and practical classification which highlights some fundamental concepts based on the clinical features of seizures and their differing pathophysiology. The classification includes three major seizure types:

1. Generalised
2. Partial
3. Unclassifiable

Generalised seizures. These are characterised by electrical discharges occurring in both cerebral hemispheres simultaneously. Despite this common electrophysiological basis, the clinical manifestations of the generalised seizures vary markedly.

A typical **tonic–clonic (grand mal) seizure** is unmistakable. The seizure begins with a tonic phase lasting 10–15 seconds, during which the patient falls to the ground with loss of consciousness. The body stiffens and there may be a piercing cry as the whole musculature is seized in a spasm. The patient clenches the teeth, may bite the tongue and becomes apnoeic. Urinary incontinence may follow. The tonic phase is followed by a clonic phase lasting 1–2 minutes, characterised by rhythmical muscular contraction involving the entire body. A postictal phase, consisting of confusion and drowsiness, follows. Tonic–clonic seizures do not always conform to this classic description, but always involve loss of consciousness.

Petit mal, or absence, seizures are characterised by brief loss of consciousness lasting 5–10 seconds. During this time the patient, usually a child, is witnessed to stare and there may be minor motor involvement such as blinking of the eyes, but the patient does not fall. Abruptly, consciousness is regained with amnesia for the event. During the seizure the EEG shows bilateral synchronous 3 Hz spike and wave activity. This EEG abnormality and the seizure may be provoked by hyperventilation.

Myoclonic seizures are relatively uncommon and are characterised clinically by brief, often single, jerking of the trunk and limbs. These may be relatively minor, involving only one limb, or may be profound, causing the patient to fall to the ground. Consciousness is retained. The EEG during a myoclonic seizure shows bilateral synchronised spike and wave activity.

Partial seizures. In contrast, in partial seizures the electrical activity begins in a well defined focus of one part of the cerebral hemisphere. Partial seizures are subdivided into:

- Simple
- Complex
- Secondarily generalised.

In **simple partial seizures** there is no alteration in the conscious state, whereas with **complex partial seizures** the conscious state is impaired. If this focus is in the motor cortex, as may occur with a parasagittal meningioma, the patient may experience a rhythmical jerking of the contralateral limb without impairment of conscious state — a simple partial seizure of motor type. When the focus is in the temporal lobe, as may occur with a temporal lobe glioma or mesial temporal sclerosis, the conscious state is usually impaired — the patient has a complex partial seizure.

Most complex partial seizures arise from a focus in the temporal lobe but some arise from the frontal lobe. Complex partial seizures of temporal lobe origin may be characterised by complex hallucinations or perceptual illusions. The patient may complain of feelings of increased reality or familiarity (déja vu) and may report an unusual taste or smell sensation or epigastric and abdominal sensations. Patients frequently complain of feelings of anxiety and fear. This may be followed by a period of unresponsiveness or confused behaviour. Automatisms, defined as a state of clouding of consciousness during which the patient performs simple and complex, often semipurposive actions, without being aware of what is happening, are frequently seen. If the seizure comprises impairment of the conscious state only, then the diagnosis may be confused with absence seizures. With both simple and complex partial seizures the focal electrical discharge may generalise and the patient may have a tonic–clonic seizure — a **secondarily generalised tonic clonic seizure**.

Classification of epilepsies

The types of epilepsy are defined on the basis of:

- Types of seizures
- Associated clinical features.

This is particularly relevant when considering the generalised forms of epilepsy. The approach to a patient with epilepsy, therefore, should comprise the sequential analysis of the seizure type or types followed by a syndrome or disease diagnosis. The epilepsies as proposed by the International League Against Epilepsy are divided into **partial epilepsies** and

generalised epilepsies (Table 21.2). Partial epilepsies are those where the seizures have either a focal structural basis (e.g. glioma), focal clinical features or a focal electrical origin shown on the EEG.

Patients seen by neurosurgeons usually have partial epilepsy. For example, a patient presenting with a tonic–clonic seizure and whose CT scan reveals a glioma, has had a partial seizure secondarily generalised and hence has a partial epilepsy. Even though the seizure may have no focal features, clearly the electrical activity begins at the site of the tumour. A patient with temporal lobe epilepsy due to mesial temporal sclerosis with both complex partial seizures and occasional secondarily generalized tonic–clonic seizures also has partial epilepsy. Benign childhood epilepsy with centrotemporal spikes is an example of idiopathic partial epilepsy — there is no underlying structural basis for the *focal* electrical and clinical features. This condition occurs in otherwise normal children and remits spontaneously during adolescence. The seizures are partial, frequently sleep-related and often characterised by orofacial or oropharyngeal involvement. The interictal EEG demonstrates a spike focus in the centrotemporal area.

There is no underlying focal structural pathology in the generalised epilepsies, and these conditions are usually managed by neurologists.

The generalised epilepsies are subdivided into primary generalised epilepsy and secondary generalised epilepsy. Primary generalised epilepsy is one of the most common conditions treated by a neurologist. In its pure form it constitutes a condition where there is no underlying pathological abnormality and the major aetiological factor is the inherited trait for the gene that is expressed electrographically as generalised 3 Hz spike wave discharges. Secondary generalised epilepsy almost always begins in childhood. In its pure form it consists of a diffuse grey matter disease, usually due to acquired factors. The former has a good prognosis but the latter is associated with a poorer prognosis. Primary generalised epilepsy is subdivided into a number of recognised clinical syndromes, the more common syndromes are shown in Table 21.2.

Table 21.2   Classification of the epilepsies

Partial epilepsies
   Symptomatic (e.g. tumour)
   Idiopathic (benign childhood epilepsy with centrotemporal spikes)

Generalised epilepsies
   Primary generalised epilepsies
      benign neonatal convulsions
      childhood absence epilepsy
      juvenile absence epilepsy
      juvenile myoclonic epilepsy of Janz
      epilepsy with tonic–clonic seizures
   Secondary generalised epilepsies
      Lennox–Gastaut syndrome
      West syndrome
      epilepsy with myoclonic absences

POST-TRAUMATIC EPILEPSY

The occurrence of epileptic seizures following a head injury is well recognised, and the first neurosurgical procedure performed by Victor Horsley in 1886, was on a 22-year-old man with intractable epilepsy following a compound depressed skull fracture in earlier life. Hence, it is clear that even at this early time the concept that trauma could produce brain changes capable of causing epilepsy was well understood.

Post-traumatic epilepsy may be classified into three types:

1. Immediate epilepsy
2. Early epilepsy
3. Late epilepsy.

Immediate epilepsy. Immediate epilepsy refers to a seizure which occurs at the time, or within minutes of the head injury. It does not recur and carries a good prognosis. Its occurrence does not predispose patients to late post-traumatic epilepsy.

Early epilepsy. Early epilepsy is defined as seizures occurring within the first week of a head injury. In adults they tend to complicate quite severe head injuries, often with intracranial haemorrhage, prolonged post-traumatic amnesia or depressed fractures. In children early seizures are relatively common and may complicate relatively minor injuries. Early seizures are often limited to focal twitching, particularly in children. 25% of adult patients with early seizures will have recurrent late seizures. In children, early seizures also predispose the patient to late epilepsy, but the risk is less than in the adult population. The incidence of late epilepsy is unaffected by the type, time and number of early seizures.

Late epilepsy. Late epilepsy is defined as seizures occurring after the first week and may appear for the first time some years after the head injury. Over 50% of those destined to develop late epilepsy will do so within the first year, the incidence then falls rapidly over the following 3 years, so that after 4 years there is only a small ongoing risk.

50% of patients with late epilepsy have seizures with focal features, which is not surprising given that in most cases they are a form of partial epilepsy. Most, however are subject to tonic–clonic seizures. Absence seizures are never the result of head trauma. Most patients with late post-traumatic seizures continue to have recurring seizures, albeit infrequently.

Factors predisposing patients to late post-traumatic epilepsy include:

- Post-traumatic amnesia of more than 24 hours
- Intracranial haemorrhage
- Occurrence of early epileptic seizures
- Depressed fracture.

Table 21.3 tabulates these clinical features and associated risks of late post-traumatic epilepsy.

Table 21.3 Influence of various factors on the incidence of late post-traumatic epilepsy

Associated clinical feature	Risk of late post-traumatic epilepsy (%)
Post-traumatic amnesia <24 hours	1
Post-traumatic amnesia >24 hours	3
Early epilepsy	25
Post-traumatic amnesia >24 hours Early epilepsy	25
Compound depressed fracture	
Dura intact	7
Dura torn	25
Extradural haemorrhage	20
Subdural haemorrhage (acute)	40
Intracerebral haemorrhage	50
Post-traumatic amnesia >24 hours Early epilepsy intracranial haemorrhage	35
Post-traumatic amnesia >24 hours Dural tear Early epilepsy Compound depressed fracture	70

Post-traumatic epilepsy is treated with phenytoin or carbamazepine. Head injuries with clinical features associated with a high risk of post-traumatic epilepsy are treated prophylactically with phenytoin or carbamazepine. If no seizures occur, treatment may be ceased after 12 months.

POSTOPERATIVE EPILEPSY

The occurrence of seizures for the first time following craniotomy is well recognised. The incidence varies depending on the type of neurosurgical procedure, but the overall incidence is 18%. Almost half occur within the first week of surgery and two-thirds occur within the first postoperative month.

Incidence of postoperative epilepsy

- Aneurysm surgery has an incidence of over 20%. Seizures are more common with middle cerebral artery aneurysms
- Cerebral abscess is associated with a 70% incidence of epilepsy
- In tumour surgery, seizures occur in 20–30% of patients
- Burr hole biopsy of tumour has an incidence of 9%
- Seizures do not occur following posterior fossa surgery.

Postoperative prophylaxis

Most studies assessing the value of seizure prophylaxis with anticonvulsants have shown a significant reduction in the incidence of postoperative seizures. Phenytoin is the drug of choice for postoperative seizure prophylaxis.

As the incidence of seizures is high during the first postoperative week, patients should receive a pre-operative loading dose of phenytoin and then continue on maintenance therapy. If seizures do not occur and the intracranial lesion has been excised, prophylactic treatment with phenytoin should be discontinued after 6 months.

If seizures occur despite adequate phenytoin plasma levels, phenobarbitone should be used. If this fails, carbamazepine should be introduced.

INVESTIGATION OF SEIZURES

Investigation of seizures includes:

- History of seizures
- General and neurological history
- Examination of the patient
- EEG
- CT scan
- MRI.

The initial step in investigating a patient presenting after an epileptic seizure is to obtain a full history from the patient and a witness to the event, and to carry out a clinical examination. The aim of the neurological examination is to determine if there is an underlying structural cause. The cause of the seizure may be apparent following the initial consultation. A history of birth trauma, together with evidence of body asymmetry suggests cerebral damage in early life. A history of febrile convulsions of infancy is important in a patient with complex partial seizures, a past history of significant head injury may suggest post-traumatic epilepsy and a strong family history of epilepsy suggest primary generalised epilepsy.

Usually however, the cause remains uncertain and specific investigations are indicated. Electroencephalography (EEG) and CT scan are the most useful investigative techniques and should be performed in all patients presenting with an epileptic seizure.

The EEG is a non-invasive and relatively inexpensive technique which may be performed as an outpatient. This involves the recording of electrical activity from the surface of the brain by the use of scalp electrodes. The electrodes are placed at multiple sites over the scalp, allowing recordings to be made from 8 or 16 anatomical sites at one time. These patterns of recording sites are known as montages.

The normal adult EEG has a background rhythm of frequency of 8–13 Hz, known as alpha rhythm. Fast activity of greater than 13 Hz is known

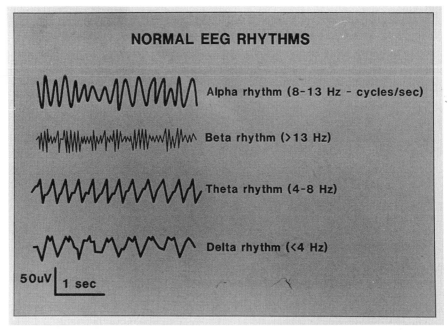

Fig. 21.1   EEG rhythms.

as beta rhythm and may be seen bifrontally or with drugs such as barbiturates and benzodiazepines. Slow activity is categorised as theta rhythm of 4–8 Hz and delta rhythm of less than 4 Hz (Fig. 21.1). The normal adult resting EEG contains only a minimal amount of theta rhythm and no delta activity. Excess slow wave activity during the resting tracing is abnormal and may be generalised, such as in an encephalopathy or focal, as with a structural lesion such as a glioma or abscess. The routine EEG comprises a resting tracing and two provocative tests, hyperventilation and photic stimulation. These provocative tests may induce epileptic activity and hyperventilation may accentuate a focal abnormality.

The EEG is of particular value in showing:

- Focal abnormalities suggesting an underlying focal structural lesion and suggesting the seizure is partial in type
- Diagnosis of absence seizures by demonstrating characteristic 3 Hz spike and wave (Fig. 21.2) and differentiating absence seizures from complex partial seizures in which the EEG may show a focal, usually temporal lobe abnormality (Fig. 21.3)
- Interictal bilateral synchronous spike and wave, spike or polyspike activity in a patient presenting with a tonic-clonic seizure, indicating a generalised epilepsy (Fig. 21.4).

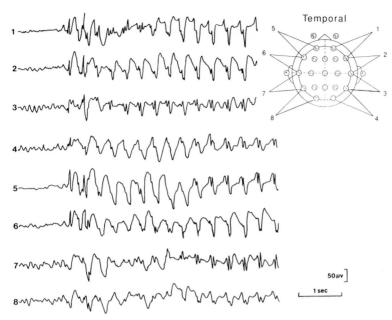

Fig. 21.2   Patient presents with absence seizures. EEG during hyperventilation shows 3Hz spike and wave activity bilaterally.

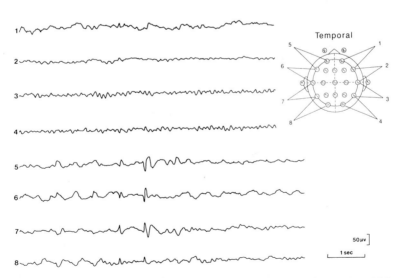

Fig. 21.3   Patient presents with complex partial seizures. EEG shows focal temporal lobe abnormality with excess slow wave activity and episodic sharp waves and sharp and slow wave complexes in the left temporal leads.

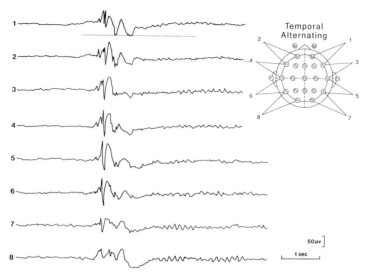

Fig. 21.4   Patient presents with tonic–clonic seizures. EEG shows bilateral synchronous spike and wave and polyspike activity.

When interpreting EEG findings, it must be remembered that:

- A normal EEG does not exclude epilepsy
- An abnormal EEG does not indicate epilepsy. Epilepsy is a clinical diagnosis
- Normal people may have an abnormal EEG

Video EEG telemetry, which involves simultaneous recording of electro-encephalographic data and clinical events, is of particular value in:

- Investigating patients in whom the type of seizure is uncertain
- Differentiating pseudoseizures, i.e. attacks which clinically resemble epileptic seizures (but which are not accompanied by an electrical disturbance in the brain) from epileptic seizures
- As part of the surgical assessment of patients with complex partial seizures of temporal lobe origin prior to temporal lobectomy.

A contrast enhanced CT scan is indicated in all adult patients presenting with a seizure. The CT scan is useful in identifying those patients with an underlying structural abnormality, such as a tumour or arteriovenous mal-formation, and in identifying long-standing benign, static and focal abnormalities, such as hemiatrophy or a porencephalic cyst.

Although the major concern, particularly to the patient who presents with a seizure, is the possibility of a cerebral tumour, tumours are responsible for late onset epilepsy (as defined by seizures occurring after the age of 25 years) in only about 10% of cases; the incidence is higher in patients presenting with partial seizures. Tumours are an uncommon cause of childhood epilepsy. The tumours most likely to cause seizures are those affecting the cerebral cortex, in particular the frontoparietal region. There is an inverse relationship between malignancy of a tumour and the risk of seizure. The incidence of seizure with meningiomas is approximately 70%, compared with only 40% in patients with a malignant glioma.

In a patient with partial seizures and a normal CT scan, a repeat CT scan 4–6 months later should be performed, as a low grade glioma may not be apparent on the initial CT scan.

Magnetic resonance imaging is a sensitive technique for demonstrating tumours and cerebral infarcts, relatively common identifiable structural causes of late onset epilepsy. It is also able to demonstrate mesial temporal sclerosis, a common cause of temporal lobe epilepsy, a finding which is not usually seen on CT scanning. All patients with complex partial seizures of temporal lobe origin in whom the CT scan is normal, should have an MR scan. If MRI is not freely available it should be limited to those with late onset epilepsy, in particular those patients with partial seizures where the risk of an underlying structural lesion is greatest.

MANAGEMENT OF EPILEPSY

Management of the single seizure

A patient presenting with a single seizure should be fully investigated with an EEG and a CT scan. If no cause is found and the EEG is normal, the question of whether the patient should be treated with anticonvulsant drugs arises. Studies of the estimated risk of subsequent seizures in a patient presenting with a single seizure vary markedly, but probably 50% of patients who have a single seizure, a normal CT scan and EEG and no family history of epilepsy, will have a further seizure within a 2 year follow-up period. In general, if the investigations reveal no abnormality, treatment with anticonvulsant drugs is not recommended following an initial seizure. In patients where the CT scan reveals a cause such as a tumour, the risk of further seizures is high and the patient should be treated with anticonvulsant medication.

Anticonvulsant drugs

Anticonvulsant therapy is the most important facet of treatment of epilepsy. Certain drugs are more effective in one type of seizure than in another and hence the need for accurate seizure diagnosis. Table 21.4 indicates the common anticonvulsant drugs and their relative specificity of action for different types of seizures. Table 21.5 lists the common anticonvulsant drugs, their daily dosages, dosage regimen, side-effects, pharmacokinetics and relative value of plasma concentrations. Table 21.6 lists the common seizure types and order of preference of anticonvulsant drugs.

Table 21.4 Relative specificity of action of anticonvulsants for different types of seizures

	Epileptic seizures					
	Generalised			Partial		
	Absence	Myoclonic	Tonic–Clonic	Simple	Complex	Secondarily generalised
Carbamazepine			+	+	+	+
Phenytoin			+	+	+	+
Valproate	+	+	+			?
Phenobarbitone			+	+	+	+
Ethosuximide	+					
Clonazepam	+	+	+			+

Table 21.5 Anticonvulsant drugs, side effects and relative value of plasma levels

Drug	Average daily dose	Regimen	Side effects	Plasma levels
Carbamazepine	600 mg	12 hourly	Initial drowsiness, leucopenia (rare), teratogenic	Some value
Phenytoin	300 mg	Once daily or 8–12 hourly	Gum hypertrophy, hirsutism, acne, teratogenic	Very useful. Note change from first order to zero order kinetics, hence only small dose increase will result in therapeutic plasma levels
Valproate	1000 mg	8 or 12 hourly	Gastrointestinal. Reduce platelet aggregation. Hepatotoxicity (rare) Teratogenic	Little value
Primidone	750 mg	12 hourly	Drowsiness. Teratogenic	Some value
Phenobarbitone	120 mg	12 hourly	Drowsiness. Teratogenic	Some value

Carbamazepine is the drug of choice in patients with secondarily generalised seizures as occurs with a tumour or vascular malformation. Sodium valproate is the drug of choice in an adult patient with primary generalised epilepsy presenting with a tonic–clonic seizure. Phenytoin is preferred in patients with post-traumatic epilepsy and postoperative seizures. Ethosuximide is the drug of choice in the treatment of absence seizures alone, but patients with both absence seizures and tonic–clonic seizures should be treated with sodium valproate. Complex partial seizures

Table 21.6   Type of seizure and order of preference of anticonvulsant drugs

Type of seizure	Drug (order of preference)
Tonic–clonic seizure (generalised)	Valproate Carbamazepine Phenytoin Phenobarbitone
Absence seizure	Ethosuximide Valproate
Myoclonic seizures	Valproate Clonazepam
Complex partial seizure	Carbamazepine Phenytoin Phenobarbitone
Simple partial seizure	Phenytoin Carbamazepine Phenobarbitone
Tonic–clonic seizure (secondarily generalised)	Carbamazepine Phenytoin Phenobarbitone Valproate

should be treated with carbamazepine and simple partial seizures with phenytoin or carbamazepine.

If, despite optimal dosage and an adequate trial of therapy, satisfactory results are not achieved with one drug, then another should be tried. Although one aims for monotherapy, in some patients better results are achieved with a combination of two drugs. Medication should always be withdrawn gradually, as the sudden withdrawal of a drug may lead to status epilepticus, even though a new drug has been substituted. This is particularly true for the barbiturates. Once an anticonvulsant or combination of anticonvulsant drugs is found to be effective, the medication should be continued for at least several years.

Teratogenicity of anticonvulsant drugs

There is a well recognised increased incidence of fetal malformations in infants born to women with epilepsy taking anticonvulsant drugs during pregnancy. How much of this increased incidence relates to epilepsy itself, and how much to the drugs, is uncertain. All the anticonvulsant drugs are thought to be teratogenic, but some appear to have a higher risk than others. At the present time, carbamazepine is thought to be the safest drug to use during pregnancy. Phenytoin has been associated with an increased risk of congenital heart disease, cleft lip and palate, and valproate has been associated with an increased incidence of spina bifida.

Although patients are always very concerned about taking anticonvulsant drugs during pregnancy, the patient should be reassured that there is at least a 90% chance they will have a normal healthy child and they should be advised that the control of the epilepsy is of the utmost importance and the fetus is probably at greater risk from seizures than from the drugs themselves.

Plasma concentrations of anticonvulsant drugs

Plasma concentrations of all the commonly used anticonvulsant drugs can be measured routinely. The plasma concentration of an anticonvulsant drug aids the physician in choosing an appropriate dosage to achieve maximum therapeutic response and avoid toxicity. Phenytoin plasma concentrations are particularly useful as there is a good correlation between plasma phenytoin concentration and therapeutic and toxic effects. Plasma concentration of carbamazepine and barbiturates are of some value but the correlation between plasma concentration of valproate and therapeutic benefit is poor (Table 21.5).

Management of status epilepticus

Status epilepticus is defined as recurrent seizures without recovery of consciousness between attacks. It occurs in a minority of patients with epilepsy and is more common in patients with an underlying structural cause than in patients with primary generalised epilepsy. It may be the first presentation of epilepsy. Status epilepticus may be precipitated by withdrawal of anticonvulsant drugs, intercurrent infection or may be spontaneous. True status epilepticus is a medical emergency and requires urgent and intensive treatment. Seizures which are multiple and frequent, but not continuous, may herald status and should be controlled rapidly.

The principles of management of status epilepticus are:

- To stop the fitting
- To prevent further seizures.

To stop the fitting use intravenous diazepam and, if this fails, intravenous clonazepam or intravenous hemineurium.

Particular care must be given to maintenance of the airway and the patient's ventilation. In postoperative patients an urgent CT scan must be performed to exclude a postoperative collection, such as an intracerebral haemorrhage.

Maintenance anticonvulsant therapy should be introduced or optimised to prevent further seizures. Patients must be investigated thoroughly to ascertain the cause of the status epilepticus.

SURGICAL TREATMENT OF EPILEPSY

In 1886, Horsley pioneered cortical exploration based on clinical seizure patterns in patients with focal epilepsy and showed that, following excision of this area, the attacks ceased.

Surgical treatment of epilepsy is indicated if the epilepsy is intractable to all anticonvulsant medication and if it can be shown that there is a focal origin for the attacks in an area of the brain that can be removed without producing a neurological deficit. Temporal lobectomy is the most common surgical procedure in the management of patients with epilepsy.

Temporal lobectomy

Assessment of patients prior to temporal lobectomy includes:

- History of seizures
- Video EEG recording with surface, sphenoidal and, if necessary, depth electrodes and subdural plates
- CT scan, MRI and single photon emission computerised tomography (SPECT) scanning
- Neuropsychology assessment
- Wada test.

Proper evaluation and selection of patients for surgical management of epilepsy is the most important factor in determining success or failure of surgical treatment. Initial assessment involves a detailed clinical history from both the patient and a witness. Video EEG recording of seizures is essential to confirm seizure type and lateralisation, based on both the clinical features of the seizure and the site of the electrical discharges. Monitoring initially involves use of surface electrodes and sphenoidal electrodes and, if necessary, temporal depth electrodes are inserted under stereotactic control to confirm the site of the epileptic discharge. If there is any doubt, then subdural electrode plates may need to be inserted to define the site of discharge and its relationship to vital brain structures.

All patients have CT and MR scans. Of particular importance is the demonstration, using MRI, of mesial temporal sclerosis in patients with temporal lobe epilepsy. Positron emission tomography, when available, is also useful in demonstrating focal abnormalities, as is SPECT using HM-PAO ictally or immediately postictally. These imaging techniques have circumvented the need for depth electrodes in many patients with complex partial seizures.

All patients undergo detailed neuropsychological evaluation. This provides an overall assessment of intellectual function and allows detection of abnormalities of temporal lobe or frontal lobe function. Verbal and non-verbal memory tests allow good discrimination between dominant and non-dominant temporal lobe involvement, respectively. Hence these tests provide lateralisation of temporal lobe abnormalities. In a patient where a temporal lobectomy is being contemplated, one clearly needs to be reassured that the contralateral temporal lobe function is normal, otherwise an amnestic syndrome may result.

The **Wada test** establishes whether or not the contralateral temporal lobe can sustain memory. This test also indicates which temporal lobe is dominant for language. The test involves unilateral intracarotid injection of sodium amytal to temporarily ablate one or other temporal lobe. The Wada test is indicated in patients in whom:

- The presumed temporal lobe epileptic focus does not coincide with the findings on neuropsychological examination. For example, a right handed patient with a verbal memory deficit suggesting a dominant or left temporal lobe abnormality and a right temporal epileptic focus based on electrographic, neuro-imaging and clinical data.
- Patients in whom there is evidence of bilateral temporal lobe dysfunction.

If the clinical history and description of seizures, electrographic data, imaging and neuropsychological testing all suggest the same localisation and lateralisation of the seizure focus, then temporal lobectomy has a high chance of success.

Callosotomy

The place of callosotomy in the management of patients with epilepsy remains unclear. At present the procedure should only be considered in patients with severe uncontrolled epilepsy, characterised by generalised seizures including tonic–clonic, tonic and atonic (drop attacks).

Hemispherectomy

Patients with severe epilepsy and hemiparesis are occasionally treated with hemispherectomy. The procedure is of most value in reducing atonic seizures.

DRIVING AND EPILEPSY

The management of a patient with a single seizure or epilepsy includes advice regarding the safety to drive. Every country has different regulations. In general a patient who has had a single seizure for which, following thorough investigation, no cause is found, should be advised not to drive for at least 3 months. Patients with epilepsy, i.e. a tendency to have recurrent seizures, must be free of seizures for 2 years before obtaining a driver's licence. Following supratentorial craniotomy patients are advised not to drive for 6 months. Similar advice should be given following a significant head injury. Most patients with a glioma should probably be advised not to return to driving, given the recognised risk of seizures and the anticipated decline in cerebral function due to the intracerebral tumour.

FURTHER READING

Goldring S 1983 Epilepsy surgery. Clinical Neurosurgery 31: 369–388
Jennett B 1975 Epilepsy after non-missile head injuries, 2nd edn. Heinemann, London
Laidlaw J, Richens A 1972 Textbook of Epilepsy, 2nd edn. Churchill Livingstone, Edinburgh
North J 1989 Anticonvulsant prophylaxis in neurosurgery. British Journal of Neurosurgery (Editorial) 3: 425–428
Ojemann G A 1989 Surgical therapy for medically intractable epilepsy. Journal of Neurosurgery 25: 153–160

Index

Page numbers in italics refer to tables and figures.